International Regimes in Global Health Governance

By analysing the roles and problems faced by international regimes as major players in global health governance, this book looks into the root causes of the often insufficient supply of global public goods for health and of the deficiencies in current global health governance.

Combining several different methods of analysis and methodologies, this book sketches out the landscape of international public health governance involving a range of international actors. These actors include the World Health Organization, the World Trade Organization, the Biological Weapons Convention and international human rights regimes. Through a novel theoretical framework that synthesises the theory of securitisation, public goods and international regimes, the author focuses on factors that have resulted in observed deficiencies in global health governance. Based on these examinations, the book also tries to explore feasible approaches for institutional refinement and innovations for greater effectiveness in global health governance.

The book will appeal to academics and policymakers interested in global health, international relations and international law.

Jiyong Jin is a professor of political science at Shanghai International Studies University. He specialises in global health governance and health diplomacy.

China Perspectives

The *China Perspectives* series focuses on translating and publishing works by leading Chinese scholars, writing about both global topics and China-related themes. It covers Humanities & Social Sciences, Education, Media and Psychology, as well as many interdisciplinary themes.

This is the first time any of these books have been published in English for international readers. The series aims to put forward a Chinese perspective, give insights into cutting-edge academic thinking in China and inspire researchers globally.

To submit proposals, please contact the Taylor & Francis Publisher for China Publishing Programme, Lian Sun (Lian.Sun@informa.com).

Titles in health and social care currently include

International Regimes in Global Health Governance
Jiyong Jin

For more information, please visit www.routledge.com/China-Perspectives/book-series/CPH

International Regimes in Global Health Governance

Jiyong Jin

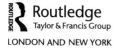
LONDON AND NEW YORK

This book's publication is under the subsidy of Chinese Fund for the Humanities and Social Sciences (中华社会科学基金).

First published 2021
by Routledge
2 Park Square, Milton Park, Abingdon, Oxon OX14 4RN

and by Routledge
52 Vanderbilt Avenue, New York, NY 10017

Routledge is an imprint of the Taylor & Francis Group, an informa business

© 2021 Jiyong Jin

Translated by Rui Li et al.

The right of Jiyong Jin to be identified as author of this work has been asserted by him in accordance with sections 77 and 78 of the Copyright, Designs and Patents Act 1988.

All rights reserved. No part of this book may be reprinted or reproduced or utilised in any form or by any electronic, mechanical, or other means, now known or hereafter invented, including photocopying and recording, or in any information storage or retrieval system, without permission in writing from the publishers.

Trademark notice: Product or corporate names may be trademarks or registered trademarks, and are used only for identification and explanation without intent to infringe.

English Version by permission of Shanghai People's Publishing House.

British Library Cataloguing-in-Publication Data
A catalogue record for this book is available from the British Library

Library of Congress Cataloging-in-Publication Data
A catalog record for this book has been requested

ISBN: 978-0-367-70791-0 (hbk)
ISBN: 978-0-367-70792-7 (pbk)
ISBN: 978-1-003-14803-6 (ebk)

Typeset in Times New Roman
by Apex CoVantage, LLC

Contents

List of figures	vi
List of tables	vii

1	Introduction	1
2	Theoretical underpinnings of global health governance	14
3	World Health Organization and global health governance	55
4	World Trade Organization and global health governance	106
5	International human rights regimes and global health governance	133
6	Biological Weapons Convention (BWC) and global health governance	171
7	China's role in global health governance	194
8	Conclusion	213
	Index	224

Figures

2.1	Three-dimensional Structure of Securitizing Health Issues	35
3.1	Proportion of Assessed Contributions and Voluntary Contributions in the WHO Budget	90
5.1	Linkages Between Human Rights and Public Health	141
5.2	Components of the Right to Health	155
5.3	National Recognition of a Right to Health	160
6.1	Linkages Between the BWC and Public Health	178
8.1	Triangle of Publicness	214

Tables

2.1	Actors and Their Functions in Global Health Governance	45
3.1	International Sanitary Conferences Between 1851 and 1897	59
3.2	Actors in Global Health Governance	88
4.1	Specific Health Issues and Most Relevant WTO Agreements	111
4.2	World Pharmaceutical Market by Region or Country	127
5.1	Current Major International Declarations and Covenants on Human Rights	140
5.2	Potential Impact of Major International Human Rights Regimes on Public Health	144
7.1	Annual Themes of the BRICS Health Ministers Meetings	202
7.2	Medical Teams Sent by Chinese Provinces to African Countries	205

1 Introduction

1.1 Practical and theoretical implications of research

Human history is a history of combatting diseases. From time immemorial, pandemic crises have plagued human society. The first-ever recorded plague in human history virtually destroyed Athens. The flu that swept the globe in 1918 killed an estimated 20–50 million people in just a few months. As of 2017, an estimated 70 million people had been infected with HIV, and 35 million had died of AIDS, making the disease the "primary killer" in Africa and the world. The September 11 terrorist attacks in the United States, as well as the subsequent anthrax virus outbreak, left the international community deeply haunted by the spectre of bioterrorism. The rapid spread of SARS in 2003 demonstrated starkly the vulnerability of human beings in an increasingly interdependent world to deadly diseases. In 2014, the raging Ebola outbreak in West Africa caused a death toll of more than 11,000 people, underscoring the serious challenges to maintaining global health security and promoting global health development. The unprecedented global health, humanitarian and socioeconomic crisis triggered by the COVID-19 pandemic has significantly reflected the vulnerability of the international community to infectious diseases. Simply put, "the state of global health is in a state of crisis" (Bradford, 2007, p. 77).

However, such astonishing public health problems have long been regarded as technical issues delegated to the biological and medical domains or to the specialised territory of epidemiologists. Public health issues within a country are also considered problems within its sovereignty with which no other nation or international organisations may interfere. In other words, public health governance in the traditional sense has always been subject to what German philosopher Ulrich Beck (2007) called rules of "methodological nationalism" (p. 286). However, as globalisation deepens, public health governance—once an issue of domestic governance—has become global. At the same time, public health crises have also risen above their status as mere medical problems and brought forth important societal, economic, and political implications. Viruses travel around the world passport-free. Many emerging and recurrent infectious diseases have made countries around the world more vulnerable and interdependent. Today, it has become a serious challenge to manage global health issues confronting the international community.

2 Introduction

Global health issues are major global problems "with potential ramifications as great as any war; yet hardly any political scientist shows scientific interest in it!" (Lanegran & Hyden, 1993, p. 247). Not even in the realm of issues regarded as "low politics" can we find discussions of these problems. As Rudolph Virchow, a German politician and doctor and revered as the "father of modern pathology" observes, "Medicine is a social science, and politics nothing but medicine at a larger scale" (1848). Indeed, public health issues are not only medical issues but also political issues. "Health is deeply political. We need to tackle the political determinants of health" (Kickbusch, 2005, p. 246). Given that transnationally transmissible diseases and potential bioterrorism pose a threat to security at individual, national, international and global levels, global health issues have been increasingly securitised in recent years. Scholars in China and elsewhere have extended some discussions about such securitisation,[1] all agreeing that global health threats have risen to the status of security issues. As Su (2000) put it,

> International Relations Studies, or the Studies of the International Society, should and in many ways has already become a discipline both aiming to explore and realize global public interest and designed to probe the meaning of 'publicness'. Only in this sense can International Relations Studies justifiably maintain its status as a unique discipline.
>
> (p. 284)

Doubtless, the "publicness" of global health issues has made global health governance a central concern for scholars in the field. It is thus not only practical but also necessary to analyse global health issues from the perspective of international relations.

The emergence of global public issues calls for global governance. The efficiency of global governance, in turn, depends on the availability of global public goods. The proper response to global health crises lies in how to effectively achieve global health governance. The approach relies on providing more global public goods for health when it comes to global health (Kaul et al., 2003; Smith et al., 2003). As main actors in global health governance, international regimes are the most important providers of global public goods for health, spanning security, trade, development, human rights and many other policy areas. Therefore, an analysis of the roles and deficiencies of global regimes in addressing global health governance, including those of the World Health Organization (WHO), the World Trade Organization (WTO), the Biological Weapons Convention (BWC) and international human rights regimes, can help identify the root causes of the insufficient supply of global public goods for health. It will also help us achieve greater effectiveness of global health governance through further regime design and innovation.

By identifying the shortcomings of these international regimes in global health governance, this book seeks to map out the deep-seated causes leading to these deficiencies. It is therefore of both theoretical and practical significance to approach the issue of global health governance from the perspective of international regimes.

1.2 Literature review

Research on global health issues is inextricably linked to the globalisation of public health issues. Since the 1990s, three major development trends have been identified in the area of public health: 1) AIDS continues to spread globally and is wielding increasing political, economic and social impact in developing countries; 2) people are increasingly concerned about the proliferation of biological weapons, especially such proliferation in terrorist groups and 3) people are increasingly aware of the vulnerability and interdependence in both rich and poor countries arising from the global spread of pathogens, products and pollutants. "In the global context, the transnational menace of infectious and non-communicable diseases in a globalizing world has immersed all of the humanity in a single microbial sea" (Aginam, 2007, p. 147). Such interdependence in global health security has been driving this line of academic research. Although international regimes play an important role in global health governance, most public health scientists choose not to view international regimes as effective tools but rather analyse global health issues from a narrowly defined medical science perspective. Scholars of international relations have thus remained quite passive in the fields of global health issues. As Lee and Dodgson (2003) point out, "Although health is a classic trans-border issue, it continues to receive limited attention in international relations" (p. 214). Scholars interested in this issue have mostly adopted a "segmented" approach and have analysed the impact of these factors on public health from the aspect of international trade and international human rights regimes separately. In general, a holistic and interdisciplinary research approach is wanting for such scholarship.

Due to the impact of emerging and recurrent infectious diseases, particularly AIDS, and threats from bioterrorism, research on global health issues from the angle of international relations has garnered increasing attention. Prominent among international relations scholars is David P. Fidler, of Indiana University, USA, who has made important contributions to interdisciplinary research in international relations and public health. One of his most representative works is *SARS, Governance, and Globalization of Diseases* (2003). Taking the SARS epidemic as an example, he analyses, in the context of globalisation, the impact brought by the public health crisis to international politics under the Westphalian system. He argues that the globalisation of public health issues requires taking a "post-Westphalian" system of public health governance—that is, a global health governance approach—and identifies the deficiencies of the International Health Regulations (IHR) as an international regime in addressing issues in global health governance. He even coined a new term, "microbialpolitik", to describe the interaction between international relations and health problems posed by pathogens (Fidler, 1998, pp. 1–11). He has placed global health issues under the framework formed by the international treaties, analysed the impact arising from the threat of viral microbes on the formation of a global health regime, and traced the history to a series of international public health conferences and public health diplomacies in the 19th century.

4 *Introduction*

In 2008, Fidler and Lawrence O. Gostin co-published their book *Biosecurity in the Global Age: Biological Weapons, Public Health, and the Rule of Law*. The two authors believe that since biosecurity threats mainly come from biological weapons and natural outbreaks, security and public health—two previously independent areas—need to be integrated and coordinated, in particular through the coordination of two international regimes, the BWC and the WHO. This approach exemplifies the securitisation of public health issues. In the book, they also emphasise the importance and difficulties of this integration strategy and maintain that the integration between safety issues and public health issues requires a change of perspective and practice to cope with, through sustainable governance, the threat from microbial pathogens. They hold that it is important to use legal channels to provide an effective global governance framework for biosafety, in particular by strengthening the legal functions of the WHO and the Biological Weapons Convention, to enhance the role of the two international regimes in global biosafety governance.

In 2001, Andrew T. Price-Smith, Professor of International Politics at Colorado College, USA, published *Plagues and Politics: Infectious Disease and International Policy*. He based his discussion on theories of international relations and analysed the impact of public health crises on global security. He argued that global health crises would pose direct and serious long-term threats to global governance and prosperity. In 2005, Obijiofor Aginam, of Carleton University, Canada, published *Global Health Governance: International Law and Public Health in a Divided World*. Through the lens of globalisation, Aginam examined the shared vulnerabilities the international community faced in the field of public health security. He also traced the history of diplomatic efforts on infectious diseases in the 19th century and the origin of public health multilateralism during the European colonial period. Through investigating contemporaneous international law, Aginam critically examined the significance and limitations of the IHR and of the right to health in global health governance. He concluded that, despite the international community's interdependence in public health security, the widening capability gap between developed and developing countries at the time meant international law could only play a limited role in global health governance.

In 2007, Andrew F. Cooper et al. co-published *Governing Global Health: Challenges, Responses, and Innovations*. The book highlighted the significance and challenges of global health governance in the 21st century and examined the evolution of global health cooperation since the 1990s. Using WHO as an example, the authors listed a number of public health challenges that had emerged in the era of globalisation and discussed the influence WTO had on public health in its quest to meet the United Nations' (UN) Millennium Development Goals (MDGs). The authors believed global health governance required innovations, particularly innovations of multilateral international regimes. These innovations involved relinquishing sovereignty to collective action, setting up accountability mechanisms and establishing effective monitoring and implementation mechanisms.

In the same year, Wolfgang Hein, in collaboration with his fellow researchers from the German Institute of Global and Area Studies (GIGA), published *Global*

Health Governance and the Fight Against HIV/AIDS (2007). The authors gave a convincing explanation on the role global health governance has in curbing HIV/AIDS. The authors started with a serious attempt to define the concept of global health governance, followed by an evaluation of the functions of international intergovernmental organisations and non-governmental organisations in global health governance. The book ended by endorsing the view that global health governance requires a "post-Westphalian" framework in which global health governance is not restricted to countries, and non-state actors can play an increasingly important role in global health governance.

In 2008, Mark Zacher and Tania Keefe, Professors of International Relations at the University of British Columbia in Canada, co-published their monograph *The Politics of Global Health Governance*. They traced the development of global health governance regimes in the 20th century and described the clashes between international patent law and the accessibility to essential medicines. They contended that global health governance requires cooperation in global politics. In addition, some Western scholars have also taken a historical approach to study how global public issues have emerged as global issues (Goodman, 1977; Hayes, 1998; Howard-Jones, 1975; McNeill, 1976; Porter, 1999; Zinsser, 1963).

At the same time, there is also research from the field of public health focusing on the mutual interactions between public health and international relations. For example, *World Health and World Politics* (1995), written by Javed Siddiqi at the School of Public Health of Western University, Canada, is the most representative work in this field of research. Using WHO as a case study, Siddiqi described the interactions between world health and world politics and their impact on each other. In particular, he gave a detailed analysis of the impact international politics has had on WHO since the establishment of the organisation in 1948. One of his conclusions was that politicisation within WHO is harmful to its functioning.

For another example, Meri Koivusalo and Eeva Ollila, two researchers at the National Research and Development Centre of Finland, co-published *Making a Healthy World: Agencies, Actors & Policies in International Health* (1997). It was a pioneering work that gave a broad view of international organisations involved in international health strategies. The authors examined the structures, policies and practices of WHO and WTO and other international regimes. They also brought other actors, particularly non-governmental organizations (NGOs), into their discussion. On top of that, they took an in-depth look into the scope of international health policies, including "Health for All", "Primary Health Care Strategies", and accessibility to essential medicines in developing countries. *Global Public Goods for Health*, written by Richard D. Smith et al. (2003), at the University of East Anglia, is yet another refreshing attempt in this line of research. By categorising and analysing the supply of global health goods from the perspective of global public goods, they propose a theoretical framework for collective action at a global level.

In addition to the books mentioned previously, there have also been several institutional reports and papers on global health and governance in the field of international relations in the West. For example, Rand published a report titled

6 *Introduction*

The Global Threat of New and Re-emerging Infectious Diseases: Reconciling US National Security and Public Health Policy. Its two authors, Jennifer Brower and Peter Chalk (2003), pointed out that due to the adverse consequences brought by globalisation, modern medical practices, agricultural activities, changes in human behaviours and environmental factors, infectious diseases and public health crises have replaced direct military threats from a hostile country to become the gravest challenge confronting the international community and national governments and the biggest threat to international security. The German Overseas Institute published a report titled *Global Health Governance: Conflicts on Global Social Rights* (Hein, 2008), which gave a detailed analysis on problems that existed in global health governance from the perspective of global social justice and civil rights (pp. 80–108).

Relative to the number of institutional reports, there is an even greater number of articles addressing global health security. For example, Caroline Thomas and Martin Weber, Professors of International Politics at the University of Southampton, co-published *The Politics of Global Health Governance: Whatever Happened to "Health for All by the Year 2000"?* (2004). The two co-authors contended that one important challenge in global health governance was to overcome the North–South Divide. They also examined some limitations of the UN system in global health governance. Mely Caballero-Anthony, a professor from Columbia University, published *Combating Infectious Diseases in East Asia: Securitization and Global Public Goods for Health and Human Security* (2006), in which she compared two possible approaches (securitising health vs. providing global public goods) that could be applied to tackle public health crises in East Asia. She also discussed at length the impact brought by public health crises on "human security" (pp. 105–127).

The severe acute respiratory syndrome (SARS) outbreak, which struck China and many other countries in 2003, marked a watershed moment in research on global health security in China. Previously, international public health cooperation had attracted little scholarly attention in China. In view of some initial setbacks China's diplomacy suffered during the SARS epidemic, Chinese scholars have conducted some research on public health challenges from perspectives of non-traditional security and international law. On the whole, relevant research is still wanting.

Li Na et al.'s book *WTO and Public Health* (2004) examined international law to investigate WTO's impact on global public health, particularly in developing countries. He also addressed the clash between global intellectual property regime and the accessibility of medicines in developing countries. Shaojun Li's book *Contemporary Global Issue* (2006) gave a broad view of global public crises that had emerged in the context of globalisation. He used Chapter 7 of the book to exclusively examine how global health threats had affected global security and national security. He also briefly analysed WHO's role in global health governance. *Plagues and Human* (Wang & Meng, 2005), a volume edited by Xudong Wang of the Chinese Academy of Social Sciences, provided a historical assessment of the impact of major infectious diseases on human society.

Xiangqian Gong's book, *Infectious Disease Control from the Perspective of International Law* (2011), used international law as a theoretical tool to analyse global health crises. Specifically, he examined the role and impact of international health laws, trade laws, and human rights laws on the control of infectious diseases. Fan He's project *The Impact of Infectious Diseases on Economic Development and International Relations* (2004) addressed international cooperation in the field of public health. He brought several inter-related topics together into his discussion, including emerging epidemic outbreaks and ensuing crises, acts of bioterrorism and China's relationship with WHO.

In addition to books, theses and edited volumes, many journal articles have also examined at varying lengths features and weaknesses of international public health regimes(Chen, 2008; Gong, 2006; Hou, 2006; Jin, 2008a, 2008b, 2008c, 2008d, 2009; Pan, 2007; Qi & Zhu, 2006; Zhu, 2006). Gong's paper "Infectious Disease Globalization and Global Health Governance" (2006), for example, briefly discusses the correlations between global health governance and some of the recent public health crises.

A literature review reveals a fair amount of Western scholarship on global health governance. Most of this research applies a national security or international security lens to analyse the impact of public health crises on national interests. Nevertheless, this approach may have been biased by pre-established Western assumptions, as few of them acknowledge the global North–South Divide and the international political and economic order as root causes for global health problems. It should be noted that since the international regimes in global health governance are mostly established by developed countries, they failed to reflect the interests and concerns of the developing countries.

1.3 Research methods and contributions

This book attempts to cover a broad field of international relations, public health and international law. Many research methods are employed to, hopefully, do justice on each of the relevant issues. On the whole, research methods used in this book include the following:

Levels of analysis. Analysis according to levels is an important and commonly used research method in the field of international relations. It was first proposed by Kenneth Waltz in his book *Man, the State, and War* (1959). In this pioneering work on the use of this method, Waltz analyses and classifies the root causes of war into the individual, state and international aspects, which he refers to as "images". Inspired by the approach, the book tries to analyse the reasons why public health crises, or public health threats, have been securitised from the aspects of individual, national and international security.

Qualitative analysis. The book intends to investigate the weaknesses and deficiencies of a number of international regimes in global health governance. Regimes analysed include WHO, WTO, and the BWC. Based on these examples, this book offers some proposals that seek to improve their functioning.

8 *Introduction*

Qualitative analysis has proven to be a particularly useful method to dissect the roles of these international regimes.

Quantitative analysis. The book tries to show, with emphasis on being concrete and objective, the damage of public health crises, such as HIV/AIDS and SARS, on individual, national and international security. The conclusion is supported by a combined use of statistics and documentation analysis. At the same time, since "public goods", a central theme of this book, is a notion borrowed from economics, quantitative analysis is thus needed to explain why global public goods must be provided in the field of global health security.

Historical analysis. Although it was not long ago that global health governance gained its name, the origin of the practice dates back a long time ago. International cooperation in public health can be identified in as early as the 18th century. It is thus necessary to put international public health governance back into its historical context to locate the historical reasons that led to their current insufficiencies.

Case analysis. Two case studies are used to flesh out relevant theoretical discussions. The first examines the conflicts between the accessibility of HIV/AIDS medicines and WTO's *Agreement on Trade-Related Aspects of Intellectual Property Rights* (TRIPS). This analysis helps illustrate the predicament that plagues the current global health governance. The second case focuses on China's global health governance strategy, seen in its responses to tackle the COVID-19 pandemic that broke out at the end of 2019.

With the combined use of the aforementioned methods, this book tries to paint a broad landscape of international public health governance comprised of different actors and then zoom in on factors that have resulted in observed deficiencies. Contributions of this book include, first, a new perspective. This book pools together several international regimes that are intimately involved in global health governance endeavours. By analysing their respective limitations in public health governance, this book aims to pinpoint the convergence of their insufficiencies. The book then proposes that China should play a role commensurate with its influence on public health governance. There has been a dearth of publications, neither in China nor in the West, with this research perspective in the field of International Relations Studies. Second, this book contributes to global health governance research with conceptual analysis. It largely builds on pre-existing notions, discusses insufficiencies thereof and develops updated definitions on concepts such as global health governance and public health diplomacy, concepts that consider current developments of contemporary global health status and international cooperation.

Finally, the book provides a novel framework for analysis. It adopts a tripartite theoretical framework consisting of securitisation theory, which is utilised to emphasise the need for global health governance; public goods theory, to explain the approach used in global health governance; and international regime theory, as a way to introduce a number of international regimes currently involved in global public governance. It concludes that one reason why these actors have failed to provide enough global public goods for health is that they lack public-ness in both decision-making and distribution of benefits. On a deeper level, their insufficiency has to do with problems of collective action, the global North–South Divide in public health and the power imbalance in global health governance.

1.4 Research framework

Chapter 1 begins with the theoretical and practical implications of the research, followed by a look at the state of the art and the contributions the book attempts to make.

Chapter 2 lays the groundwork for the whole book by introducing the back-ground, concepts, necessity and approaches of global health governance. Based on previous studies, Section 2.1 defines and delineates global health governance and analyses its characteristics. Section 2.2 uses Copenhagen School's securitisation theory to analyse the securitisation of global health issues. Global health issues have implications for individual, national and international security, prompting these issues to be securitised and demonstrating the necessity and urgency of global health governance. By analysing the global "externality" of public health security, that is the "non-rivalry" and "non-excludability" features of consump-tion, Section 2.3 illustrates the qualities of public health security as a global public good. This further shows that to achieve global health governance, we must pro-vide public goods of global health. Section 2.4 gives a brief overview of how each of the international regimes covered in the book have contributed to global health governance. These regimes are themselves intermediate global public goods for health. They also serve as suppliers of global public goods for health. This chapter ends by pointing out the root causes for the insufficiencies of these regimes to play out such dual roles.

In Chapter 3, WHO, the most prominent actor of global health governance, is put under the microscope. The chapter starts with an overview on the history of international public health cooperation. An attempt is made to divide this timeline into different phases based on their respective characteristics. For an international organisation, its organisational structure is crucial to its agenda. Section 3.2 thus describes the structure of WHO and its three regulatory functions. This is fol-lowed by an in-depth look at the newly revised IHR, a legally binding instrument of international law adopted by WHO, and its weaknesses in Section 3.3. These discussions lay the ground for Section 3.4's discussion on the factors restraining WHO's role in global health governance and the root causes for such limitations. In Section 3.5, we examine to what degree historical and current reforms have succeeded in redressing such limitations.

Chapter 4 dives into the relationship between trade and global health. Section 4.1 studies the close connections between WTO and global health governance. The chapter continues through a discussion of the conflict between WTO's *Agree-ment on Trade-Related Aspects of Intellectual Property Rights* (TRIPS) and the accessibility of medicines, with an end goal to reveal TRIPS's negative impact on global health governance and the limitations of WTO's flexible measures in

10 *Introduction*

response to the TRIPS Agreement. Section 4.3 ends the chapter by investigating the root causes that restrain WTO's role in global health governance.

Chapter 5 first assesses the connections between the current international human rights regimes and public health. Section 5.1 briefly describes the evolution and stages of development of these international human rights regimes and then focuses in more detail on how human rights protections have contributed to global health governance. In Section 5.2, two important human rights conventions, the International Covenant on Civil and Political Rights and the International Covenant on Economic, Social and Cultural Rights, are put under scrutiny to reveal their impact on public health governance. This author argues that global health governance can be achieved only if human rights are promoted and protected in all dimensions. Section 5.3 is organised around the key concept of the right to health. Discussions include the scope of the concept, its evolution and its goals. Section 5.4 examines and summarises limitations of the current international human rights regimes in global health governance and probes into reasons behind such insufficiency.

Chapter 6 begins with a quick historical overview of the BWC, followed by a detailed analysis of the relationship between the BWC and public health. Today, the blurred lines between biological terrorism and natural outbreaks suggest that development of biological weapons and biological defence is not only a military issue but also a public health issue. As the only international regime in the world that governs the use of biological weapons, BWC is of special significance to global health governance. How to enhance BWC's efficiency has become an important goal of global health governance. Therefore, Section 6.3 closely examines the three dilemmas that lead to the BWC's dysfunction.

Chapter 7 is devoted to an assessment of China's contribution to the current global health governance, in particular its public health diplomatic endeavours and achievements made at the global and regional level. It then sheds light on China's health diplomacy with a case study on China's response to the COVID-19 pandemic.

Chapter 8 summarises the main findings of the previous chapters. Based on Inge Kaul's "Triangle of Publicness" model on the supply of public goods, the chapter first summarises the reasons why each of the previously analysed international regimes has failed to provide enough global public goods for health. A common theme is that all of them lack publicness in both decision-making and distribution of benefits. On a deeper level, their insufficiency has to do with the North–South Divide in public health, the power factor in international regimes and their interest-driven orientation in global health governance. To achieve better global health governance, the international regimes must work to democratise, add publicness to global health policymaking and narrow the North–South Divide.

Note

1 According to Barry Buzan, in "securitization" a securitizing actor performs a "speech act" to portray an issue to have highest priority and then labels it as a "security threat" after it

Introduction 11

gains collective acceptance and identification. An issue will be securitised or partly securitized if the audiences accept this statement and international norms will be formulated through social and inter-subjective endeavours. For more references on the securitization of global health issues, see: Alexander, K. (2006). Securitization of International Public Health: Implications for Global Health Governance and the Biological Weapons Prohibition Regime. *Global Governance: A Review of Multilateralism and International Organizations*, 13(2); Leboeuf, A. (n.d.). Securitization of Health and Environmental issues. Retrieved from www.ifri.org/files/Sante_env/Securitization_Health_Environment.pdf; Sheehan, C. C. (2008). *Securitizing the HIV/AIDS Pandemic in U.S. Foreign Policy* (Unpublished doctoral dissertation). American University. Davies, S. E. (2008). Securitizing Infectious Disease. *International Affairs*, 84(2), 295–313; Caballero-Anthony, M. (2006). Combating Infectious Diseases in East Asia. *Journal of International Affairs*, 59(2), 109; Christian, E. (2005, March 5). Securitizing Infectious Diseases. *Paper presented at the annual meeting of the International Studies Association*, Hilton Hawaiian Village, Honolulu, Hawaii. Retrieved from www.allacademic.com/meta/p69269_index. html; Pan, Y. (2007). Life Cycle of International Norms and Theory of Security: Taking Securitization of HIV/AIDS as an Example. *Chinese Journal of European Studies*, 1(4).

References

Aginam, O. (2005). *Global Health Governance: International Law and Public Health in a Divided World*. Toronto: University of Toronto Press.

Aginam, O. (2007). Diplomatic Rhetoric or Rhetoric Diplomacy. In A. F. Cooper, J. J. Kirton, & T. Schrecker (Eds.), *Governing Global Health: Challenge, Response, Innovation*. Hampshire: Ashgate Publishing Ltd.

Beck, U. (2007). The Cosmopolitan Condition: Why Methodological Nationalism Fails. *Theory, Culture & Society*, 24(7–8), 286.

Bradford Jr., C. I. (2007). Reaching the Millennium Development Goals. In A. F. Cooper, J. J. Kirton, & T. Schrecker (Eds.), *Governing Global Health: Challenge, Response, Innovation*. Hampshire: Ashgate Publishing Ltd.

Brower, J., & Peter Chalk, P. (2003). *The Global Threat of New and Re-Emerging Infectious Diseases: Reconciling U.S. National Security and Public Health Policy*. Santa Monica, CA: Rand.

Caballero-Anthony, M. (2006). Combating Infectious Diseases in East Asia: Securitization and Global Public Goods for Health and Human security. *Journal of International Affairs*, 59(2), 105–127.

Chen, Y. (2008). On the Expansion of Functions of United Nations Specialized Agencies Issues: WHO as an example. *Foreign Affairs Review*, (2), 72–78.

Cooper, A. F., Kirton, J. J., & Schrecker, T. (Eds.). (2007). *Governing Global Health: Challenge, Response, Innovation*. Hampshire: Ashgate Publishing Ltd.

Fidler, D. P. (1998). Microbialpolitik: Infectious Diseases and International Relations. *American University Law Review*, 14, 1–11.

Fidler, D. P. (2003). *SARS, Governance and the Globalization of Disease*. New York: Palgrave Macmillan.

Fidler, D. P., & Gostin, L. O. (2008). *Biosecurity in the Global Age: Biological Weapons, Public Health, and the Rule of Law*. Redwood City, CA: Stanford University Press.

Gong, X. (2006). Infectious Disease Globalization and Global Health Governance. *International Review*, (3), 24–29.

Gong, X. (2011). *Infectious Disease Control from the Perspective of International Law*. Beijing: Law Press·China.

12 Introduction

Goodman, N. M. (1977). *International Health Organizations and Their Work* (2nd ed.). London: Churchill Livingstone.

Hayes, J. N. (1998). *The Burdens of Disease: Epidemics and Human Response in Western History*. New Brunswicks, NJ: Rutgers University Press.

He, F. (2004). The Impact of Infectious Diseases on Economic Development and International Relations. *Academic Monthly*, (3), 34–42.

Hein, W. (2008). Global Health Governance: Conflicts on Global Social Rights. *Global Social Policy*, 8(1), 80–108.

Hein, W., Bartsch, S., & Kohlmorgen, L. (2007). *Global Health Governance and the Fight against HIV/AIDS*. New York: Palgrave Macmillan.

Hou, S. (2006). International Cooperation Principles in Global Public Health. *South Forum*, 2.

Howard-Jones, N. (1975). *The Scientific Background of the International Sanitary Conferences*. Geneva: WHO.

Jin, J. (2008a). Securitization of Global Health Issues: WHO as an Example. *International Forum*, (2), 20–24, 79.

Jin, J. (2008b). A Probe into Public Health Diplomacy. *Foreign Affairs Review*, (4), 82–88.

Jin, J. (2008c). Public Health Security: A Global Public Goods for Health Analysis Framework. *Health and Society*, (9), 7–9.

Jin, J. (2008d). International Institutions and Global Health Governance. *Contemporary International Relations*, (5), 21–99.

Jin, J. (2009). Politicization of United Nations Specialized Agencies: WHO as an Example. *International Forum*, (1), 12–17.

Kaul, I., et al. (Eds.). (2003). *Providing Global Public Goods: Managing Globalization*. Oxford: Oxford University Press.

Kickbusch, I. (2005). Tackling the Political Determinants of Global Health. *Brazilian Journal of Microbiology*, (331), 246.

Koivusalo, M., & Ollila, E. (1997). *Making a Healthy World: Agencies, Actors & Policies in International Health*. London: Zed Books Ltd.

Lanegran, K., & Hyden, G. (1993). Mapping the Politics of AIDS: Illustrations from East Africa. *Population and Environment*, 14(3), 247.

Lee, K., & Dodgson, R. (2003). Globalization and Cholera: Implications for Global Governance. In K. Lee (Ed.), *Health Impacts of Globalization*. New York: Palgrave Macmillan.

Li, S. (2006). *Contemporary Global Issues*. Hangzhou: Zhejiang People's Publishing House.

McNeill, W. H. (1976). *Plagues and Peoples*. New York: Doubleday.

Na, L., He, Z., & Wang, Y. (2004). *WTO and Public Health*. Beijing: Tsinghua University Press.

Pan, Y. (2007). Life Cycle of International Norms and Theory of Security: Taking Securitization of HIV/AIDS as an Example. *Chinese Journal of European Studies*, (4), 68–82.

Porter, D. (1999). *Health, Civilization and the State: A History of Public Health from Ancient to Modern Times*. London and New York: Routledge.

Price-Smith, A. T. (2001). *Plagues and Politics: Infectious Disease and International Policy*. New York: Palgrave Macmillan.

Qi, F., & Zhu, X. (2006). An Investigation into China-ASEAN Public Health Security Cooperation Mechanism. *Southeast Asian Studies*, 1.

Siddiqi, J. (1995). *World Health and World Politics*. Columbia: University of South Carolina Press.

Smith, R. D., Beagleole, R., Woodward, D., & Drager, N. (2003). *Global Public Goods for Health*. Oxford: Oxford University Press.

Su, C. (2000). *Global Public Issues and International Cooperation: An Institutional Analysis*. Shanghai: Shanghai People's Publishing House.

Thomas, C., & Weber, M. (2004). The Politics of Global Health Governance: Whatever Happened to "Health for All by the Year 2000"? *Global Governance: A Review of Multilateralism and International Organizations*, 10(2), 187–205.

Virchow, R. (1948). Der Armenarzt. *Medicinische Reform 1848*, (18), 125–127.

Waltz, N. K. (1959). *Man, the State, and War: A Theoretical Analysis*. New York: Columbia University Press.

Wang, X., & Meng, Q. (2005). *History of World Plague*. Beijing: China Social Sciences Press.

Zacher, M., & Keefe, T. (2008). *The Politics of Global Health Governance: United by Contagion*. New York: Palgrave Macmillan.

Zhu, X. (2006). An Investigation into Southeast Public Health Cooperation Mechanism. *Southeast Asian Studies*, (1), 88–91.

Zinsser, H. (1963). *Rats, Lice and History: A Chronicle of Pestilence and Plagues*. New York: Black Dog and Leventhal.

2 Theoretical underpinnings of global health governance

International cooperation on public health can be traced back to the mid-19th century. At the time, two cholera epidemics, one in 1830 and the other in 1847, made it necessary for European countries to confront their vulnerability to each other in the event of public health crises; Europe's trade and business also demanded that countries adopt a consistent set of quarantine regulations. These two conditions paved the way for "multilateralization" in early collaborative public health practices and marked the beginning of international public health cooperation. On July 23, 1851, at France's initiative, 12 European countries convened the first International Health Conference in Paris.[1] The agenda of the meeting was control and coordination of quarantine efforts from various ports. Another crucial topic on the agenda concerned international collaboration to contain cholera, epidemic disease and yellow fever. From 1851 to the end of the 19th century, a total of ten international health conferences were held and eight agreements and conventions reached (Fidler, 2000, p. 327). Since international collaboration on public health policies centred around Europe, such collaboration was notably Eurocentric. Further, as countries had shifting priorities between development of business interest and multilateral collaboration on disease containment, most conventions ended up not being ratified and consequently were not enforced, let alone contribute towards the establishment of an international public health institution. International public health cooperation at the time was thus additionally very non-institutionalized.

By the end of the 19th century, European countries gradually realized that international conventions and treaties alone could neither address common vulnerabilities nor "put an end" to the threat of infectious diseases. To implement and enforce the international public health conventions reached, countries across the world began to coordinate diplomatically to establish formal international regimes. By the beginning of the 20th century, multilateral public health initiatives were no longer confined to Europe and became a concerted global effort through the establishment of a series of international health organisations, including in particular the formation of the League of Nations after the end of World War I. Article 23 of the *Covenant of the League of Nations* states that members "will endeavour to take steps in matters of international concern for the prevention and control of disease" (The League of Nations, 1920). In 1923, more international health organisations were put in place, including the League of Nations Health Organization

Theoretical underpinnings 15

and the International Veterinary Agency. WHO came into being on April 7, 1948. This was a landmark event in the history of international public health cooperation and marked the globalisation and institutionalisation of international public health cooperation in the true sense of the word.

As globalisation deepens, countries around the world become more interdependent upon each other in public health security. "Globalization is changing the public health landscape" (Drager & Beaglehole, 2001, p. 803). The rapid movement of people as well as the increasingly interdependent and interconnected world has also sparked countless new risks for diseases. As Laurie Garrett (1995) puts it in her pioneering book *The Coming Plague: Newly Emerging Diseases in a World out of Balance,*

> To some extent, each of these processes has been occurring throughtout history. What is new, however, is the increased potential that at least will generate large-scale, even worldwide epidemics. The global epidemics of human immunodeficiency virus is the most powerful and recent example. Yet, AIDS doesn't stand alone, it may well be just the first of the modern, large-scale epidemics.
>
> (p. xv)

Infectious diseases are now spreading across countries at unprecedented rates. Newly found emerging infectious diseases are also rising with unparalleled variety. Since the 1970s, each year has seen the spread of at least one or more new type of emerging infectious disease. Nearly 40 types of infectious diseases today were unknown a generation ago, including SARS and the avian flu. The anthrax attacks in the United States in 2001 have also made the threat of bioterrorism a stark reality. "The fact is however that national health has become an international challenge. An outbreak anywhere must now be seen as a threat to virtually all countries" (WHO, 1996, p. 17). Since public health crises pose serious threats to security on individual, national and international levels, public health issues have risen to a security-level concern. In other words, they have been securitised. "The solution to global public problems calls for multilateral joint action rather than unilateral action; it requires global public policies and cooperation-based planning rather than individual unilateral decision-making" (Su, 2000, p. 6). In the same vein, the solution to global health issues requires global health governance. The ultimate goal is to provide more global public goods for health. One of the main approaches to achieving this aim is through global health governance regimes based on principles of multilateralism.

2.1 Global health governance: concepts, context and features

2.1.1 Key concepts in global health governance

Over the past few years, global health governance has become increasingly prominent in the global agenda. For instance, out of the eight UN MDGs, three

16 Theoretical underpinnings

of them directly concern public health, and the other five are also connected to public health issues.[2] Promoting better health is also seen as an important aspect of ensuring "human security". There is a growing global awareness of the importance of public health as a cross-cutting issue. "The growth in the importance of health in world politics over the past decade constitutes an unprecedented transformation" (Fidler, 2007a, p. 1). Although global health governance is now featured in the discourse of International Relations Studies, the concept behind the term has rarely been properly elucidated. It is essential to start by defining and clarifying the concept of global health governance.

Wolfgang Hein, from the Centre for Global and Regional Studies at the University of Hamburg, Germany, was the first person to analyse the concept of global health governance. In 2005, he defined global health governance as "the totality of collective regulations to deal with international and transnational interdependence in the context of health issues" (Hein, 2008, p. 84). Another interpretation comes from Delroy S. Beckford of the Global Trade Development Centre. He defines global health governance as the rules and codes of conduct established in order to govern health protection and the roles played by both national and non-governmental organisations in the formulation and implementation of these rules (2008). Although these definitions roughly illustrate the idea of global health governance, they do not fully explain the complexity involved in global health governance today. There is a clear need to define the meaning of global health governance. One of the ways to do so is to break down "global health governance" into "governance", "global governance", and "global public health". Only with a clear understanding of these individual concepts can we come to truly appreciate the concept of global health governance.

First, what is "governance"? The word originates from a classical Latin/ancient Greek verb meaning "to steer", mainly used to convey a sense of governing, guiding and directing. It is often used in conjunction with "government". The World Bank was the first to use the term "crisis in governance" in 1989. According to a study published by the Global Governance Commission titled *Our Global Neighbourhood*, governance is the sum of the many ways individuals and institutions, public and private, manage their common affairs. The concept covers formal institutions and regimes empowered to enforce compliance and informal arrangements that people and institutions either have agreed to or perceive to be in their interest (Commission on Global Governance, 1995, pp. 2–3). "Governance" essentially describes the ways official or private public management organisations use their public authority to maintain order within a given scope. It is both a public management activity and public management process. The central value of governance is to provide certain range of public goods more effectively.

Regarding "global governance", scholars worldwide diverge in their views and have not yet come to an agreed-upon definition. Some scholars see it as an extension of governance at the national level, the result of which is the expansion of national public goods into global public goods (Yu, 2003). German scholar Sonja Bartsch defines global governance as "the totality of collective regulations to deal with international and transnational interdependence problems" (Hein et al., 2007, p. 9), whereas Chinese scholar Keping Yu (2003) believes that global governance should be understood as "an effort intended to solve issues concerning global conflict, ecology, human rights, immigration, drugs, smuggling, and infectious diseases through legally-binding international regulations (regimes) in order to maintain a normal international political economy" (p. 13). In short, global governance is one response to the negative effects of globalisation and a way to control *global public bads* by means of global cooperation to promote the supply of global public goods. There are in general three types of actors that can play the role of global governance: governments, formal international regimes (such as WTO and WHO) and global civil society organisations.[3]

The object of public health research is "the health of societies" rather than the health of individuals in medical research. Global health as a concept derives from the expansion of globalisation in the field of public health. Global health research focuses on the political and social determinants and consequences of health issues worldwide (Baum, 2002, p. 7). Robert Beaglehole and Ruth Bonita (2008) think that "global health is the collective action we take worldwide for improving health and health equity" (p. 1998). Collective action requires decision-making regimes leading to governance. According to a document titled "Health is Global" (2008) published by the UK Department of Health, "global health" refers to

> health issues where the determinants circumvent, undermine or are obvious to the territorial boundaries of states, and are thus beyond the capacity of individual countries to address through domestic institutions. Global health is focused on people across the whole planet rather than the concerns of a state. Global health recognizes that health is determined by problems, issues and concerns that transcend national boundaries.
>
> (p. 5)

The *World Health Report 2007* defines "global health security" as "the activities required, both proactive and reactive, to minimize vulnerability to acute public health events that endanger the collective health of populations living across geographical regions and international boundaries" (WHO, 2007a, p. 1). In other words, the purpose of these proactive and reactive activities is to reduce or to lower mutual vulnerabilities people face across the globe in the event of emergencies to public health.[4] The purpose of global health governance is to ensure global health security. Having analysed the previous concepts ("global governance", "public health", "global public health"), we may now define global health governance as a process to reduce global common vulnerability in public health security through the development and implementation of binding international regulations in areas that determine global public health.

2.1.2 The context for the rise of global health governance

Global health governance rises because of several factors. As the tide of globalisation deepens interdependence among countries in the world, public health

18 *Theoretical underpinnings*

security is no exception to this trend. While non-traditional security theories offer us theoretical support to analyse global health issues from a "security" perspective, the emergence of global governance theories in turn provides an analytical framework under which to analyse global health governance.

2.1.2.1 Influence of globalisation

As Lee and Dodgson (2005) argue, "an understanding of the linkages between globalization and health depends foremost on one's definition of globalization and precise dating of the process" (p. 214). Most people regard globalisation as a process in which countries are increasingly connected. As a result, "events occurring in one country will have repercussions in other countries and consequently their people" (Smith & Baylis, 1997, p. 2). The essence of globalisation is the "transcendence of boundaries and the disappearance of spatial distance" (Aron, 1967, p. 7). Fidler believes that globalisation refers to processes or phenomena that undermine the ability of the sovereign state to control what occurs in its territory (1997), while Gordon R. Walker and Mark A. Fox (1996) contend that a basic feature characterising globalisation is the constant erosion and loss of relevance of national borders in the context of market globalisation.

Various proposals on the precise timing of globalisation exist, all invariably falling into two competing schools: the "recent" school and the "ancient" school. The recent school holds that globalisation did not start until the 1990s and is mainly propelled by the activities of multinational corporations. The ancient school, on the other hand, believes that, notwithstanding the emergence of the new forces of globalisation in the past few decades, globalisation has historical roots tracing back to the 15th century (Giddens, 1990; Robertson, 1992). If globalisation is characterised by the disappearance of geographical and physical geopolitical boundaries, then these historical antecedents to the transnational spread of disease make the notion that globalisation "is the concept of the 1990s" less persuasive. In his account of the plague that ravaged Athens during the Peloponnesian War, Thucydides writes:

> It is said that the plague first originated in Ethiopia and then descended into Egypt and Lebanon and much of the Persian Empire. It fell suddenly upon Athens and attacked in the first instance the population of the port city of Piraeus. Later it also arrived in the upper city and by this time the number of deaths was greatly increasing. The question of the probable origin of the plague and the nature of the causes capable of creating so great an upheaval, I leave to other writers, with or without medical experience. . . . I caught the disease myself and observed others suffering from it.
>
> (Longrigg, 1992, p. 21)

When European colonists conquered the Americas, they also imported European disease that decimated the population of native American Indians. Europeans then began to sell slaves purchased from Africa to replace the lost labour, but the West

Theoretical underpinnings 19

African slaves in turn brought falciparum malaria to the Americas. A transnational process of infectious diseases is thus completed between the "New World" and the "Old World". The tripartite exchange between Europeans, Native Americans, and Africans raised mutual vulnerability in ways not known in human history (Crosby, 1972; Porter, 1999; Watts, 1997). Keohane and Nye (2000) also side with the "ancient" school. They write:

> One of the most important forms of globalization is biological. The first smallpox epidemic is recorded in Egypt in 1350 B.C.; it reached China in 49 A.D.; Europe after 700; the Americas in 1520; and Australia in 1789. The plague or Black Death originated in Asia, but its spread killed a quarter to a third of the population of Europe between 1346 and 1352. When Europeans journeyed to the New World in the fifteenth and sixteenth centuries, they carried pathogens that destroyed up to 95% of the local indigenous population.
>
> (p. 2)

In short, the whole world has been getting smaller since the 16th century, and microbes have had more opportunities to spread quickly across borders.

The developments in science and technology in the 20th century accelerated the process of globalisation. Globalisation in an irreversible fashion continues to drive the expansion of trade and travel. Many of the previous domestic issues are increasingly being externalised internationally. As Nakajima (1997) argues:

> In the late twentieth century, an era characterised by the globalization of the world's political economy, the threat of infectious disease transmission across national borders and the expansion of the trade and promotion of harmful commodities, such as tobacco, represent transnational health problems. The fact that the political boundaries of sovereign states do not represent natural barriers to infectious agents or to harmful products underscores the need for interstate cooperation to address these global health issues.
>
> (p. 317)

It is as if globalisation has opened Pandora's box, with infectious diseases flying out like ominous bats. In 1992, the Institute of Medicine published a landmark report titled *Emerging Infections: Microbial Threats to Health in the United States*, in which it is argued that, as a result of increases in global population movements, more drug-resistant strains of viruses and mounting damage to the ecology and environment, diseases such as cholera, plague, malaria, tuberculosis and diphtheria have all, despite their former containment, risen in the number of cases. New types of infectious diseases, such as AIDS, Ebola, Legionnaires' disease, avian flu and SARS, also joined the fray. Over the past 60 years, the number of infectious diseases has increased at an unprecedented rate. For example, in the 1940s, only 20 types of new infectious diseases had been identified; in the 1980s, the number jumped to 90 (Jone et al., 2008, p. 990). Infectious diseases as "global bads" do not respect national borders in their path of transmission. Given

20 *Theoretical underpinnings*

that an estimated 2.1 billion passengers chose to travel by air in 2006, once a disease strikes an area, it only takes a few hours for it to descend upon another place (WHO, 2007, p. ix). "Globalization has directly caused or contributed to transnational health risks posed by emerging and recurrent infectious diseases, various non-communicable diseases, and environmental changes" (Dodgson & Lee, 2002, p. 98). "Globalization has changed the global health landscape" (Drager & Beaglehole, 2001, p. 803). It has also widened the gap between the rich and the poor in the world. Some poorly governed or "failed" countries now find their economy deteriorating day by day. As these countries do not have the means to invest in their public health provision, malnutrition is a serious challenge. At the same time, the global health crisis is compounded by the globalisation of poor living habits, the degradation of ecological environments and the abuse of antibiotics. WHO believes that the globalisation of infectious diseases represents a world crisis manifested by the increasing vulnerability of national borders to transnational microbial threats. G. Berlinguer aptly describes this phenomenon as "the microbial unification of the world" (1999, p. 18). The process of globalisation is in this sense the process of "de-nationalization". On one hand, globalisation has released the ills of infectious diseases: Microbes can now travel passport-free; they do not respect geopolitical or sovereign boundaries; they have weakened the ability of any single sovereign state to govern its own public health. On the other hand, personal and public health within a country has become a matter of global concern; health issues across borders become more dependent on each other because of their common vulnerability in public health security. "The national and international dimensions of public health policies are increasingly intertwined and inseparable" (Yach & Bettcher, 1998, p. 735). "Global health is indivisible" (Berlinguer, 2003, p. 61). To meet the challenges of global public health, international collaboration and global cooperation efforts must be strengthened. This requires that we no longer stick to the traditional concept of national sovereignty but rather yield part of domestic sovereignty power to global health governance regimes. A country cannot solve all public health security issues on its own. The solution to globalisation problems is not to avoid the process but to learn to manage globalisation There is an urgent need for better global governance. In the same vein, we must build up effective global health governance to solve global health security issues.

2.1.2.2 Rise of non-traditional security studies

It is difficult to pinpoint the exact time when the notion of "non-traditional security" was first proposed. It emerged sometime in the early 1970s after the publication of the Club of Rome report. The *Brandt Report*, published in 1980, first proposed that security issues should be addressed through a "non-traditional approach" and suggested that one of the important ways for countries to address international security was to pay more attention to "non-traditional security" (Salmon, 2000, pp. 61–62). Later on, in his book *People, States, and Fear*, Barry Buzan (1983) elevated economic, social and environmental issues to the same

Theoretical underpinnings 21

status as political and military ones and contended that security threat affects more than the military dimension. Security issues affect not only countries but also societies and individuals. After the end of the Cold War, British scholar Ken Booth (1991) proposed that security should achieve "social emancipation" and "human emancipation." He held that in the post–Cold War era, security should not only forego military technology's control over people but also reflect the ties of nations in the world as an inseparable community and that all social phenomena should be "people-centred" (pp. 313–326). The concept of global security and "human security" gradually became popular. "Human security" was even featured in the UN's *Human Development Report 1994*, which addressed seven major security issues. In the same year, then UN Secretary-General Boutros Boutros-Ghali wrote *An Agenda for Peace* for the UN, which also highlighted the threats facing humanity brought by unlimited population growth, debt, drugs, the gap between rich and poor, poverty, disease, famine and refugee settlement. This report also reminded people to note that the harm caused by these threats amounted to no less than the traditional threats of war. Most traditional international political theories tend to emphasise peace and conflict issues between nations and overlook tremendous disruption of infectious diseases on human security. These traditional theories hold that the main actors of security are the sovereign states who project their sovereign independence and territorial integrity through the means of military force. "Defining national security merely (or even primarily) in military terms conveys a profoundly false image of reality. It causes states to concentrate on military threats and to ignore other and perhaps even more harmful dangers" (Ullman, 1983, p. 129). In comparison, non-traditional security theory tries to bring changes to people's understanding of the source, the object and the means to achieve security. The object of security research in the field of international politics shall no longer be dominated by military and ideological challenges confronting the state as an actor.

Indeed, the non-traditional view holds that people and society should maintain their economic, health- and human rights–related security, etc., through consultation, legal system building and governance. The non-traditional security theory epitomises the human-centred approach and marks the return of human-centred thinking. An important aspect of achieving human-centred security is to protect people's lives from various threats and promote long-term human development. Global infectious diseases have a grave impact on human security. As a matter of fact, more people die each year from infections than from war. According to the World Bank report *Investing for Health*, the global death toll from infectious diseases was 16.69 million in 1990, accounting for 34.4% of total deaths, almost 50 times more than 320,000, the number of people dying from warfare, occupying 0.64% of the total population (World Bank, 1993). The bioterrorism of the anthrax virus after the September 11 attacks in the United States is clear evidence that not even the most affluent nation in the world is immune to viral weapons. In addition to bioterrorism, the global spread of AIDS also poses a serious threat to human security. Former UN Secretary-General Kofi Annan once described AIDS as "a real weapon of mass destruction" (Yu, 2006, p. 250). "HIV/AIDS is creating

22 *Theoretical underpinnings*

a September 11 every day in Africa" (Cooper et al., 2007, p. 230). According to *The Global Threat of New and Re-emerging Infectious Diseases: Reconciling US National Security and Public Health Policy*, a report issued by the US Rand Corporation, the threat posed by the emergence of new and recurrent infectious diseases worldwide to human and national security has risen to a point that even the current US policies cannot adequately cope (Brower & Chalk, 2003). According to a report by *Boston Globe* on June 30, 2000, at a hearing held by the House International Relations Committee on June 29, some CIA officials stated that the spread of infectious diseases would increasingly constitute a global health issue, possibly at a catastrophic level. They also considered it possible those infectious diseases may seriously damage US national security. In a speech given at Fudan University on January 9, 2006, Robert Keohane also expressed his belief that one major threat facing the international community in the future would be the outbreak of infectious diseases. To conclude, grim threats to public health security in the world today have made it necessary to make public health security concerns a high priority in the security agenda.

2.1.2.3 Rise of global governance

Since the 1990s, many international relations scholars have adopted the concept of "global governance". Global governance is in some sense an extension of domestic governance to international contexts as well as a globalisation process of domestic public goods. The main target of global governance concerns "global pubic bads" that grow with globalisation, such as international terrorism, ecological degradation and transnational infectious diseases. The goal of global governance is to provide more global public goods by actors that span individual countries, international organisations, non-governmental organisations, multinational corporations and individuals. The fate of all nations is tied to the same string when it comes to global health and safety with ever-deepening interdependence. This mutual vulnerability to the threat of infectious diseases calls for collective action by individual countries to promote global governance. The global health crisis calls for global health governance. "The crisis in global health is not a health crisis, but a governance crisis" (Kickbusch, 2004, pp. 463–469). Global governance theory provides a theoretical perspective and framework to analyse global health governance. Global health governance is a process to resolve the global health crisis through international public health regimes. Its ultimate goal is to provide the global community with more global public goods for health. Only through active public health diplomacy and multilateral cooperation can countries reach consensus and take collective actions so awareness of the global health crisis can be raised. This is the only path towards the establishment and implementation of an effective global health governance regime. The TRIPS Agreement and the Doha Declaration on Public Health adopted by WTO and the IHR, revised and adopted in 2005, are examples of such efforts.

Theoretical underpinnings 23

2.1.3 Features of global health governance

2.1.3.1 Flexibility of (formal/informal) regimes

Global health governance has flexible regimes whose international components include both formal and informal counterparts. Formal regimes are binding on all member states. This in some ways addresses issues concerning coordination vis-à-vis collective action in the field of public health and make public health governance behaviours of various countries more predictable. Formal regimes include the IHR, and the Agreement on Trade-Related Aspects of Intellectual Property Rights, both of which were revised in 2005, and the Framework Convention on Tobacco Control, concluded in July 2005. Informal regimes include, among others, the International Red Cross Organization, The Ottawa Charter for Health Promotion, the Health for all by the Year 2000 initiative proposed by WHO in 1981 and the Global Fund to Fight AIDS, Tuberculosis and Malaria. Informal regimes can take advantage of their flexibility, thereby compensating for the shortcomings of formal regimes.

2.1.3.2 Multilateralism

The multilateralism of global health governance is reflected at national, regional and global levels. Such multi-level agents complement each other and together make up a multidimensional effort of global health governance. On a national level, one country can provide unilateral medical assistance or global health public goods to another country. For example, China has in the past dispatched medical teams to African countries. The United States also launched the President's Emergency Plan for AIDS Relief (PEPFAR) in 2007. Bilateral cooperation to promote global health governance is also on the rise. For example, through the China–UK Global Health Support Programme (GHSP), jointly launched by the Chinese and British governments in 2012, the two countries have established a new type of Sino-British health partnership to enhance China's ability to participate in global health development, strengthen cooperation in the field of global health and jointly promote global health governance and the improvement of global health. In recent years, with the rise of regionalism, public health governance actions at the regional level have also increased. For example, at the St. Petersburg Summit in 2006, the G8 countries put the control of infectious diseases as one of its three priority goals and held its first G8 Health Ministers' Meeting. Likewise, the Asia-Pacific Economic Cooperation (APEC) has put public health issues into its area of focus. The organisation also published the APEC Strategy to Fight Epidemics at the 2001 Shanghai Summit. At the Mexico Summit in 2002, APEC countries unanimously agreed to establish a regional public health surveillance network and an early warning system tasked to provide a response to major disease epidemics, especially one arising from bioterrorism. The agenda of the 2006 Ha Noi Declaration contained a discussion on control of the bird flu and

24 *Theoretical underpinnings*

epidemics. In November 2004, ASEAN and China, Japan and South Korea issued the Bangkok Statement on the Prevention of Avian Influenza in Asia, emphasising cooperation between governments, international organisations and social groups to contain the spread of the bird flu. In October 2003, China and ASEAN launched the "10+1" health ministers' meeting mechanism; in March 2004, the China-ASEAN Special Meeting on Avian Influenza Control was held in Beijing, and a China-and-ASEAN Public Health Fund was also set up. In 2006, China, Japan and South Korea signed a Memorandum of Cooperation on a joint response to epidemics and established a cooperation mechanism for health ministers from the three countries to meet annually. Emerging countries are also increasingly involved. For example, in July 2011, the BRICS countries held their first health ministers' meeting in Beijing and established a long-term dialogue mechanism for BRICS countries' health ministers. The mechanism seeks to enhance the role of BRICS countries in global health governance by promoting access to medical resources and strengthening multisectoral coordination to address antibiotic resistance. In comparison, public health governance efforts are more wide ranging at the global level. Notable examples include the Declaration of Alma-Ata signed in 1978,[5] the Millennium Development Goals (MDGs) adopted by the United Nations in September 2000, the 2030 Agenda for Sustainable Development adopted in September 2015 and the relevant articles on public health made by WHO and WTO.

2.1.3.3 Diversity of actors in global health governance

Actors of global health governance are diverse. Diverse political, economic and social impact of public health issues lead to increasing involvement from more organisations and sectors. "Any efforts that seek to divide policies and politics between 'domestic' and 'foreign', 'hard' and 'soft', and 'high' and 'low' categories are out of place" (Kickbusch, 2003a, p. 192). The multisectoral nature of public health includes participation of a wide range of actors, including not only governmental and non-governmental organisations but also individuals and multinational companies, such as the Gates Foundation; the Rockefeller Foundation; the Global Fund to Fight AIDS, Tuberculosis and Malaria and Doctors Without Borders. Each of these organisations has played an important role in global health governance. As far as international regimes in global health governance are concerned, there exist traditional development regimes, such as WHO, traditional security regimes, such as the Convention on the Prohibition of Biological Weapons and WTO and international human rights regimes, such as the International Covenant on Civil Economic, Social and Cultural Rights. Just as Fidler (2007a) argues, "Governance of global health issues has shifted from a Westphalian to a post-Westphalian context in which both States and non-State actors shape responses to transnational health threats and opportunities" (p. 2). Only through the participation of such diverse actors can we achieve better global health governance. For example, NGOs are more flexible because they are not bound by political constraints. Some of them have contributed substantial funding for public health programs run by WHO. Some government organisations have also established global public-private partnerships with NGOs. There are currently approximately 80 global public-private partnerships in public health (Buse, 2004, p. 225), of which notable players include the Accelerated Access Initiative, the Global Alliance for Vaccine Initiative and the Roll Back Malaria Global Partnership. The participation of so many actors promotes effective governance of global health issues.

2.1.3.4 High level of professionalism

Global health governance inevitably involves medical issues, especially vis-à-vis control of transnational communicable diseases, making it a highly specialised area. Nevertheless, requirements of professional knowledge should not cut off the link between the health sector and other sectors. As Aginam, legal adviser for WHO, states, "Public health is no longer the prerogative of doctors and infectious disease scientists" (2002a, p. 946). The purpose of global governance is to serve global security and development. Some public health issues are security and development issues. When it comes to global health security, all countries in the world have shared interests in which benefit to one means benefit to all, whereas harm to one means harm to all. The public health sector alone cannot solve public health security issues, whose solution requires the political commitment and will of every country as well as the integration of health issues and diplomatic issues. However, given the level of professional knowledge required, some countries have chosen to set up specialised departments under their Ministry of Foreign Affairs to tackle public health issues. For example, the US National Security Council has set aside a special post for the public health security strategy advisor to coordinate technical issues between health and diplomacy. The combination of policies regarding public health issues and diplomacy will help global health governance gain political commitment from every country in the world.

The previous characteristics of global health governance fully illustrate the complexity involved in today's international affairs, as well as the arduous nature of the challenges confronting global health governance. Therefore, we need to continue to innovate at the institutional and regime levels to effectively provide more global public goods for health for the sake of individual security, national security and by extension global security.

2.2 Necessity of global health governance: securitisation

The parochialism in the scope of security research is a well-recognised fact in the study of international relations. The nuclear arms race during the Cold War only further brought this observation to the fore. Scholars of mainstream security research rarely expand their agenda from national security to other fields, let alone scholars who subscribe to neorealism and neoliberalism. The securitisation theory proposed by the Copenhagen School re-examines and criticises this

26 *Theoretical underpinnings*

narrowness. The school contends that any issue can be securitised so long as it is portrayed as an existential threat, is addressed by unconventional measures, receives inter-subjective construction or identification and triggers the formation of relevant international norms.

Global health issues have long been considered biomedical and developmental issues whose importance is eclipsed by traditional "security" threats. However, the global spread of infectious diseases has brought numerous risks to individual and social security, even to national and international security. "The nexus between health and security has become increasingly clear" (WHO, 2002b). The SARS crisis, which affected more than 30 countries in 2003, the prevalent HIV/AIDS epidemic, and the lurking "bird flu", are all classic examples in this regard. The Tokyo subway sarin attack by Aum Shinrikyo cult members in March 1995 and the anthrax attacks in the United States in 2001 fuelled more concerns over public health security crises. All such threats prompted the academia to engage in the "discourse" of bioterrorism. Given the prominence of "existential threats" posed by the transnational spread of infectious diseases and bioterrorism, there is also a tendency to securitise public health crises in security research. The securitisation of global health issues testifies to the necessity and urgency of global health governance.

2.2.1 Securitisation: content and concepts

While the end of the Cold War breathed new life into security research, it also made the field even more contentious. Security research has become a field where the most challenging new perspectives on international politics thrive and the most intense theoretical debates take place (Hopf, 1998). As globalisation proceeds, issues that can be securitised have diversified. Traditional security research, which uses nation-states as basic units of analysis, is no longer up to date; military security can no longer monopolise the discourse of security research. Issues previously dismissed in security studies, such as the impact of Third World countries on security, that include the challenges of their domestic political and social-cultural factors to security, ethnic and religious conflicts due to lack of protection for individual rights, refugees and wide-spread epidemics, etc., have all become focal points in security-related discussions. The securitisation theory, developed by Ole Wæver and Barry Buzan, has become an influential school in security research.

2.2.1.1 Content of the securitisation theory

The content of the securitisation theory closely relates to the definition of security. How to demarcate security issues from non-security ones is the key in security research. Traditionally, the defining feature of a security agenda is the likelihood of military conflicts or the use of force, but Buzan criticised this type of understanding in *Security: A New Framework for Analysis*. He argued that the concept of security was apt for a re-definition. Security is not only a perception but is more conspicuously a "speech act". In fact, there is no pre-existing formal definition

Theoretical underpinnings 27

of security. Anything can be a security issue if it is considered as one (Buzan & Wæver, 2003). In short, in order to securitise an issue, a securitising actor performs a speech act to portray an issue as having the highest priority and then labels it as a "security threat" after it gains collective acceptance and identification. "Thereby, the actor has claimed a right to handle the issue through extraordinary means" (Buzan & Wæver, 2003, p. 25). Securitisation "is constituted by the intersubjective establishment of an existential threat with a saliency sufficient to have subsitential political effects" (Buzan & Wæver, 2003, p. 25).

In the process of securitisation, a securitising actor identifies the threat to a specifically marked object through speech acts and explains that containing the existing threat requires extraordinary means. If the audiences accept this statement, then relevant international norms would be formulated through social and inter-subjective endeavor. In so doing, this problem becomes 'securitized'.

In other words, it becomes a security issue or a part of security issue. Of course, this does not mean that the securitisation theory holds that all speech acts will lead to securitisation. According to Buzan and Wæver, a successful securitisation consists of three steps: 1) identification of existential threats, 2) taking emergency action and 3) effects on inter subjective relations by breaking free of normal procedures (Buzan & Wæver, 2003). Each step is indispensable for the success of securitisation and the establishment of relevant international norms.

2.2.1.2 Core concepts of securitisation theory

Core concepts provide the substance for any theory; this observation also applies to the securitisation theory underpinned by the following key concepts.

EXISTENTIAL THREAT

They are threats to the referent objects in a specific area. These threats are so serious "that [they] should not be exposed to the normal haggling of politics but should be dealt with decisively by top leaders prior to other issues" (Buzan & Wæver, 2003, p. 29). They may warrant emergency measures and actions outside the normal bounds of political procedure. For example, as a referent object, one of the "existential threats" China faces in its sovereign security is its relationship with Taiwan. There is absolutely no room for Taiwan to haggle with sovereignty issues, and the Chinese government has never ceded the extraordinary option of using military intervention to address the threat of Taiwan's independence.

SPEECH ACT

This is an analytical tool the securitisation school borrowed from linguistic constructivism. Approaching security from a speech act perspective raises questions about the relationship between actors and analysts in defining and understanding the security agenda. A successful speech act combines interlocution with societal norms and gives nod to the inherent relationship between the two in speech, thus

28   *Theoretical underpinnings*

winning collective approval. Of all internal conditions to the speech act, the most important is to stick to the security regime and security grammar rules. A speech act must include a secret plan pointing to "existential threats", setting limit points and providing a viable way out of the dilemma under discussion. These constitute the catalysts for an issue to be securitised. The external form of a speech act has two main conditions: 1) the social resources of the speaker—the securitising actor must be in an authoritative if not official position, and 2) the speech act must be linked to threats. For example, the raging HIV/AIDS epidemic is an existential threat for countries in Africa. However, these countries cannot securitise this public health issue due to their less advantageous position in the international community. The United States, on the other hand, is in an authoritative position. The Clinton administration first described AIDS as an existential threat to US national security in 1999. At the United States' initiative, on January 10, 2000, the UN Security Council specifically addressed the impact of AIDS on Africa's peace and security and on international security, thereby signalling the successful securitisation of HIV/AIDS. In July of the same year, the Security Council passed Resolution 1308 on HIV/AIDS, marking the official establishment of the first set of international norms on the securitisation of the disease.

INTERSUBJECTIVITY

Speech acts made by the securitising actor provide a necessary but not sufficient condition for issues to be successfully securitised. *Intersubjectivity* refers to the extent to which an existential threat is recognised by securitising actors. It emphasises the actual construction of securitisation. Whether a certain issue is a security matter is not determined only through identification of a participatory agent since securitisation involves both intersubjectivity and sociality. Successful securitisation is not only determined by a securitising actor but also by the "audience" of the security speech act. Or rather, it is determined by whether the audience accepts that an issue as an existential threat has threatened a shared value. In other words, securitisation is a process in which a securitising actor adapts its perception to other agents' understanding of certain existential threats and thus involves security-related interaction under the international system. For example, the United States has successfully promoted the securitisation of terrorism. This whole process was based on the international community's shared identification of the current threat of terrorism. Moreover, through a series of counter-terrorism resolutions the UN has passed, countries around the globe have confirmed their support of relevant international norms.

2.2.2 *How global health issues are securitised*

Public health is often considered a biomedical as well as a technical issue belonging to a specialised territory for epidemiologists. National public health authorities and international regimes for public health (e.g. WHO) are given the exclusive and narrow responsibility to manage the prevention and control of diseases. However, as globalisation proceeds, existential threats that originally emerged from the field of public health have been linked to the concepts of human security, national security, regional security and global security. "Public health is the basic tenet upon which all other forms of security rest" (Randy, 2004, p. 24). Public health issues have gone beyond the scope of medical science and become securitised after entering the political realm. As Ilona Kickbusch, an expert at Geneva Graduate Institute of International and Development Studies, states, health protection is no longer just a humanitarian and technical issue related to UN specialized agencies. It is more widely accepted as an issue linked to economic, political, and security questions in a complex, interdependent, post-Cold War world (2005, p. 192). In general, global health issues are securitised according to the following steps.

2.2.2.1 Existential threats: external conditions for securitising global health issues

According to Kenneth Waltz's theory of international politics, security can be defined at individual, national and international levels. Current public health crises pose major threats to security at all three of these levels.

First, public health crises pose a threat to individual security. The United Nations Development Programme first introduced the concept of "human security" in its *Human Development Report* in 1994. Former UN Secretary-General Kofi Annan held that,

> At the dawn of the twenty-first century, a new understanding of security is emerging. Human security, in its broadest sense, embraces far more than the absence of violent conflict. It encompasses human rights, good governance, access to education and health care and ensuring that each individual has opportunities and choices to fulfill his or her potential.
>
> (Annan, 2000)

Human security is a human-centred concept that involves both individuals and communities with focuses on human life and dignity. The *Human Development Report* listed seven key types of human security: health, personal, food, economic, environmental, community and political. Clearly, public health crises may threaten each of these elements. Many historians and biologists point out that between 1918 and 1919, almost a third of the world's population was infected with the flu, from which 100 million died (Garrett, 2006). At the end of the 20th century, approximately one-quarter of the global deaths each year were due to infectious diseases. In Africa, more than 60% of the deaths were caused by infectious diseases. Diseases that have been under control in the past, such as cholera, plague, tuberculosis and diphtheria, are resurfacing. In 1993, WHO declared tuberculosis a global crisis. On top of that, some new infectious diseases are still cropping up. According to WHO statistics, since the 1970s, as many as 35 new types of human infectious diseases have been detected. Current epidemiological techniques are useless in the face of most of these highly toxic pathogens, such

30 *Theoretical underpinnings*

as dengue fever and HIV/AIDS (Caballero-Anthony, 2006, p. 109). Since the first case of HIV/AIDS identified in the United States in 1983, 40 million people worldwide have been infected. Every year, 3 million people die from HIV/AIDS, and 40 million become newly infected (UNAIDS, 2007). "[The] HIV/AIDS crisis is no longer just a public health or humanitarian issue. It not only threatens the economic and social development of the poorest regions in the world, but also poses a grave threat to human security" (Karns et al., 2003, p. 499). In 2003, the SARS virus, which originated in China, became serious in just a few months. The sporadic outbreaks of the bird flu were like the sword of Damocles hanging over people's heads. According to World Bank estimates, if the bird flu epidemic were to last one year, the world's total loss could be as high as US\$800 billion (Doyle, 2006, p. 401). Due to the high HIV infection rate, economic growth in some African countries has already come to a halt. In recent years, the rapid development of biotechnology has greatly improved a country's ability to manufacture lethal biological weapons, enlarging too the potential threat of biological terrorism. Most biological agents are highly contagious pathogenic microorganisms that can easily spread and cause massive outbreaks of infectious diseases to threaten human security. "In the post-Cold War world, infectious diseases present the greatest potential threat to human security in the world" (Pirages, 1995, p. 5).

Second, public health crises threaten a country's internal and external security. National security is defined as the ability for a government to protect its citizens, territorial integrity, national sovereignty, politics, society, economy and defence mechanisms from direct or indirect threats. Achieving national security relies on national strength. National strength is "government at all levels of power and/ or capability to maximize its prosperity and stability, to protect its population from predation, and to adapt to diverse crises" (Burkle, 2006, p. 246). A country's prosperity and power depend on the health of its people. The degree to which a country's public health is secured constitutes an important metric of its national strength. According to Andrew Price-Smith (2004), an important measure of national strength is whether a country has the ability to cope with outbreaks of infectious diseases. Clearly, outbreaks of large-scale infectious diseases and potential biological terrorist attacks could cripple a country's national strength. A country's failure to protect the health of its citizens is a failure to fulfil its basic responsibility. This failure undermines its legitimacy and destabilises the domestic situation. The HIV/AIDS epidemic in Africa has somewhat contributed to the emergence of "failed states". "The total defense which [a] nation seeks involves a great deal more than building airplanes, ships, guns and bombs. We cannot be a strong nation unless we are a healthy one" (Franklin Roosevelt, as cited in Fallows, 1999). Public health crises not only weaken a nation's economic competitiveness but also its military vitality. This is especially true in sub-Saharan African countries, where HIV/AIDS infection rates in the armies can be as high as 50% on average and even higher at 75% to 80% in Malawi and Zimbabwe and possibly even 90% in South Africa (Heinechen, 2003, p. 784). As South African scholar Peter Fourie and senior managing legal officer for the Open Society Justice Initiative Martin Schönteich point out, "Armed forces form the basis of a country's defense and constitute the underpinning of stability within states and between them. If they become debilitated by disease, national security is compromised" (2001, p. 37). The armies' vulnerability to HIV/AIDS may present a serious external threat to national security.

Third, public health crises threaten global security. The globalisation of the public health crises has made the international community mutually vulnerable. According to Dr Brundtland (2003), former director-general of WHO,

> In today's interdependent world, the spread of viruses and bacteria is almost as fast as sending e-mails and transferring money. Globalization has connected Bujumbura to Mumbai, as well as Bangkok to Boston. There is no such thing as virus-free shelter anymore, and there is no impenetrable wall between a healthy and happy world with an adequate food supply and another weak, poorly subsisted and impoverished world. While globalization has shortened distances, knocked down obstacles, and built people-to-people connection, the problem that appears in one place has also become a shared problem for other places worldwide.
>
> (p. 417)

The world is becoming more and more integrated in many ways, a significant aspect of which is the "integration of microorganisms". Global integration has proven that outbreaks of infectious diseases pose a threat to international security. Since public health issues have become a global challenge, outbreaks of diseases in any place must be considered a threat to all countries. This is especially true for major international transport hubs. As Garrett (2005) states, "The mutual vulnerability of weak and powerful nations at the moment has never been so obvious. Even the security of the richest nations might be subject to the ability of the poorest nations to control infectious diseases" (p. 55). Some analysts even predict that "the spreading AIDS epidemic in Europe and Asia will break the global military balance" (Eberstadt, 2002, p. 22). In some places, infectious diseases have engendered failed states. For example, some countries may plunge into anarchy due to high HIV infection rates, thus becoming a breeding ground for terrorism and a contributor to the emergence of international terrorism. The refugee problem caused by outbreaks of infectious diseases has also disrupted regional stability. Public health crises also hamper UN peacekeeping operations because peacekeeping forces are usually deployed at places with high HIV/AIDS infection rates. Peacekeepers would be at risk of contracting HIV/AIDS and are likely to become carriers of HIV/AIDS to spread the disease to other areas. "Peacekeeping forces have become one of the main carriers of HIV/AIDS" (Singer, 2002, p. 152). If a large number of peacekeepers were infected with HIV/AIDS, their combat effectiveness and efficiency would be compromised to the detriment of international security. "HIV/AIDS is more destructive than any military force, any conflict, and any weapon of mass destruction" (Powell, 2003). Some analysts pointed out that while focusing on the global war on terrorism and nuclear proliferation, we should not forget that the threat of HIV/AIDS to the world is not less dangerous

32 Theoretical underpinnings

than furnishing terrorists with nuclear weapons. The international community must arrive at the consensus that HIV/AIDS is already a global security issue and that it poses the same threat to both developed and developing countries (Piot, 2001). "Global health is an investment in global security" (Schrecker & Labonte, 2007, p. 298). Therefore, global health threats present security implications.

2.2.2.2 Speech acts: initiatives in the securitisation of global health issues

"In the global health discourse, 'securitization' encompasses various challenges to health and disease control and their connections with national or global security" (Cooper et al., 2007, p. 7). Existential threat is just an external condition for public health issues to be securitised. The securitisation of public health issues cannot proceed without certain speech acts, which involves putting these threats high on the agenda by a securitising actor. In 1993, WHO declared tuberculosis a global crisis. In January 2000, the UN Security Council took unprecedented action to address the threat posed by the HIV/AIDS epidemic to international peace and security. In July 2000, the UN Security Council convened the first ever conference on health. The UN Security Council passed Security Council Resolution 1308 and Security Council Resolution 1983 on July 17, 2000, and June 7, 2011, respectively. These two resolutions emphasised that "without proper containment, HIV/AIDS could pose a threat to stability and security" (UN Security Council, 2000a, p. 1). They also called on all member states to make political commitments to implement the relevant Security Council resolutions and address the threat of the HIV/AIDS epidemic (UN Security Council, 2011a, p. 1). In view of the raging Ebola outbreak in West Africa in 2014, the UN General Assembly convened a special meeting on Ebola on September 19, 2014, and passed resolution 69/1 Measures to Contain and Combat the Recent Ebola Outbreak in West Africa (United Nations General Assembly, 2014). Moreover, the UN secretary-general set up the UN Ebola Emergency Mission, the first ever UN public health mission, to ensure that all organisations under the UN system could effectively respond to the Ebola epidemic. The UN Security Council had successively passed Resolutions 2176 and 2177 in September 2014, expressing its grave concern for the potential security threats caused by the Ebola epidemic (UN Security Council, 2014), and believed the epidemic had constituted an unprecedented threat to international stability and security (UN Security Council, 2011b). In a report titled *A More Secure World: Our Shared Responsibility*, the UN High Level Panel on Global Security Threats, Challenges and Change emphasised: "If any event or process results in mass death or shortened lifespan, damages the very existence of a country, the basic unit in the international system, it would be a threat to international security". Infectious diseases and other social threats (e.g. poverty) are listed as one of the six types of threats (The High-level Panel of UN, 2004, p. 23). Kofi Annan noted, "AIDS is causing a socio-economic crisis, which in turn threatens political stability" (UN Security Council, 2000b, p. 1).

Theoretical underpinnings 33

In 2003, Rand Corporation published *The Global Threat of New and Reemerging Infectious Diseases Reconciling U.S. National Security and Public Health Policy*. The report pointed out that biological terrorism or biological weapons could even bring about strategic threats and that infectious diseases had replaced direct military threats from a hostile country to become the most serious challenge facing the international community and governments. These views were reemphasised in the 2006 *World Economic Forum's Global Risks Report* in Davos, Switzerland, which listed epidemics and natural disasters as among the greatest dangers facing the international community at that time. On World AIDS Day in 2005, China's former president Hu Jintao pointed out that "Health security is part of national security." On January 18, 2017, during his visit to WHO, China's president Xi Jinping again emphasised that "health issues are a global challenge and promoting global health is an important part of implementing the 2030 Agenda for Sustainable Development" (Xi, 2017). On the 2007 World Health Day, former UN Secretary-General Ban Ki-moon affirmed that "health, development, and global security are intertwined." In February 2017, the Munich Security Conference, one of the most important forums in the world to discuss international security policy, named health security a central theme for one of the three roundtable forums.[6] Bill Gates also stated his belief that outbreaks of infectious disease, climate change, and nuclear wars are the three most serious security threats facing the world today (2017). In short, there are countless examples of speech acts about health security.

2.2.2.3 *Inter-subjective construction in the securitisation of global health issues: establishing international norms*

The securitisation theory holds that the process of securitising a problem is also a process of intersubjective construction. In other words, the audience accepts the speech acts of the securitising actors and agrees to set up relevant norms. In view of the threats brought by public health issues to human security and national security, actors in the international community have agreed through cooperation to set up international norms on how to securitise public health issues. The UN Security Council is mandated to supervise traditional security issues, but with the deepening global health crises, the council has also started to pay more attention to the potential threats of global health crises to the international security and has passed a number of resolutions to address global health security issues.

The establishment of the Joint United Nations Program on HIV/AIDS (UNAIDS) in 1995 marked the beginning of the securitisation of public health issues. On July 17, 2000, the UN Security Council passed Resolution 1308 on AIDS. On November 14, 2001, the Fourth WTO Ministerial Conference adopted the Declaration on the TRIPS and Public Health. In 2003, the SARS crisis prompted the revision of the IHR. The Global Health Security Conference, which concluded on January 8, 2005, issued the Rome Declaration, in which member states agreed on a set of norms to strengthen bird flu control through cooperation.

34 *Theoretical underpinnings*

On January 31, 2006, the International Alliance of National Public Health Institutes (IANPHI) was established.

As a neutral and technical international organisation, WHO has also begun to securitise public health issues by collaborating with international traditional security regimes, such as the UN Security Council and the BWC. For example, the UN secretary-general's High-level Panel issued a report titled *A More Secure World: Our Shared Responsibility* in December 2004, which emphasised the potential role WHO could play in the fight against bioterrorism. In the report, the panel also recommended that "when a new infectious disease or malicious release of infectious agent causes a serious threat, it is necessary to cooperate with WHO and the Security Council to establish an effective epidemic prevention measure".[7] Meanwhile, WHO has achieved securitisation of public health issues by extending its own functions. For example, following the anthrax attacks in the United States, the WHO Secretariat prepared a report titled *Deliberate Use of Biological and Chemical Agents to Cause Harm* in the spring of 2002 in preparation for the 55th World Health Assembly (WHO, 2002a). The report stated that to respond to these incidents, WHO should "enhance public health disease early warning systems at all levels because such systems can detect and respond to deliberately created diseases" (ibid., p. 2). Similarly, in response to potential biological attacks, WHO published *Public Health Response to Biological and Chemical Weapons* in 2004.

At the moment, to achieve biosecurity and prevent bioterrorism, the international community is also working to reach a consensus on how to ensure better compliance with the BWC and on how to enhance trust measures and promote the universality of the convention.

In addition, international regimes such as WTO and national human rights institutions (NHRIs) have taken unprecedented measures to ensure global health security. For example, the Fourth WTO Ministerial Conference in November 2001 specifically addressed the conflict between intellectual property agreements and accessibility to medicines and published the Declaration on The TRIPS Agreement and Public Health. In addition, it has become a new area of interest to study public health from the perspective of human rights. For example, the United Nations issued comment No. 14 on the right to health,[8] and the United Nations appointed its first-ever rapporteur on the right to health.[9] All of these endeavours illustrate the growing prominence of health security issues and increasing concern for the right to health by international human rights regimes.

Based on the previous analysis, the securitisation of public health issues is seen as a social construction process in which public issues rise to become political issues and ultimately to security issues, thereby making up an interactive three-dimensional structure (see Figure 2.1).

"Public health has entered a post-security era" (Fidler, 2007b, p. 41). In other words, global health issues have been securitised. Viewing public health issues from a security perspective has become an integral part of public health governance in the 21st century. The implications of such a dramatic change for global health governance call for attention. Within the post-security era, it has become an established trend in public health governance to design and solve problems

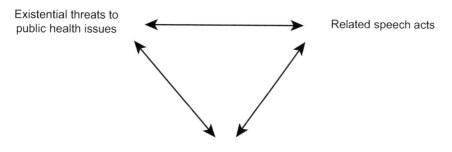

Figure 2.1 Three-dimensional Structure of Securitizing Health Issues

through security-related tactics and strategies for the promotion of public health. Moreover, one of the biggest impacts of the securitisation of public health is on the setting of priorities. The process of public health securitisation is also a process in which public health problems are prioritised. It should be noted that securitisation is not for its own sake. Today's securitisation is for tomorrow's de-securitisation. The only way to de-securitise global health threats is to prioritise securitised threats on the global agenda and give full play to the role of international regimes. Only in so doing can we give more political and policy support to global health as well as be more effective in global health governance.

2.3 Approach for global health governance: providing global public goods for health

> He who receives an idea from me, receives instruction himself without lessening mine; as he who lights his taper at mine, receives light without darkening me.
> —Thomas Jefferson (Lipscomb & Bergh, n.d.)

The notion of "public goods" is important for analysing the economic consequences of public policies at the state level. In fact, public goods are often defined as goods provided by national governments. That governments should provide such goods is one of the reasons why governments exist. To some extent, a legitimate government can overcome the "free-rider" problem and the "prisoner's dilemma" by supplying public goods in an effective way. However, against the backdrop of deepening globalisation, some issues, which in the past were solved by domestic policies, have become global issues due to their growing global impact. No single country has the capacity or incentive to single-handedly solve these global problems. The interdependence among countries makes public goods which were once confined by national borders into global public goods. In a sense, globalisation has also given rise to "global pubic bads" that transcend

36 *Theoretical underpinnings*

borders. This makes the supply of global public goods an urgent necessity. The way in which the global public goods are supplied determines whether globalisation is more of an opportunity or a threat to mankind, while the amount of such provision will determine the success or failure of global governance as well as its performance. Since there is no international entity that can undertake equivalent functions of institutions of national power, the "free-rider" problem or the problem of "collective action" in the supply of global public goods becomes more intractable. Effective global governance requires proper management of these problems. The globalisation and securitisation of public health issues highlights the necessity and importance of global health governance. The inefficiency of global health governance can be attributed to problems of global collective action and the "democratic deficit" in the policymaking process. On a deeper level, the root causes have to do with the global North–South Divide in public health and a nation's fixation with the traditional concept of sovereignty. Therefore, if we use global public goods as a lens through which public health security is examined, we might have a thorough assessment of collective action at the international level and a deeper understanding of global public goods used for public health. This knowledge will help us achieve effective global health governance.

2.3.1 Global public goods: definitions and classifications

In the current era of globalisation, almost all global issues are related to the provision of global public goods. Public goods have been discussed by many scholars both in China and in the rest of the world (Fan, 2006; Mueller, 1999; Samuelson, 1954; Smith, 1994). The notion was first introduced into the study of global issues in the 1960s. The discussion on global public goods was part of the analysis of global problems in both *The Tragedy of the Commons* written by Garrett Hardin (1968) and *Collective Goods and International Organizations* co-authored by Bruce M. Russett and John D. Sulivan (1971). It is Mancur Olson (1971) who first used the term "international collective goods", a concept with which he studied ways to increase the incentives for international cooperation (pp. 866–874). In 1981, Todd Sandler (1980) adopted the concept of international collective goods in his edited *The Theory and Structures of International Political Economy*, in which he applied the notion to examine some international political economy issues, such as the international environment and global health. Charles P. Kindleberger (1986) was also one of the early scholars to have brought international collective goods into the study of international political economy. He attributed the Great Depression in the 1930s to the absence of global public goods, such as the absence of an open trading system and an international lender of last resort.

2.3.1.1 Definitions of global public goods

Although the aforementioned scholars have more or less addressed global public goods, they have failed to provide a clear definition of the term. It was not until

Theoretical underpinnings   37

the publication of Inge Kaul et al.'s book *Global Public Goods: International Cooperation in the 21st Century* that a relatively broad definition began to appear. Kaul and colleagues defined "global public goods" as goods that have strong universality in terms of countries (covering more than one group of countries), people (accruing to several, preferably all population groups) and generations (extending to both current and future generations, or at least meeting the needs of current generations without foreclosing development options for future generations) (Kaul et al., 1999, pp. 509–510). Later, in her edited *Providing Global Public Goods: Managing Globalization*, Kaul revised her definition into "goods with benefits that extend to all countries, people, and generations" (Kaul, 2003, p. 23). However, this definition is also inadequate under closer scrutiny.

First, it does not make a clear distinction between cross-border externalities of global public goods and more limited externalities of domestic public goods. Instead, this definition of public goods includes products that are universally provided but whose beneficiaries include only the providers. For instance, water conservancy facilities are constructed in virtually all countries and thus provide a prime example for the provider–beneficiary relationship of the aforementioned problem. China, for one, has many water conservancy facilities, yet we are hardly warranted to call this provision a true global public good. Second, the requirement of "strong universality" on beneficiary groups means that some women's health programmes, programmes that only affect certain ethnicities or target only the poor, are excluded from global public goods. Last, in Kaul's definition, the requirement to protect the rights of present generations or those of future generations from being compromised would lead to a "temporal stalemate" because only programs that benefit both present and future generations are recognised as global public goods. At the same time, based on this definition, many disease eradication programmes would also be excluded because they require resources of the present generation be redistributed so the next generation would benefit. For example, the Global Polio Eradication Initiative, launched by WHO in the 1980s, does not fit this definition because it mainly uses resources of the present generation to benefit the next. For these reasons, global public goods should be considered goods that transcend national boundaries (not necessarily group and generational boundaries) and exhibit a high degree of publicness (i.e. non-excludability and non-rivalry). In addition, the World Bank has provided a more comprehensive definition:

> Global public goods are commodities, resources, services, and also systems of rules or policy regimes with substantial cross-border externalities that are important for development and poverty-reduction, and that can be produced in sufficient supply only through cooperation and collective action by developed and developing countries.
>
> (Development Committee, 2000, p. 2)

In short, all these definitions show that the provision of global public goods is the very purpose of global governance.

38 *Theoretical underpinnings*

2.3.1.2 Classification of global public goods

Pedro Conceicao (2003) listed seven categories of global public goods: international financial stability, multilateral trade regime, global communications networks and the Internet, communicable disease control, reducing the excessive disease burden, climate stability and peace and security. In *Road Map Towards the Implementation of the United Nations Millennium Declaration*, a report from the UN secretary-general published in 2001, there are ten categories of public goods that are of concern to the international community. They are fundamental human rights, respect for national sovereignty, global health security, international security, international peace, cross-border communications and transportation systems, institutional infrastructure to coordinate cross-border actions, centralised knowledge management, centralised management of global commons and effectiveness of international forums for multilateral negotiations (United Nations, 2001). According to the International Task Force on Global Public Goods, the provision of the following six public goods is critical: achieving peace and security, preventing the emergence and spread of infectious diseases, managing global commons, enhancing international financial stability, strengthening the international trading system and opening the exchange of knowledge (International Task Force on Global Public Goods, 2006).

According to the degree of publicness, global public goods can be divided into pure global public goods and quasi-public goods. The former refers to public goods that are fully non-excludable and non-rivalrous. For example, international peace is a pure global public good. The latter are global public goods that have only one of the two qualities. The protection of the ozone layer and the Internet are examples of the latter. Based on stages of their provision, there are final global public goods and intermediate global public goods. The former are outcomes rather than goods in the standard sense. They may be either tangible, such as the environment or the common heritage of mankind, or intangible, such as peace or financial stability. The latter refer to the provision regime of global public goods, such as formal or informal international regimes. The term "intermediate global public goods" were coined to highlight fields that require international intervention for the provision of a particular public good. For example, to protect the ozone layer, the required intermediate global public goods are international regimes such as the *Montreal Protocol* and the *Kyoto Protocol*; whereas to achieve public health security, the required intermediate global public goods are international regimes relevant to public health, such as WHO and WTO.

These classifications of global public goods not only help countries to better understand, examine and solve relevant problems but also to spell out current global challenges. This will help us make feasible and widely applicable policies and strategies to ensure a more reliable supply of global public goods, an end goal committing us to innovating international regimes that act as intermediate global public goods.

2.3.2 Characteristics of global public goods for health

Public health issues have accompanied human beings throughout history, causing suffering and hardship that are defining elements of our past. Throughout history, infectious diseases have caused more deaths than wars have. The Black Death in the 14th century wiped out almost a third of Europe's entire population. The SARS outbreak in 2003 brought home to people the severity of public health crises. The "bird flu" (H5N1) virus lurks and may become the severest global health crisis since the flu pandemic that killed 50 million people in 1918. Experts estimate that, if an avian flu pandemic were to occur with medical resources at the status quo, at least 7.5 million people could die, with Asia being the epicentre of the disaster (Chen, 2007, p. 4). Globalisation has many undertones, one of which fuels the international spread of infectious diseases and global health crises. According to the International Air Transport Association's 2017 Annual Review, thanks to improving global economic conditions and lower ticket prices, air travel passengers around the world exceeded an unprecedented 4 billion in 2017. Thus, if there was a disease outbreak or epidemic, it would take just a few hours for it to spread to any location on the planet.

The age of globalisation is "the age of universal contagion" (Hardt, 2003, p. 138). A public health crisis is no longer just a medical problem. SARS has become "a formidable enemy at every level—medical, political, economic and even psychological" (Kaib, 2003, p. 28). Globalised public health crises and their severity call for global health governance. The provision of public goods is often driven by national and international crises. "Action on global public goods will happen only to the extent that the international community faces a crisis and must respond" (Desai, 2003, p. 74). In view of current public health crises facing the international community, it is necessary to analyse the nature of global public goods for public health security. This will help the international community fulfil the important role it plays in the global agenda and help it achieve more effective global health governance. In general, global public goods for public health security are marked by the following three qualities.

2.3.2.1 Globalised negative externalities of public health crises

In a world with open borders and a wide range of cross-border activities, public health crises, especially outbreaks of epidemics, have worldwide ramifications wherever they occur. Traditional fortifications along national borders cannot prevent the invasion of diseases or their vectors. In today's interdependent world, "distinctions between domestic and international health problems are losing their relevance and often mislead" (Institute of Medicine, 1997, p. 8). Globalisation has made domestic public bads global. Public health security was originally a public good provided by sovereign nations to their nationals. However, poverty and poor governance in some countries have given rise to *public health bads* that include the emergence of epidemics. In the context of globalisation these negative

40 *Theoretical underpinnings*

externalities are shared by the whole world. The negative externalities of global health crises manifest in the following three aspects.

First, public health crises occurring within one country can spread and evolve into regional or even global health crises. Viruses can travel passport-free. Since the first AIDS patient was diagnosed in the United States in 1981, the HIV virus has been spreading at an alarming rate around the world. According to UNAIDS, the HIV/ADIS epidemic had been detected in 210 countries and regions around the world as of 1997 (Chen, 2007, p. 134). Despite the spread of AIDS, experts still believe the HIV epidemic has not yet peaked in terms of rate of contagion and severity of consequences (UN Calls on Developed Countries to Help Developing Countries Fight AIDS, 2003). First detected in Foshan, Guangdong province of China in November 2002, the SARS virus spread to 32 countries in just five months, infected 8,098 people and claimed 774 lives (Caballero-Anthony, 2006, p. 109). The "bird flu" (H5N1) virus evolved into an infectious disease that spread rapidly around the world in the 21st century. WHO officials believe the conditions are ripe for the human-to-human chain of transmission; it may be just a matter of time before the avian influenza strikes. There is no doubt that if one country cannot handle and control an influenza epidemic properly, all countries will suffer.

Second, national public health crises can cause global economic losses. "When one part of the human body is sick, the whole body can hardly function properly; especially, when one part of the global village is a reservoir of preventable diseases, the entire neighbourhood may be perpetually endangered" (Aginam, 2005, p. 45). A domestic public health crisis not only affects a country's own economy but also takes a toll on the global economy. It is extremely difficult to calculate the direct and indirect economic losses that SARS inflicted on the world, but it is clear that it must have exceeded US$100 billion (Prystay, 2003). Sherry Cooper (2006, p. 22), an American economist, estimated that a mild avian flu pandemic lasting three months would cause economic losses of US$1.1 trillion globally. The global damage from the rampant spread of AIDS is even more difficult to estimate.

Lastly, national public health crises endanger global security. Outbreaks of infectious diseases in an integrated world have proved to be a threat to global security. Reflecting on SARS in 2003, Heymann and Rodier (2004), two WHO officials, stressed that "the SARS experience made one lesson clear early in its course: inadequate surveillance and response capacity in a single country can endanger national populations and the public health security of the entire world" (p. 173). Due to the spread of infectious diseases, some countries became "failed states" and breeding grounds for terrorism, thus fuelling the rise of terrorism around the globe. A refugee problem caused by the outbreak of an infectious disease can engender regional instability. For example, in the bubonic and pneumonic plague in India in 1994, people were so frightened that they fled in large numbers, causing a large wave of refugees. Pakistan in response banned all air and sea traffic with India. Ships entering Pakistan could only be moored 12 kilometres offshore, and all personnel on board were required to undergo sanitary inspections that could last three to five days. This caused great grievances in India, which

Theoretical underpinnings 41

later claimed the plague was the result of a biological attack launched by Pakistan against India. The dispute between the two countries further aggravated the regional situation. In addition, public health crises are not conducive to UN peacekeeping operations. If a large number of peacekeepers are infected with AIDS, their combat effectiveness will decrease and peacekeeping operations will lose effectiveness, both to the detriment of global security.

2.3.2.2 Non-excludability of public health security

Global health security is a form of collective security on a global scale. All countries in the world will benefit if public health security is ensured globally. Even countries not making any contribution to global health security actions will not be deprived of such benefits. For example, "in the early 1950s, an estimated 50 million smallpox cases occurred globally each year with an estimated 15 million deaths. Through the success of the global eradication campaign that began in 1967, the global eradication of smallpox was certified in 1979" (WHO, 2007, p. 5). Although some countries did not contribute to the eradication of smallpox that ensures global health security, they would still enjoy the benefits of being protected from the smallpox virus, which meant they no longer needed to immunise their citizens with smallpox vaccines. Since its establishment in 2001, the Global Fund to Fight Aids, Tuberculosis and Malaria (GFATM) has been promoting global health security, benefiting all countries around the world without leaving any behind.

2.3.2.3 Non-rivalry of public health security

Public health security is a non-traditional type of security. The public health security in one country does not come at a cost to the public health insecurity in another country. That is to say, there is no so-called security dilemma in public health security. Instead, public health security in one country is conducive to regional and even global health security. Global health security depends on close cooperation among all countries in the world. One country's efforts to secure its own public health security do not undermine the public health security in other countries. In other words, global health security is the result of cooperation, not competition, among the actors in global governance. For example, if a country works hard to bring the spread of SARS under control, it will boost its own public health security. Such security does not undermine efforts of other countries in fighting SARS; instead, it would provide a favourable external environment for them to fight the disease and achieve their national public health security as well. In other words, public health security in one country is not at the expense of public health security in other countries but rather promotes other countries' domestic health conditions. In short, in the field of public health security, countries are in win–win relationships instead of competition with each other.

"Global health is in the national interests of the major state powers" (Gostin, 2008, p. 331). The negative externalities of public health crises on a global scale

42 *Theoretical underpinnings*

as well as the non-excludability and non-rivalry of public health security indicate that public health security is a global public good, that is, a global public good for health. Given the globalised nature of public health security as a public good, the self-interests of countries around the world are built into an adequate supply of public goods for health. "Investing in health as a global public good is the best policy to ensure domestic health" (Kickbusch, 2003b). If all countries become stakeholders in global health security, they would be less incentivised to be "free riders", thus making global health governance more effective. The non-excludability and non-rivalry of global public goods for health suggest that the provision of global health goods, like provision of any other global public good, inevitably suffers from problems of collective action, including "tragedy of the commons" and the "free-rider" problem. In the absence of a global government, there exists a chronic shortage of global public goods. To provide more global public goods for health, the international community must formulate global health policies and plans on the basis of mutual cooperation and carry out effective global health governance. In the state of virtual anarchy at the international level, it should be obvious that international regimes will serve as the coordination centre of global health policies and play an indispensable role in the provision of global public goods for health.

2.4 Actors of global health governance: international regimes

In an increasingly interdependent world, global public issues have increasingly gained prominence in international studies. Responding to increasingly complicated global public issues has become the main challenge confronting scholars of international relations in today's world. The rise of global public issues has made the world even more interdependent, while such interdependence in turn demands the supply of global public goods. The provision of global public goods must be based on collective cooperation. "The solution to global public problems calls for multilateral joint action rather than unilateral action; it requires global public policies and cooperation-based planning rather than individual unilateral decision-making" (Su, 2000, p. 6). Global public goods must be provided through global governance. The availability of global public goods depends on the efficiency of global governance, which in turn depends on the proper functioning of international regimes. Given the threat posed by global health issues in different dimensions and global interdependence in the field of health security, international regimes must fully play their provision roles to achieve effective global health governance.

2.4.1 Significance of international regimes in global governance

The notion of international regimes is closely related to interdependence among countries. As countries become increasingly interdependent on each other in various fields, almost every global public affair requires management from some "international regime". International regimes are derivative products of such interdependence. As Keohane and Nye (2002) have observed, "Relationships of interdependence often occur within, and may be affected by, networks of rules, norms, and procedures that regularise behaviour and controls its effects; We refer to the sets of governing arrangements that affect relationships of interdependence as international regimes" (p. 22). The prevailing view defines international regimes as sets of implicit or explicit principles, norms, rules and decision-making procedures around which actors' expectations converge in an area of international relations. Within this definition, principles are beliefs of fact, causation and rectitude; norms are standards of behaviour defined in terms of rights and obligations; rules are specific prescriptions or proscriptions for action; and decision-making procedures are prevailing practices for making and implementing collective choice (Krasner, 1983, p. 2).

"An interdependent world calls for international regimes" (Su, 2000, p. 126). In a sense, international regimes are at the core of global governance. If there were no international regime to restrain and regulate the behaviours of countries, the "tragedy of the commons" would occur, putting global governance in an unimaginable mess. As a set of binding institutional arrangements, international regimes can raise the expectations for the actions of various countries and reduce transaction costs. A well-balanced state of interdependence can provide institutional support for global collective action. The governance of global public issues cannot be achieved without international regimes. As Keohane (2001) noted, "if global institutions are designed well, they will promote human welfare" (p. 12). Even if national states retain many of their present functions, effective governance of an increasingly globalised world will require more extensive international institutions. International regimes mostly play the following functions in global governance.

First, international regimes are important providers of global public goods. Oran Young pointed out that "international regimes, like other social institutions, will ordinarily exhibit the attributes of collective goods to a relatively high degree" (Young, 1980, p. 353). In fact, international regimes are intermediate global public goods whose role is to provide ultimate goods in the global public domain. "International meetings and agreements are often focused on global public goods" (Albin, 2006, p. 227). Even in the absence of a centralised authority, such as a governing body, in the international community, it is still possible to supply global public goods. Although global public issues can only be solved through global collective action, they do not automatically trigger global collective action. If the benefits of a community are publicly owned, shared, and indivisible, every member of that community has an incentive to be a "free rider". As a result, no community member is still willing to provide public goods. Although the supply of global public goods would encounter the "free-rider" problem or problems of collective action, the provision of global public goods is "completed through relative international regimes out of the choices made by individual countries" (Su, 2000, p. 124). Only through universally binding norms or decision-making procedures can we overcome problems of collective action associated with the provision of global public goods. An adequate supply of global public

44   *Theoretical underpinnings*

goods does not so much depend on whether there is a global government in the international community as on whether countries in the world can surmount problems of collective action and design appropriate international regimes balancing both self- and collective interest. More importantly, only when such international regimes achieve publicness in decision-making and in the distribution of benefits can they achieve "ideal" provision of global public goods, thereby avoiding the global "tragedy of the commons".

Second, international regimes can effectively reduce the cost of international transactions, thereby promoting international cooperation on global public issues. International regimes can help reduce uncertainties from incomplete and asymmetric information. In response to risks arising from opportunism in the process of international exchanges, international regimes can change the utility curve of the member states through principled and standardised moral principles as well as "issues linkage", so their member states would be more incentivised to comply with such norms. In other words, international regimes can provide a "platform" for member states and in this way serve for international cooperation.

Third, international regimes provide common norms and values for global governance. International regimes are guided by the overarching goal to achieve global governance of public issues. The success of global public governance will affect the shared future of mankind. International regimes, through their standardised discourse and decision-making procedures, in some degree warrant the joint participation of all countries in global governance. They bring a certain degree of order and justice to international relations. In addition, international regimes raise global awareness by advocating the importance of resolving global public issues. For example, by advocating people's right to health, international human rights regimes call on all countries to be cognizant of human rights problems within public health so countries may further take due notice to improve the health conditions of their citizens. Therefore, notions surrounding "the right to health" have gradually become part of global consensus as well as common norms and values.

2.4.2 *International regimes in global health governance*

Global health governance requires the cooperation of all actors of governance in the international community. The synergy forged would promote the provision of global public goods for health (see Table 2.1). "To secure the best provision of international public goods, it is essential to have collective action based on cooperation and to put in place generally-accepted international norms" (Su, 2000, p. 125). Similarly, the supply of global public goods for health cannot be achieved without international regimes, important actors in global health governance.

Researchers describe deepened connection and interaction among problems from diverse fields in global public issues, including public health, trade and human rights, fields traditionally considered independent from each other, as "issues linkage" (Trachtman, 2002, pp. 77–93). For example, WTO's TRIPS

Theoretical underpinnings 45

Table 2.1 Actors and Their Functions in Global Health Governance

Actors	Main functions
Existing multilateral international regimes(e.g. WHO and WTO)	Coordinate international cooperation in public health of the health and trade departments of the member countries
Global public-private partnerships(e.g. The Global Fund to Fight AIDS, Tuberculosis and Malaria)	Integrate the comparative advantages of global public and private sectors in disease development and funding
Philanthropic foundations(e.g. the Bill & Melinda Gates Foundation and the Rockefeller Foundation)	Pool global public resources and provide medical resources with low commercial value
NGOs(e.g. the Red Cross)	Support or advocate special global public goods for health or global actions
National institutions(e.g. the Chinese Centre for Disease Control and Prevention)	Collect domestic epidemic information, coordinate vaccine development, be responsible for domestic prevention and control of communicable diseases, etc.

Agreement may have brought a negative impact on the accessibility of medicines in developing countries. Human rights protection in international human rights regimes has also played an important role in promoting public health. With the deepening of globalisation, issues linkage means global health governance is no longer only about cooperation and coordination of public health measures. In other words, global health issues are no longer research areas reserved only for the public health experts. Instead, such issues encompass all aspects of the international community. So far, due to the effect of issues linkage, a great number of international regimes, including WTO, international human rights regimes, the World Bank, the International Monetary Fund (IMF) and the Food and Agriculture Organization of the United Nations (FAO), have now engaged themselves with issues of global health governance. Based on the global universality of their members states and the degree of their connection to global health issues, the most important global health regimes are WHO, WTO, international human rights regimes, and the BWC. Some of these regimes are discussed next.

First, the World Health Organization. The Constitution of the World Health Organization, adopted at the International Health Conference in 1946, marked the official establishment of WHO. The first International Sanitary Conference convoked in Paris witnessed the beginning of international health cooperation. The League of Nations Health Organization (HOLN), which was established in 1920, made international health cooperation more institutionalised during its lifespan but ceased to exist after the outbreak of World War II. In 1945, the United Nations Conference on International Organization unanimously approved a proposal by Brazil and China to "establish a new international health organization". WHO's establishment marked a milestone in the history of international public health

46   *Theoretical underpinnings*

cooperation. Thanks to its decision-making procedures, organisational structure and the broad representation of member states, international public health cooperation has become globalised and institutionalised. However, WHO is also afflicted with inherent problems. A tendency of functionalism and internal politicisation have restricted it from playing a bigger role. The World Health Assembly adopted the IHR, which "aims to prevent, protect against, control and respond to the international spread of disease while avoiding unnecessary interference with international traffic and trade". The IHR has become "the only international health agreement on communicable diseases that is binding on member states" (WHO, 2000, p. 10). However, for the next three-and-a-half decades after its birth in 1969, the IHR had not been amended or revised. As global economy, health and security became integrated, the IHR turned increasingly ill-equipped for the current public health security challenges, particularly during the spread of SARS in 2003. For these reasons, WHO revised and adopted a new IHR at the 2005 World Health Assembly. Nevertheless, due to problems of collective action in international cooperation and the weak compliance with the IHR, WHO has been restrained from playing a bigger role in global health governance.

Second, the World Trade Organization. "If, in the old colonial days, it was true that 'trade follows the flag', it was equally true that the first faltering steps towards international health cooperation followed trade" (Howard-Jones, 1975, p. 12). The quote illuminates the close connection between trade and public health. In a sense, early international public health cooperation was marked by connections and conflicts between economic interests and public health security. Driven by the unstoppable momentum of economic globalisation the cross-border flow of economic factors will have an unprecedented impact on global public health. How can the clash between health protection and trade promotion be resolved? We might need to look to the current international economic and trade system, notably WTO, also widely known as the "Economic United Nations", to find the answer. The Marrakesh Agreement, signed in 1994, marked WTO's official establishment. Many parts of this agreement addressed the provision of public health services in developing countries. WTO's advocacy of a free trade system and rules directly or indirectly affected public health governance in many ways. WTO officially brought public health issues into the Doha Declaration on the TRIPS Agreement and Public Health issued in July 2002. The Doha Declaration sought to resolve the conflict between the accessibility and patent protection of medicines. In addition, WTO has been working to redress issues of trade protection policies adopted in the name of protecting domestic public health. WTO's free trade measures have also had a huge impact on the public health systems of developing countries. How to integrate free trade and public health policies under the WTO system and how to coordinate global trade policies and global health policies are issues that require immediate attention in global health governance.

Third, the international human rights regimes. After World War II, the international community set up a series of international human rights covenants. The close relationship between public health and human rights protection received growing attention from the international community. The right to health also became a focus of international human rights conventions. With the emergence of the human rights crisis caused by HIV/AIDS, people came to realise that respecting, protecting, and fulfilling human rights are not only international obligations of each member state but also important strategies for global health governance. As a result, the international human rights law on both civil and political rights as well as economic, social and cultural rights have "become one of the most important areas of international law for public health in general and for infectious disease control in particular" (Fidler, 2001, p. 18). According to the International Bill of Human Rights, each member state should take responsibility for the health of its citizens, but governments should refrain from restraining their citizens' civil and political rights for the purpose of controlling communicable diseases. Put differently, governments shall not exercise control of communicable diseases at the expense of citizens' economic and political rights. In fact, the protection and promotion of the aforementioned human rights are themselves important building blocks for effective public health governance. In addition, the "right to health" itself illustrates the close link between human rights regimes and public health. Adopting a human rights approach to achieve global health governance illustrates the human-based philosophy and the essence of public health governance.

Finally, the Biological Weapons Convention. BWC is the first international norm in the history of mankind to ban an entire category of weapons: weapons of mass destruction (WMD). It is also an important part of the international disarmament system and the international collective security framework with the UN at its centre. At first glance, issues related to biological weapons have nothing in common with public health issues, as the two come from completely different areas of concern. Security issues related to biological weapons and public health security are governed by different international regimes. Since biological defence and biological weapons arms control belong to the traditional field of security, they are governed by the BWC, whereas disease prevention and control belong to the field of public health and are therefore governed by WHO. However, given the development of biological science and technology and the emergence of biological terrorism, the once-clear distinction between the two is increasingly blurred. Some national biological weapons programmes have become targets of terrorists. BWC's provisions on international cooperation in biotechnology have strangled countries' capacity, especially that of developing countries, to respond to public health crises. Therefore, implementing the BWC and strengthening its effectiveness has become an important aspect of global health governance.

"International organizations are neither irrelevant nor omnipotent in global politics" (Diehl, 1997, p. 3). Although these international regimes have played important roles in global health governance, their limitations are also obvious. They do not have publicness in the decision-making process and in the distribution of benefits when it comes to global health policies, resulting in the undersupply of global public goods for health. On a deeper level, the problems of collective action are caused by member states' adherence to the traditional concepts of

48 *Theoretical underpinnings*

sovereignty, their different priorities, and the growing North–South Divide. Democratic deficits, power politics and interest-driven orientation are also important reasons for their dysfunction in global health governance.

Summary

Globalisation has spawned globalised public health crises. Interdependence in global health security calls for global health governance. The growing securitisation of global health issues underscores not only the need for global health governance but also the need to put public health issues on the security agenda and the need to show political commitments for global health governance. Global health governance can only be achieved through the provision of global health goods. International regimes, such as WHO and WTO, are important actors in global health governance as well as important providers of global public goods for health. By examining their institutional defects and the deep-rooted reasons for their insufficiency in the supply of global public goods for health, we may have a chance to identify and resolve the root of these problems. This is the ultimate purpose of global health governance.

Notes

1 The countries represented at the first International Health Conference include four Italian nation states (Sardinia, Tuscany and the two Sicilies), Austria, the United Kingdom, Greece, Portugal, the Russian Empire, Spain, France and Turkey.
2 See United Nations Millennium Development Goals. Retrieved from www.un.org/millenniumgoals/
3 Actors in global governance can also be divided into governments which work in politics (through diplomacy and international regimes such as WTO, WHO, etc. and international law), private markets which work in economics (multinational corporations, international chamber of commerce and industrial associations) and civil society which works in social cultural fields (NGOs and professional associations). See Axford, B. (1995). *The Global System: Economics, Politics and Culture*. New York: St. Martin's Press.
4 "Mutual vulnerability" was first used to describe political economic issues and development and non-development issues in North–South relations. See Head, I. L. (1991). *On a Hinge of History: The Mutual Vulnerability of South and North*. Toronto: University of Toronto Press; Nef, J. (1999), *Human Security and Mutual Vulnerability: The Global Political Economy of Development and Underdevelopment (2nd ed)*. Ottawa: National Library of Canada. pp. 13–26.
5 The Declaration of Alma-Ata analysed the social and political determinants of global public health, reiterated the right to health and proposed the basic goals of global health governance. See Chan, M. (2008). *Return to Alma-Ata*. Retrieved from www.who.int/dg/20080915/en/.
6 See Munich Security Conference 2017 Agenda. Retrieved from www.securityconference.de/fileadmin/MSC_/2017/Sonstiges/170218_MSC2017_Agenda.pdf.
7 See Article 70 of the *Report of the High-level Panel on Threats, Challenges and Change* (2004).
8 See United Nations Human Rights website, Economic and Social Council: Substantive Issues Arising in the Implantation of the International Covenant on Economic, Social

and Cultural Rights: General Comment No. 14 (2000). Retrieved from www.unhchr.ch/tbs/doc.nsf/(Symbol)/40d009901358b0e2c1256915005090be.

9 For the first report of the United Nations special rapporteur, see Hunt, P. (2003, February 13). *Report of the Special Rapporteur: The Right of Everyone to the Enjoyment of the Highest Attainable Standard of Physical and Mental Health*, U.N. ESCOR, 59th Sess., Agenda Item 10, U.N. Doc. E/CN.4/2003/58. Retrieved from www.unhchr.ch/Huridocda.nsf/0/9854302995c2c86fc1256cec005al8d7.

References

Albin, C. (2006). Getting to Fairness: Negotiations over Global Public Goods. In I. Kaul (Ed.), *Providing Global Public Goods: Managing Globalization* (C. Zhang et al., Trans.). Beijing: People's Publishing House.

Aginam, O. (2002). International Law and Communicable Diseases. *The Bulletin of the World Health Organization*, 80, 946.

Aginam, O. (2005). *International Law and Public Health in a Divided World*. Toronto: University of Toronto Press.

Annan, K. (2000). *Secretary-General Salutes International Workshop on Human Security in Mongolia*. Retrieved from www.un.org/press/en/2000/20000508.sgsm7382.doc.html

Aron, R. (1967). *The Industrial Society: Three Essays on Ideology and Development*. New York: Praeger Press.

Baum, F. (2002). *The New Public Health* (2nd ed.). Melbourne: Oxford University Press.

Beaglehole, R., & Bonita, R. (2008). Global Public Health: A Scorecard. *The Lancet*, 372, 1988.

Beckford, D. S. (2008, March 26–29). *Global Health Governance in the WTO: A Preliminary Assessment of the Appellate Body' Interpretation of the SPS Agreement and the Legitimacy of SPS Measures*. Paper prepared for ISA'S 49th Annual Convention: Bridging Multiple Divides. San Francisco, CA, USA.

Berlinguer, G. (1999). Health and Equity as a Primary Global Goal. *Development*, 42(4), 18.

Berlinguer, G. (2003). Bioethics, Human Security, and Global Health. In L. Chen, J. Leaning, & V. Barasimhan (Eds.), *Global Health Challenges for Human Security*. Cambridge, MA: Harvard University Press.

Booth, K. (1991). Security and Emancipation. *Review of International Studies*, 17, 313–326.

Brower, J., & Chalk, P. (2003). *The Global Threat of New and Re-Emerging Infectious Diseases*. Santa Monica, CA: Rand.

Brundtland, G. B. (2003). Global Health and International Security. *Global Governance*, 9, 417.

Burkle Jr., F. M. (2006). Globalization and Disasters: Issues of Public Health, State Capacity and Political Action. *Journal of International Affairs*, 59(2), 246.

Buse, K. (2004). Governing Public-Private Infectious Disease Partnerships. *The Brown Journal of World Affairs*, 10(2), 225.

Buzan, B. (1983). *People, State and Fear*. Chapel Hill: University of North Carolina.

Buzan, B., & Wæver, O. (2003). *Security: A New Framework for Analysis* (N. Zhu, Trans.). Hangzhou: Zhejiang People's Publishing House.

Caballero-Anthony, M. (2006). Combating Infectious Diseases in East Asia. *Journal of International Affairs*, 59(2), 109.

Chen, K. (2007). *Public Health Security*. Hangzhou: Zhejiang University Press.

The Commission on Global Governance. (1995). *Our Global Neighbourhood*. Oxford: Oxford University Press.

50 Theoretical underpinnings

Conceicao, P. (2003). Assessing the Provision Status of Global Public Goods. In Kaul, I. (Ed.), *Providing Global Public Goods*. Oxford: Oxford University Press.

Cooper, A. F., Kirton, J. J., & Schrecker, T. (2007). *Governing Global Health: Challenge, Response, Innovation*. Hampshire: Ashgate Publishing Ltd.

Cooper, S. (2006). *The Avian Flu Crisis: An Economic Update*. Toronto, ON: BMO Nesbitt Burns, Inc.

Crosby, A. W. (1972). *The Columbian Exchange: Biological and Cultural Consequences of 1492*. Westport: Greenwood Press.

Department of Health. (2008). *Health Is Global*. A UK Government Strategy 2008–13. HM Government, London.

Desai, M. (2003). Public Goods: A Historical Perspective. In I. Kaul et al. (Eds.), *Providing Global Public Goods: Managing Globalization*. Oxford: Oxford University Press.

Development Committee. (2000). *Poverty Reduction and Global Public Goods: Issues for the World Bank in Supporting Global Collective Action*. DC/2000–16. Washington, DC, p. 2.

Diehl, P. F. (1997). *The Politics of Global Governance*. Boulder: Lynne Rienner Publishers, Inc.

Drager, N., & Beaglehole, R. (2001). Globalization: Changing the Public Health Landscape. *Bulletin of the World Health Organization*, 79(9), 803.

Dodgson, R., & Lee, K. (2002). Global Health Governance: A Conceptual Review. In R. Wilkinson & S. Hughes (Eds.), *Global Governance: Critical Perspectives*. London: Routledge.

Doyle, G. S. (2006). An International Public Health Crisis: Can Global Institutions Respond Effectively to HIV/AIDS. *Australian Journal of International Affairs*, 60(3), 401.

Eberstadt, N. (2002). The Future of AIDS. *Foreign Affairs*, 81(6), 22.

Fallows, J. (1999, June 7). The Political Scientist. *The New Yorker*.

Fan, Y. (2006). *Public Economics*. Shanghai: Fudan University Press.

Fidler, D. P. (1997). The Globalization of Public Health: Emerging Infectious Diseases and International Relations. *Indiana Journal of Global Legal Studies*, 11(7).

Fidler, D. P. (2000). A Kinder, Gentler System of Capitulations? International Law, Structural Adjustment Policies, and the Standard of Liberal, Globalized Civilization. *Texas Law Journal* (35), 327.

Fidler, D. P. (2001). *International Law and Global Infectious Disease Control*. CMC Working Paper Series Paper No.WG2: 18.

Fidler, D. P. (2007a). Architecture Amidst Anarchy: Global Health Quest for Governance. *Global Health Governance*, 1(1).

Fidler, D. P. (2007b). A Pathology of Public Health Securitism. In A. F. Cooper, J. J. Kirton, & T. Schrecker (Eds.), *Governing Global Health: Challenge, Response, Innovation*. Hampshire: Ashgate Publishing Ltd.

Fourie, P., & Schönteich, M. (2001). Africa's New Security Threat: HIV/AIDS and Human Security in Southern Africa. *African Security Review*, 10(4). Retrieved from www.iss.co.za/Pubs/ASR/10No4/Fourie.html

Garrett, L. (1995). *The Coming Plague: Newly Emerging Diseases in a World out of Balance*. New York: Penguin Books.

Garrett, L. (2005). The Next Pandemic. *Foreign Affairs*, 84(4), 2.

Garrett, L. (2006, September). *HIV and National Security: Where Are the Links?* New York: Council on Foreign Relations, p. 55. Retrieved from www.cfr.org/content/publications/attachments/HIV_National _Security.pdf

Gates, B. (2017, February 18). *A New Kind of Terrorism Could Wipe Out 30 Million People in Less Than a Year- and We Ae Not Prepared*. Bill & Melinda Gates Foundation. Retrieved from www.businessinsider.com/bill-gates-op-ed-bio-terrorism-epidemic-world-threat-2017-2?r=UK&IR=T

Giddens, A. (1990). *The Consequences of Modernity*. London: Polity Press.

Gostin, L. O. (2008). Meeting Basic Survival Needs of the World's Least Healthy People: Towards a Framework Convention on Global Health. *The Georgetown Law Journal*, 96, 331.

Hardin, G. (1968). The Tragedy of the Commons. *Science*, 162, 1243–1248.

Hardt, M., & Negri, A. (2003). *Empire* (J. Yang & Y. Fan, Trans.). Nanjing: Jiangsu People's Publishing.

Hein, W. (2008). Global Health Governance: Conflicts on Global Social Rights. *Global Social Policy*, 8(1), 84.

Hein, W., Bartsch, S., & Kohlmorgen, L. (2007). *Global Health Governance and the Fight against HIV/AIDS*. London: Palgrave Macmillan.

Heinechen, L. (2003). Facing a Merciless Enemy: HIV/AIDS and the South African Armed Forces. *Armed Forces and Society*, 29(2), 784.

Heymann, D. L., & Rodier, G. (2004). Global Surveillance, National Surveillance, and SARS. *Emerging Infectious Diseases*, 10(2), 173.

The High-Level Panel of UN. (2004). *A More Secure World: Our Shared Responsibility: Report of the High-Level Panel on Threats, Challenges and Change*. New York: United Nations.

Hopf, T. (1998). The Promise of Constructivism in International Relations Theory. *International Security*, 23(1), 171–200.

Howard-Jones, N. (1975). *The Scientific Background of the International Sanitary Conferences 1851–1938*. Geneva: WHO.

Institute of Medicine. (1997). *American's Vital Interest in Global Health*. Washington: National Academy Press.

International Task Force on Global Public Goods. (2006). *Meeting Global Challenges: International Cooperation in the National Interest*. Final Report. Stockholm, Sweden.

Jone, K. et al. (2008). Global Trends in Emerging Infectious Disease. *Nature*, 451, 990.

Kaib, C. (2003, May 5). The Battle to Contain SARS. *News Week*, 28.

Karns, M. P., Karen, A., & Mingst, K. A. (2003). *International Organizations: The Politics and Processes of Global Governance*. London: Lynne Rieenner Publishers.

Kaul, I. (Ed.). (2003). *Providing Global Public Goods: Managing Globalization*. Oxford: Oxford University Press.

Kaul, I., Grunberg, I., & Stern, M. A. (1999). *Global Public Goods: International Cooperation in the 21st Century*. Oxford: Oxford University Press.

Keohane, R. O. (2001). Governance in a Partially Globalized World. *American Political Science Review*, 95(1), 1–13.

Keohane, R. O., & Nye, J. S. (2000). Introduction. In J. S. Nye & J. D. Donahue (Eds.), *Governance in a Globalizing World*. Washington, DC: Brookings Institution Press.

Keohane, R. O., & Nye, J. S. (2002). *Power and Interdependence: World Politics in Transition* (M. Lin et al., Trans.). Beijing: China Renmin University Press.

Kickbusch, I. (2003a). Global Health Governance: Some New Theoretical Considerations on the New Political Space. In K. Lee (Ed.), *Globalization and Health*. London: Palgrave Macmillan.

Kickbusch, I. (2003b, April 25). SARS: Wake-Up Call for a Strong Global Health Policy. *Yale Global*. Retrieved from http://yaleglobal.yale.edu/display.article?id=1476

52 *Theoretical underpinnings*

Kickbusch, I. (2004). The Leavell Lecture: The End of Public Health as We Know It: Constructing Global Health in the 21st Century. *Public Health*, 188(7), 463–469.

Kickbusch, I. (2005). Global Health Governance: Some Theoretical Considerations on the New Political Space. In K. Lee (Ed.), *Health Impact of Globalization: Towards Global Governance*. London: Palgrave Macmillan.

Kindleberger, C. P. (1986). *The World in Depression, 1929–1939* (C. Song & W. Hong, Trans.). Shanghai: Shanghai Translation Publishing House.

Krasner, S. (1983). *International Regimes*. New York: Cornell University Press.

The League of Nations. (1920). *The Covenant of the League of Nations*. Retrieved from https://avalon.law.yale.edu/20th_century/leagcov.asp

Lee, K., & Dodgson, R. (2005). Globalization and Cholera: Implications for Global Governance. *Global Governance*, 6(2), 213–224.

Lipscomb, A. A., & Bergh, A. E. (n.d.). *The Writings of Thomas Jefferson* (Volume 3, Article 1, Section 8, Clause 8, Document 12). Washington: Thomas Jefferson Memorial Association, 1905. Retrieved from http://press-pubs.uchicago.edu/founders/documents/a1_8_8s12.html

Longrigg, J. (1992). Epidemic, Ideas and Classical Athenian Society. In T. Ranger & P. Slack (Eds.), *Epidemics and Ideas*. Cambridge: Cambridge University Press.

Mueller, D. C. (1999). *Public Choice* (X. Han & C. Yang, Trans.). Beijing: China Social Sciences Press.

Nakajima, H. (1997). Global Disease Threats and Foreign Policy. *Brown Journal of World Affairs*, 4(1), 319.

Olson, M. (1971). Increasing the Incentives in International Cooperation. *International Organization*, 25(4), 866–874.

Piot, P. (2001, October 2). *AIDS and Human Security: A Lecture at United Nations University*. Tokyo: United Nations University.

Pirages, D. (1995). Microsecurity: Disease Organisms and Human Well-Being. *Washington Quarterly*, 18(4), 5.

Porter, D. (1999). *Health, Civilization and the State: A History of Public Health from Ancient to Modern Times*. London and New York: Routledge.

Powell, C. (2003, June 12). *Speech to the Global Business Coalition on AIDS 2003 Awards for Business Excellence*. Retrieved from www.kintera.org/atf/cf/{EE846F03-1625-4723-9A53-B0CDD2195782}/gbc_awards_transcript_2003.pdf

Price-Smith, A. T. (2004). Downward Spiral: HIV/AIDS, State Capacity, and Political Conflict in Zimbabwe. *Peaceworks*, 53, 13–14.

Prystay, C. (2003, May 16). SARS Squeezes Asia's Travel Sector. *Wall Street Journal*.

Randy, C. (2004, December). Public Health as a Global Security Issue. *Foreign Service Journal*, p. 24.

Robertson, R. (1992). *Globalization: Social Theory and Global Culture*. London: Sage.

Russett, B. M., & Sulivan, J. D. (1971). Collective Goods and International Organizations. *International Organization*, 25(4), 845–865.

Salmon, C. T. (2000). *Issues in International Relations*. London and New York: Routledge.

Samuelson, P. A. (1954). The Pure Theory of Public Expenditure. *The Review of Economics and Statistics*, 36(4), 387–389.

Sandler, T. (1980). *The Theory and Structures of International Political Economy*. Boulder, CO: Westview Press.

Singer, P. W. (2002). AIDS and International Security. *Survival*, 44(1), 152.

Schrecker, T., & Labonte, R. (2007). What's Politics Got to Do with It? Health, the G8, and the Global Economy. In I. Kawachi & S. Wamala (Eds.), *Globalization and Health*. Oxford: Oxford University Press.

Smith, A. (1994). *An Inquiry Into the Nature and Causes of the Wealth of Nations*. New York: Modern Library.

Smith, S., & Baylis, J. (1997). *The Globalization of World Politics*. Oxford: Oxford University Press.

Su, C. (2000). *Global Public Issues and International Cooperation: An Institutional Analysis*. Shanghai: Shanghai People's Publishing House.

Trachtman, J. P. (2002). Institutional Linkage. *American Journal of International Law*, 96, 7–93.

Ullman, R. (1983). Redefining Security. *International Security*, 8(1), 129.

UN. (2001, September 6). *Road Map towards the Implementation of the United Nations Millennium Declaration*. Report of the Secretary-General. A/56/326. Retrieved from www.un.org/documents/ga/docs/56/a56326.pdf

UNAIDS. (2007). *About UNAIDS*. Retrieved from www.unaids.org/en/AboutUNAIDS/default.asp

UN Calls on Developed Countries to Help Developing Countries Fight AIDS. (2003, July 2). *Xinhua News*. Retrieved from http://news.xinhuanet.com

United Nations General Assembly. (2014, September 23). *69/1: Measures to Contain and Combat the Recent Ebola Outbreak in West Africa*. Retrieved from www.un.org/en/ga/search/view_doc.asp?symbol=A/RES/69/1&referer=www.un.org/en/ga/69/resolutions.shtml&Lang=C

UN Security Council. (2000a, January). *The Impact of AIDS on Peace and Security in Africa* (Press Release SC/6781), p. 1. Retrieved from https://www.un.org/press/en/2000/20000110.sc6781.doc.html

UN Security Council. (2000b, July 17). *Resolution 1308 (2000)*, p. 1. Retrieved from www.securitycouncilreport.org/atf/cf/%7B65BFCF9B-6D27-4E9C-8CD3-CF6E4FF96FF9%7D/CC%20SRES%201308.pdf

UN Security Council. (2011a, June 7). *Resolution 1983 (2011)*, p. 1. Retrieved from www.securitycouncilreport.org/atf/cf/%7B65BFCF9B-6D27-4E9C-8CD3-CF6E4FF96FF9%7D/HIV%20SRES%201983.pdf

UN Security Council. (2011b, September 18). *Resolution 2177 (2014)*. Retrieved from www.securitycouncilreport.org/atf/cf/%7B65BFCF9B-6D27-4E9C-8CD3-CF6E4FF96FF9%7D/S_RES_2177.pdf

UN Security Council. (2014, September 15). *Resolution 2176 (2014)*, p. 1. Retrieved from http://undocs.org/S/RES/2176(2014)

Walker, G. R., & Fox, M. A. (1996). Globalization: An Analytical Framework. *Indiana Journal of Global Legal Studies*, 375(3).

Watts, S. (1997). *Epidemics and History: Disease, Power and Imperialism*. New Haven: Yale University Press.

World Bank. (1993). *World Development Report 1993: Investing in Health*. New York: Oxford University Press.

WHO. (2000). *Division of Emerging and Other Communicable Diseases Surveillance and Control, Strategic Plan 1996–2000*, WHO/EMC/96.1, p. 10.

WHO. (2002a). *Deliberate Use of Biological and Chemical Agents to Cause Harm*. Retrieved from www.who.int/gb/ebwha/pdf_files/WHA55/ea5520.pdf

WHO. (2002b) *WHO-NTI Establish Global Emergency Outbreak Response Fund*. Retrieved from www.who.int/mediacentre/news/releases/pr92/en/

WHO. (2007). *World Health Report 2007: A Safer Future: Global Health Security in the 21st Century*. Retrieved from www.who.int/whr/2007/en/

Xi Jinping Visits the WHO Headquarters, Highlighting the Fact That China Attaches Importance to and Provides Support for the Global Health Cause. (2017, January 19).

54 *Theoretical underpinnings*

China News Network. Retrieved from www.chinanews.com/gn/2017/01-19/8129173. shtml

Yach, D., & Bettcher, D. (1998). The Globalization of Public Health: Threats and Opportunities. *American Journal of Public Health*, 88, 735.

Young, O. (1980). International Regimes and Concept Formation. *World Politics*, 32 (2), 1980.

Yu, K. (2003). *Globalization: Global Governance.* Beijing: Beijing Social Sciences Academic Press.

Yu, X. (2006). *Non-Traditional Security Theories.* Hangzhou: Zhejiang People's Publishing House.

3 World Health Organization and global health governance

By the end of World War II, countries arrived at a mutual understanding that "the health of all nations is the foundation for peace and security and relies on cooperation at the individual and national level" (WHO, 1946, p. 1). To achieve "the attainment by all peoples of the highest possible health" (WHO, 1946, p. 2), WHO was established to build on the progress brought by the International Sanitary Convention. A specialised agency of the United Nations, WHO acts as the directing and co-ordinating authority on international health work and has played an important role in the formulation and implementation of global health policies. The founding of the organisation is a landmark in the history of global health governance.

3.1 Background of the World Health Organization

The Constitution of the World Health Organization, adopted at the International Health Conference in 1946, marked the official establishment of WHO. The Constitution is the fruit of century-long public health diplomacies. Its establishment officially marked the institutionalisation of global health cooperation. Events that led to the creation of WHO roughly fall into the following stages.

3.1.1 Early International Sanitary Conferences (1851–1897)

A crucial observation characterising the international spread of disease is that "it follows the path of human transportation" (Siegfried, 1965, p. 16). Maritime transport grew rapidly in the middle of the 19th century with total tonnage of maritime transport in the world surging from 700,000 tons in 1850 to 2.62 million tons in 1910 (Headrick, 1981, p. 167). The Suez Canal opened in 1869, significantly raising the amount of goods transported, cutting costs and providing opportunities for Western travellers, Muslim pilgrims and migrants looking for better working and living conditions. Between 1815 and 1915, 46 million people had left Europe for different parts of the world, mainly North America. In the 19th century, 50 million people left China and India to settle in Latin America, Africa and various island territories (Headrick, 1988, p. 26). Accompanying the rising flow of people and goods was the settlement of serious diseases (such as malaria and cholera) in their new homes.

56 *WHO and global health governance*

European countries dominated international commerce at the time, contributing 70% of the world's total trade volume. A major trading country, the United Kingdom alone took up 20% (Foreman-Peck, 1983, p. 3). Yet despite the high volume of goods traded between Europeans and North Americans, the fastest growing international trade routes were between Europe and Asia. The volume of international travel to and from Asia, with its own share of indigenous contagious diseases, made international public health a major policy agenda in Europe. Rather than "disease importing countries" in southern Europe and the Middle East, the main initiators of public health cooperation in the mid-19th century were industrialised countries with significant maritime interests concerned with the delay of shipments from "quarantines".[1] Fidler (1999) holds that the main purpose of developing multilateral health cooperation in the 19th century was to protect "civilised" countries, mostly European ones, from being tainted by "uncivilised"—in particular Eastern—countries (p. 28). In other words, the initial international health cooperation among European countries was not intended to improve the state of international health but to protect their own economic interests and whose main priority was preventing the spread of diseases originating in Asia, Africa and Latin America.

Prior to 1851, nation states took three main measures to cope with the spread of disease. The first was through prayer and sacrificial offerings. A lack of scientific understanding for epidemiology made people regard an epidemic as a form of divine retribution to which no other response than prayer and sacrifices would suffice. The second approach was to isolate healthy people from unhealthy people through the practice of *cordon sanitaire* to prevent either an importation or exportation of disease. The third was to set up quarantine policies under which goods and people coming from areas suspected of having an outbreak would be isolated to reduce the risk from contracting diseases. For example, the Italian port of Ragusa in 1377 demanded all people from areas affected by the plague to stay at a designated place outside the port for 40 days. During the 14th and 15th centuries, many European countries had taken some type of mandatory quarantine measures, targeting ships, crews, passengers and cargo from foreign ports believed to be places prone to epidemic outbreaks, especially to plagues, yellow fever and cholera. Yet the differences in the mechanisms adopted had unintentionally strangled the flow of people and goods. An Italian government memorandum described this state of segregation as "anarchy through and through" (Goodman, 1971, p. 65). Disorganised policies such as these also found their way into contemporaneous literary works.[2]

In the following centuries, it became increasingly common to place infected people in quarantine along the Mediterranean coast. But such practice impeded the flow of goods and people between countries, leading to international conflicts. Quarantine policies then became dependent on cooperation between countries to be effective. European countries, prompted by a cholera scourge in 1830 causing thousands of deaths and widespread panic, decided to set up an international public health regime to cope with the spread of infectious diseases. In 1851, at France's initiative, the first International Sanitary Conference convened in Paris, opening the history of international public health cooperation. The purpose of the conference was to coordinate and resolve inconsistent and costly maritime quarantine policies of different countries in Europe, especially those with ports along the Mediterranean coast. Austria, France, Great Britain, Greece, Portugal, Russia, Spain, Turkey and four sovereign states that later united into Italy (the Papal States, Sardinia and the two Sicilies), attended the meeting. Most participants wanted to reach an agreement to standardise quarantine policies aimed at preventing cholera, plague and yellow fever. However, partly due to the lack of solid scientific evidence of the aetiology of the disease, partly because major shipping countries held their maritime commercial interests as a more urgent priority, countries had difficulty achieving consensus on specific texts of the International Sanitary Convention. In particular, they found it hard to standardise policies that were detrimental to international trade and transportation aimed at containing the transnational spread of disease.[3] Eventually, the motion to coordinate quarantine measures due to various inherent and insurmountable difficulties did not pass. Members of delegations, many of whom were physicians and diplomats, were equally baffled for their lack of pathogenic knowledge and ignorance on the transmission modes of the pathogens. Their ignorance of the disease manifested in renewed debate on whether the disease was caused by "miasma" or by "contagion". Miasmatists believed the disease was caused by the local dirty and foul air, whereas contagionists believed it was directly transmitted from infected people to healthy people. The views held by each country turned out to be closely aligned with their own economic interests. "Miasma theory" was in Britain's interest. As the leading maritime power at the time, the United Kingdom held that cholera was not a contagious disease; therefore, no quarantine or international management measures would help contain the disease. France seconded this view as the country benefited from merchant ships that sailed through the Suez under French jurisdiction. Quarantines, whether at the national or international level, were bound to harm French's shipping interests. At the meeting, Britain strongly opposed the provision granting countries the right to enforce quarantines. Countries along the Mediterranean and Black Sea coasts, on the other hand, supported port authority's right to quarantine. Unable to strike a compromise between public health and maritime and commercial interests, the participant countries had not one who ended up ratifying the draft International Sanitary Convention.

A second International Sanitary Conference was held in Paris in 1859, repeating the fate of the previous meeting. Dismissing quarantine measures as useless, the United Kingdom even more vehemently denied the use of quarantine policies. The Ottoman Empire and Greece, however, insisted they had the right to enforce quarantines on ships and personnel travelling their ports. The resulting draft treaty, which took five months to develop, looked identical to the previous one in 1851. Little was accomplished.

In 1864, a fourth cholera epidemic broke out in India and soon spread to other regions, lasting until 1872. After pilgrims who contracted cholera in Hejaz (the provincial name of the present Saudi Arabia) returned to the Ottoman Empire and Egypt, they brought devastating consequences to these places. In response, at the

58 *WHO and global health governance*

initiative of the Ottoman Empire, Britain, France, Russia and other countries held the third International Sanitary Conference. Although all participants agreed the cholera originated in India and was transmitted to other countries through infected travellers, Britain still maintained that cholera would not spread from person to person. Of the 21 countries represented at the conference, Britain, Russia, the Ottoman Empire and Persia all voiced oppositions to quarantines with varied motivation. Britain and Russia worried that their merchant ships passing through the Black Sea might be affected, did not want to compromise their commercial interests. The other two countries were more concerned about the high medical expenses they would have to bear if quarantine measures were to be implemented at their own ports. In summary, conflicts of interest, especially among bigger countries, made it virtually impossible for any collective action in international public health cooperation to take place. The fifth International Sanitary Conference, held in Washington in 1881, in turn reflected the conflict of interest between the United States and the rest. The agenda concerned ways to control yellow fever, but the central point of contention was not about members' rights to impose quarantine restrictions or sanitary inspections on passing ships but rather about the request from the United States to allow its own consuls, as opposed to local authorities, to issue a Bill of Health to ships destined for the United States. This requirement of extraterritoriality was met with strong opposition from other countries, especially from Latin America. The subsequent sixth Conference, held in Rome in 1885, and the seventh Conference, held in Venice in 1892, once again demonstrated the Anglo-French commercial rivalry. France, claiming that cholera was transmitted from British India, particularly Mumbai, to Europe wanted to impose more stringent sanitary measures on ships crossing the Suez Canal of the Red Sea en route to the West. France had profited handsomely from these ships, of which four-fifths were British. In 1884 alone, as many as 770 ships passed the canal sailing for British ports from India. Taking advantage of this fact, the British threatened to divert their shipping away from the French-run Suez Canal to force France to make concessions. Javed Siddiqi (1995) observed, "Persian and Turkish sensitivities were offended by the claim that cholera was endemic within their borders and considered any calls for tougher quarantines of ships leaving from Persian and Turkish ports an infringement of their sovereignty" (p. 17). Conflict of interest stymied any progress achieved through such conferences.

By the end of the 19th century, European countries held several more International Sanitary Conferences. In the course of nearly half a century, Europe's effort to coordinate public health policies resulted in frequent conclusions and replacements of conventions on infectious disease control, a process known as "a flurry of international conventions" (Carvalho & Zacher, 2001, p. 240). (see Table 3.1). Most of the cooperation were failures rather than successes. Only one international convention (targeting cholera) went into effect in 1892, the first and the only substantive outcome out of seven international conferences held in a span of 41 years. All these international conferences focused only on cholera, more specifically on the sanitary control of ships sailing westwards through the Suez Canal, most of which were British. Continental Europe was deeply concerned that

WHO and global health governance 59

Table 3.1 International Sanitary Conferences Between 1851 and 1897

Year	Venue	Initiator	Result
1851	Paris	France	The first International Sanitary Convention is signed.
1859	Paris	France	The convention to simplify the first International Sanitary Convention is adopted.
1865	Paris	Ottoman Empire	Discussions on maritime quarantine measures are held.
1874	Vienna	Russia	A convention to set up an international standing committee on infectious diseases is adopted.
1881	Washington D.C.	United States	A convention to set up an international health regime is adopted.
1885	Rome	United Kingdom	Discussions on quarantine measures related to cholera control are held.
1887	Brazil	United Kingdom	An international quarantine convention is adopted.
1892	Venice	France	The 1892 International Sanitary Convention is adopted.
1897	Venice	Austria-Hungary	The 1897 International Sanitary Convention is adopted.

the Suez Canal might become a path for cholera to spread from India to Europe. "History has proved that these concerns were groundless" (Howard-Jones, 1975, p. 65). In 1874, the fourth International Sanitary Conference adopted a convention to set up an international standing committee on infectious diseases but had no follow-up policies. In essence, most of the International Sanitary Conferences in the 19th century were mere formalities and not institutionalised in any way. It is true that ignorance concerning infectious diseases may have held countries back from reaching consensus; the more fundamental reason, though, had to do with their primary occupation with business interests rather than public health concerns. The deep-rooted conflicts of interest between countries made it difficult to reach a common ground in the negotiations of global health conventions. Notwithstanding this sequence of events,

> From the point of view of practical results, the first International Sanitary Conference was a fiasco. Everyone went on doing in their own way what they had done before. Yet there was more to it than that. The fact that the conference took place established the principle that health protection was a proper subject for international consultations even though international health cooperation was for many years to be limited to defensive quarantine measures. The French Government of the time had planted a seed that was not to germinate for some forty years and then, after a complicated cycle of development, to blossom more than half a century later into WHO.
>
> (Howard-Jones, 1975, p. 16)

60 WHO and global health governance

3.1.2 Institutionalisation of international health cooperation

By the end of the 19th century, European countries gradually realised that international conventions and treaties alone could neither address common vulnerabilities nor "put an end" to the threat of infectious diseases. Global health governance required formal regimes through which they could implement and enforce the international conventions. The institutionalisation of global health governance went through three important stages.

Stage 1: Establishment of the Office international d'hygiène publique (OIHP) (1903–1938). At the beginning of the 20th century, international public health cooperation picked up the pace. On the one hand, although conventions reached in the 19th century had been ratified by some countries, regulations and rules on international public health issues remained vague, and their enforcement was a controversial topic. Most countries did not comply with existing regulations. On the other hand, infectious diseases had become more disruptive. In 1902, a plague in Kenya and a cholera in the Philippines killed 100,000 people (Beck, 1970, p. 7). But much progress had also been made in epidemiological research in the last two decades of the 19th century. On the whole, these two factors opened the door to more effective international public health cooperation in the 20th century. Building on the progress of the previous conferences, the international community held its first International Sanitary Conference of the 20th century in 1903. The conference discussed ways to test for diseases (mainly regarding notification and quarantines measures for cholera and plague) and the resulting International Sanitary Convention required member states to report information on malaria and plague.[4] Participating countries also drafted International Sanitary Regulations, which set sanitary standards concerning ships and ports, inspections of ships, inspection certificates, segregation of infected ships and travellers and health checklists for people onboard. In fact, as Fidler (1999) maintained, 71% of the provisions were targeted at developing countries in the Middle East, Asia and Africa (p. 19). The main concern of participating countries was about preventing the spread of disease from developing countries to developed countries and how to coordinate isolation measures. The ultimate purpose was to prevent economic losses of the maritime interests of Western powers (Goodman, 1971, p. 389).

Participants of the 1903 Conference asked France to support an ensuant meeting to focus on establishing an international organisation that would facilitate the sharing of information on outbreaks. As a result, countries around the world adopted the Rome Agreement on the Establishment of an Office international d'hygiène publique at the International Sanitary Conference in 1907, and subsequently set its headquarters in Paris. The Office had a permanent secretariat and a permanent committee of senior public health officials from 12 member states, nine of which were from Europe. The reason for the establishment of this permanent body was that at an international conference in Washington in 1902, led by the United States, the governments of the Americas had already joined together to set up the International Sanitary Bureau, a regional intergovernmental organisation. One of the most important features of the OIHP was its responsibility to

WHO and global health governance 61

collect information on diseases listed in the International Sanitary Regulations. In a way, "the Office international d'hygiène publique functions primarily as an international clearinghouse" (Stern & Markel, 2004, p. 1476). By the end of 1908, the permanent committee of the OIHP had hosted a total of two meetings and continued to host meetings biannually thereafter, though interrupted for five years due to World War I. The OIHP also prepared the International Sanitary Conference in 1926, which added provisions for the control of smallpox and typhus to the International Sanitary Regulations and expanded the OIHP's scope of disease control. In short, the founding of the OIHP marked the beginning of the institutionalisation of international public health governance.

Stage 2: Establishment of the League of Nations Health Organization. After the scourge of World War I, countries around the world were eager to create a formal organisation to extend peace. As a result of the efforts, the international community established the League of Nations in 1919. Article 23 of its Charter states that member states "will endeavour to take steps in matters of international concern for the prevention and control of disease".[5] To implement this provision, the International Community established the Health Organisation of the League of Nations (HOLN) in 1920. The founders believed that the HOLN should play a more prominent role in the management of typhus and influenza outbreaks after World War I. They also held that at that time all international public health regimes, including the International Sanitary Bureau and the Office international d'hygiène publique, should be placed under the supervision of the League of Nations. As the United States, being a member of the OIHP, refused to join the British- and French-led League of Nations, it naturally opposed any proposal to merge OIHP into the HOLN. As a result, in the years between the two world wars, two independent international health organisations co-existed in Europe— the OIHP and the HOLN. In 1923, the International Sanitary Bureau was renamed the Pan-American Sanitary Bureau, the predecessor of the Pan-American Health Organization. As the United States ascended as the biggest power in the Americas since the end of the 19th century, the nation had always attempted to implement the Monroe Doctrine and establish a hegemon in America. They resisted Europe's interference in American affairs and always opposed any attempt to fuse the Pan-American Sanitary Bureau into global health organisations. Not until the end of World War II did the Pan-American Sanitary Bureau become one of the six regional offices of WHO.

During the two world wars, the international health regimes were paralysed by hostilities on both sides of the war. Three autonomous organisations, the HOLN in Geneva, the Pan-American Sanitary Bureau in Washington, and the Office international d'hygiène publique in Paris, coexisted and did not hold affiliations with one another. Each regime implemented conventions or treaties within its own sphere of influence. According to Javed Siddiqi, between 1920 and 1936 the League of Nations had suggested on four occasions that the Office international d'hygiène publique reform its international activities, eliminate overlapping functions and establish a single international health organisation. These recommendations were all rejected by the Office international d'hygiène publique.[6] After

62   *WHO and global health governance*

the outbreak of World War II, with the dissolution of the League of Nations, the HOLN ceased to exist. Other international health regimes continued to operate independently until the Office international d'hygiène publique merged with the newly established World Health Organization in 1948. On the whole, despite the setbacks these health mechanisms endured and the protracted process through which international health conventions were settled, all the international health cooperation efforts demonstrate an irrefutable fact: Multilateral cooperation is an effective tool to jointly deal with the threat of micro-organisms.

Stage 3: Establishment of WHO. In 1945, after World War II ended, world leaders all agreed to hold an international conference on international organisations in San Francisco. The call for a new International Health Organization received increasing support. The meeting provided a wonderful opportunity to start discussions on setting up an effective world health organisation and formalised this organisation as a component of the United Nations system. Since representatives of the United States and the United Kingdom did not agree to include public health issues on the agenda, the proposal to establish a UN specialised health agency was not originally included in the charters of relevant international organisations of the United Nations reached at the San Francisco meeting. Only eventually and with strong support from the Brazil and China delegations holding that "medicine is one of the pillars of peace", was the proposal added to the Charter of the United Nations. A declaration was finally adopted at the meeting mandating health to be an area in which the United Nations shall participate (Lee, 1998, p. 4). However, writing the framework for the WHO charter was easier said than done. The United Nations Economic and Social Council agreed in February 1946 to convoke an international health conference in New York to "discuss the scope of international action in the public health field, appropriate approaches, and recommendations for a single United Nations World Health Organization" (ibid., p. 4). The meeting was prepared by a technical preparatory committee composed of 16 experts in the field of international health. From March to April 1946, the committee met in Paris to draw up a schedule and recommendations for discussion and prepared proposals on the governance structure, management, finances, trusteeships and even names of the new organisation. The International Health Conference was finally held between June 19 and July 22, 1946. Fifty-one Member States of the United Nations and 13 Non-member States participated in the meeting. In addition, observers from Germany, Japan, the Korean Allies management authorities and from relevant United Nations organisations also participated in the meeting. The delegations reached a consensus on the Constitution of the new organisation, the draft concerning the suspension of the Office international d'hygiène publique, the establishment of an interim commission to continue the work previously undertaken by the HOLN and the interim United Nations Relief and Rehabilitation Administration (UNRRA) (ibid., pp. 4–5). On April 7, 1948, WHO was officially established, making the day the annual "World Health Day". The first Health Assembly opened in Geneva on June 24, 1948, with delegations from 53 of the 55 Member States. The interim commission ceased to exist on August 31, 1948, after the completion of its mission. Afterwards WHO took over international public health work, making it the first health organisation with a global dimension in the history of international public health cooperation.

3.2 Governance structure of the World Health Organization

A structure describes the inner connection and organisation of a system. In extension it may mean the framework governing interconnected components. An analysis of an organisation's structure will help us better understand its mechanism. Behaviourism holds that the structure can influence and even determine the outcome of an organisation (Hammond, 1986, pp. 379–420). A brief analysis of WHO's structure is thus in order to better understand its governance agenda.

3.2.1 Structure of the World Health Organization

The principal bodies of WHO are the World Health Assembly, the Executive Board and the Secretariat. Although they share the same goals in global health governance, they have different decision-making functions and follow different sets of procedures.

3.2.1.1 The World Health Assembly

As mandated by the Constitution of the World Health Organization, the World Health Assembly is the highest governing or the highest policymaking body of WHO. With respect to its role in the adoption of global health regulations and recommendations, WHO is also often referred to as a legislative organ. Article 13 of the Constitution stipulates that the World Health Assembly shall meet in regular annual sessions. If necessary, special sessions shall be convened at the request of the Board of WHO or upon a majority vote of the members. The Board, after consultation with the secretary-general of the United Nations, shall determine the date of each annual and special session. The World Health Assembly shall at each annual session select the country or region where the next annual session is to be held, with the Board subsequently fixing the specific location. The Board shall determine the place where a special session shall be held. Regarding the frequencies of the Health Assembly, in 1950, the Norwegian and Swedish delegations submitted a report to the Health Assembly recommending that the Assembly meet from once a year to every two years to be economical with resources and time. They also held that one year was not sufficient for a careful formulation of a new agenda to be submitted to the next Assembly. However, their recommendation was not adopted. Since then, the time provision has remained unchanged, though the length of each assembly has been shortened. In 1996, the length of each meeting was stipulated not to exceed six days.

The World Health Assembly is made up of delegates from member states:

> Each Member shall be represented by no more than three delegates, one of whom shall be designated by the Member as chief delegate. These delegates

64   *WHO and global health governance*

should be chosen from among persons most qualified by their technical competence in the field of public health, preferably representing the national health administration of the Member.

(Constitution of the World Health Organization, p. 5)

Delegates, as spokespersons for member states, can express the views of their governments. Delegates of the Executive Board, the United Nations, other specialised agencies, intergovernmental organisations that have special relations with WHO and observers from non-member countries as well as NGOs can participate in the World Health Assembly without voting rights. Article 18 of the Constitution of WHO stipulates the functions of the World Health Assembly, which include, among others, the right to review and approve of reports of the director-general and the budget as well as the right to participate in the discussion for other important issues.

3.2.1.2 Executive Board

The Executive Board is the executive organ of the World Health Assembly. The Board is composed of 34 technical experts in the field of health, each designated by a member state and approved by the World Health Assembly. Members are elected for a three-year term; one-third of the membership is replaced every year. The five permanent members of the UN Security Council are naturally members of the Executive Board, each of them is rotated out for a year once every three years. Article 28 lays out specific provisions on the functions of the Executive Board (Constitution of the World Health Organization, p. 8), whose main duty is to implement all the policies and work of WHO in cooperation with the World Health Assembly. On one hand, the Board's role includes preparing the agenda for the World Health Assembly meetings; advising the assembly on questions and matters assigned to WHO by conventions, agreements and regulations and submitting to the assembly for consideration and approval a general programme of work covering a specific period. On the other hand, the Board also assumes the role of an executive body of the World Health Assembly. In other words, it enforces decisions and policies of the World Health Assembly and performs any other functions entrusted to it by the assembly. The World Health Assembly is thus closely related to the Executive Board.

3.2.1.3 Secretariat

The Secretariat is the third organ to implement the work of WHO under the Constitution of the World Health Organization. Its origin traces back to the transitional committee before WHO formally came into being. The Secretariat is led by a director general and six regional directors and consists of technical as well as administrative staff. Since the World Health Assembly and the Executive Board convene respectively once and twice per year, they are unfit to implement all the work of WHO in the brief duration when they meet. It is therefore

WHO and global health governance   65

necessary to establish a permanent body to handle the day-to-day affairs of WHO, a role assumed by the Secretariat. It has six regional offices (see Table 2.1). Its regional arrangement has proved to be the most controversial issue with respect to WHO's organisational structure, especially regarding the issue of whether the Pan-American Health Organization should be merged into WHO. WHO finally solved the controversy by adopting the principle of "progressive and ultimate merger": The Constitution of WHO stipulates that the regional committees shall be designated as "an integral part of the Organization" in accordance with the Constitution of the World Health Organization. In other words, WHO shall have supreme authority worldwide in the governance of future intergovernmental international public health issues. After painstaking negotiations, the Pan-American Health Organization finally agreed in 1949 to become WHO's regional office in the Western Hemisphere,[7] making WHO the most authoritative global intergovernmental organisation in the field of public health.

3.2.2 Objective of the World Health Organization

Generally speaking, an international regime upholds its own constitution. This constitution has a function similar to the corresponding legal corpus in the Chinese legal system. It not only stipulates the legal status, objective, operating principles, organisational structure, procedures and rights and obligations of member states but also serves as a basis for granting the legitimacy for power of the overarching organisation (Rao, 1996, pp. 254–255). The Constitution of WHO opens by laying out explicitly the principles by which WHO abides: Health is defined not as the mere absence of disease or infirmity but rather as the state of complete physical, mental and social well-being. The enjoyment of the highest attainable standard of health is one of the fundamental rights of every human being without distinction of a fundamental human right and regardless of race, religion, political belief or economic or social condition. The health of all peoples is fundamental to the attainment of achieving peace and security and is dependent upon the fullest cooperation of individuals and states. The objective of WHO is "the attainment by all peoples of the highest possible health".

Driven by this objective, WHO defines health as "a state of complete physical, mental and social well-being and not merely the absence of disease or infirmity." This grants WHO an active role in a wide range of public health issues, not just to health care in the narrow sense. The preamble to the Constitution of WHO not only entails considerations for trade, biosafety and human rights but also indicates the importance of other areas of the international regimes to the mission of WHO and the "implicit power" of it to participate in the work of other international regimes.

3.2.3 Functions of the World Health Organization

Article 2 of the Constitution of WHO defines the organisation's functions. It not only stipulates WHO's extensive responsibilities in the control of global infectious

66 *WHO and global health governance*

diseases but also establishes its quasi-legislative functions, including the intro-duction of international conventions, international agreements, public health governance regulations and the establishment of international terms and stan-dards. In addition, Article 2 establishes the authority of WHO as the directing and coordinating authority on international health work, indicating that WHO has the authority to coordinate inconsistent international public health rules adopted by different international organisations (Constitution of the World Health Organiza-tion, pp. 2–3). In general, the functions of WHO fall into the following categories.

First, WHO has the power to adopt a convention or an agreement. An inter-national convention, like an international law, is a multilateral treaty achieved through meetings involving international organisations or presided over by an international organisation. A convention can help make a member state's behav-iour predictable in increasingly wide-ranging and close international exchanges. Therefore, since its establishment, WHO, drawing on the practices of the Interna-tional Labour Organization, the Food and Agriculture Organization of the United Nations (FAO) and other international organisations, regulates international actions of member states in the field of public health through convention-making.[8] The World Health Assembly has the authority to adopt public health conventions or agreements. Article 19 of the Constitution stipulates that "the Health Assembly shall have authority to adopt conventions or agreements with respect to any matter within the competence of the Organization" (p. 7). A convention or an agreement will be adopted if it can secure a two-thirds majority of the Health Assembly and legally bind member states once procedurally adopted by due constitutional pro-cesses within each sovereignty.

Second, WHO may ratify international public health regulations. Article 21 of the Constitution stipulates that the Health Assembly shall have authority to adopt regulations concerning: 1) sanitary and quarantine requirements and other proce-dures designed to prevent the international spread of disease; 2) nomenclatures with respect to diseases, causes of death and public health practices; 3) stan-dards with respect to diagnostic procedures for international use; 4) standards with respect to the safety, purity and potency of biological, pharmaceutical and similar products moving in international commerce and 5) advertising and label-ling of biological, pharmaceutical and similar products moving in international commerce. Regulations adopted pursuant to Article 21 shall come into force for all members after due notice has been given of their adoption by the Health Assembly except for such members as may notify the director-general of rejec-tion or reservations within the period stated in the notice. As a result, WHO has advanced the amendment procedure of a treaty to its conclusion procedure and formally established a "contracting out" method. In other words, although regu-lations proposed according to Article 21 of the Constitution shall be discussed and negotiated by member states and shall only pass after receiving a simple majority vote, the minority member states who vote against can still choose not to comply with part or all of these regulations based on their special circum-stances. This flexibility in enforcing regulations prevents treaties adopted by the Health Assembly from being nullified due to the reservations of a minority of countries.

Finally, WHO is authorised to make recommendations to ember states. Article 23 of the Constitution stipulates that "the Health Assembly shall have authority to make recommendations to Members with respect to any matter within the competence of the Organization" (p. 8). Such recommendations shall not be conceived of as a form of interference in the domestic affairs of its member states. Member states are also under no obligation to bring such recommendations to the attention of their national functional authorities within a specified period to make appropriate legislative or administrative arrangements. In other words, such recommendations are not legally binding on member states. It is noteworthy that with the increasing interdependence in the field of global health security, WHO's recommendation has expanded in scope, and the "right to knowledge" of WHO has made such recommendations influential in global health governance. For example, during the SARS epidemic in 2003, WHO had issued recommendations to individual tourists, rather than to member states, urging them not to travel to Toronto, Canada, or to China.

3.3 The power of "soft law" of the World Health Organization: International Health Regulations (2005)

The previous iteration of the IHR was born as an international health legal document originally adopted by WHO to coordinate international disputes arising from conflicting priorities between managing health issues and protecting trade interests. It replaced various health conventions implemented before 1951. In fact, it was the only binding instrument ratified by the World Health Assembly from 1948 to 2000 with the objective to ensure maximum security against the international spread of disease with minimal interference with world traffic. Despite the progress made by the IHR in global health governance, its failures overshadowed its successes. Drawing on lessons learned, the current IHR (2005) amended some of the defects of the original document. For example, it expanded the scope of disease control, incorporated human rights principles, expanded information channels from non-governmental actors, and increased its involvement in the capacity building of domestic health systems in state parties. These added features enable the IHR (2005) to be more responsive in addressing current global health issues and in promoting global health governance. However, the IHR (2005) still have shortcomings. They lack a mechanism for mandatory dispute settlement. Certain provisions are inconsistent with other international treaties. The regulations also fail to specify whether WHO has the right to monitor biological weapons. A deep reason contributing to such shortcomings is that member states still adhere to concepts of national sovereignty according to the Westphalian framework and are thereby unwilling to relinquish control of public health affairs considered within their individual sovereignty. That adherence foreshadows limitations of the IHR (2005) to function as the main regime in global health governance.

3.3.1 Background and birth of the IHR (2005)

At the first World Health Assembly in 1948, the newly formed International Committee of Experts on Epidemiology and Quarantine consolidated multiple versions

68 *WHO and global health governance*

of the International Sanitary Convention (1903) to form the International Sanitary Regulations (1948). The fourth World Health Assembly adopted the Regulations (1948) in 1951 and rolled out preliminary international rules for managing infectious diseases. In 1969, the 22nd World Health Assembly adopted, revised and consolidated the International Sanitary Regulations (1969) and renamed it the International Health Regulations (1969). The 26th World Health Assembly amended the IHR (1973) concerning provisions on cholera. In light of the global eradication of smallpox, the 34th World Health Assembly amended the IHR (1981) to exclude smallpox from the list of notifiable diseases.

However, with the deepening of globalisation and the rise of new global health crises, the IHR (1981) fell out of date for global health governance. The call for revision was gaining momentum. Concerns that the regulation was ineffective had existed long before 1995 (Dorelle, 1969; Roelsgaard, 1974; Velimirovic, 1976), including its unduly narrow scope of notifiable diseases (cholera, plague, yellow fever) and acquiescence for breaches and non-compliance by member states. The resurgence of infectious diseases in the 1980s and 1990s made the IHR fall further behind the challenges of the time. WHO also came to the realisation that in an era of accelerated globalisation, a revised IHR must break the mound of traditional approaches and introduce new agents, processes and norms to build a new public health security governance frame. For these reasons, the World Health Assembly recommended the director-general amend the IHR in 1995 (World Health Assembly, 1995). In January 1998, WHO prepared a draft amendment to the IHR, expanding the scope of diseases to be controlled and allowing the use of data from non-governmental actors. A new, more innovative framework was beginning to take shape (WHO, 1998a). In 2002, some WHO officials suggested WHO should play a more active role in dispatching working groups to countries reporting outbreaks and helping member states to improve their surveillance capabilities (Grein et al., 2000, pp. 97–102). The anthrax attacks in the United States in 2001 and the SARS crisis in 2003 accelerated the revision process of the new IHR. WHO regarded the response to SARS as a precursor to drafting the IHR (2005). In January 2004, WHO issued a full text of the recommendations as the basis for discussions in the spring and summer of that year. Following regional discussions, WHO issued a fully revised version in September of the same year. After two rounds of intergovernmental consultations, the revised IHR (2005) were adopted by the World Health Assembly in May 2005 and came into effect on June 15, 2007.

3.3.2 Transformative features of the IHR (2005)

The IHR (2005) consist of 66 articles and 9 annexes. The objective was "to prevent, protect against, control, and provide a public health response to the international spread of disease in ways that are commensurate with and restricted to public health risks, and which avoid unnecessary interference with international traffic and trade." The regulations seek to balance a nation's right to protect its people's health and "obligations to take health actions in ways that do not interfere with international travel". The new IHR stipulate that

States have, in accordance with the Charter of the United Nations and the principles of international law, the sovereign right to legislate and to implement legislation in pursuance of their health policies. In doing so they should uphold the purpose of the Regulations."[9]

By recalibrating health and trade interests, the IHR were made consistent with international trade law under WTO, which recognises the state's right to restrict trade for health purposes but limits this right t cases of absolute necessity (WHO & WTO, 2002, p. 59). The synergy between the new IHR and international trade law demonstrates that public health is de facto embedded in an international system that facilitates economic activity through globalised markets. Finding effective means to balance public health and international economic activity has assumed critical importance in finding ways to balance international trade and global health governance.

The IHR (2005) revolutionarily depart in their approach from traditions that are exemplified by previous versions of the IHR. They transform the international legal context in which states will exercise their public health sovereignty in the future. They expand the scope of the previous IHR's application, incorporate international human rights principles, contain more demanding obligations for state parties and establish important new powers for WHO. There is growing consensus on the importance of global health governance in the 21st century; changes in the IHR are closely related to this fact. Over the ten years when the IHR were revised, public health issues became increasingly important to global governance, national and international security, trade and economic development and environmental and human rights protection. The IHR (2005) not only transformed international health governance into global health governance but also elevated the political status and importance of public health issues in global governance. In general, they have promoted global health governance in the following aspects.

First, the list of goals pursued by the IHR has expanded. The objective of the IHR (1983) and prior versions was to limit the international spread of infectious disease with minimum interference with international business. The IHR (2005), in addition to these two goals, also urged member states to promote human rights, environmental protection and security. Fidler (2005) refers to the expansion of these political or value goals as "integrated governance" (p. 344). The expansion of this mechanism's goals is arguably the biggest change in global health governance. For example, in the IHR (2005), the provisions on the cooperation between WHO and traditional international security regimes reflect the securitisation of public health issues. Article 6 on the notification of public health events provides that "if the notification received by WHO involves the competency of the International Atomic Energy Agency (IAEA), WHO shall immediately notify the IAEA". At the same time, Article 14(2) of the IHR (2005) stipulates that

> in cases in which notification or verification of, or response to, an event is primarily within competence of other intergovernmental organisations or international bodies, WHO shall coordinate its activities with such organisations

70 *WHO and global health governance*

or bodies in order to ensure the application of adequate measures for the protection of public health.

The implication is that should biological weapons be used with a malicious intent and cause international health crises, WHO should consult and cooperate with the UN Security Council considering its close connections to the BWC.

Second, scope of the IHR (2005) has been expanded with the adoption of an all-risks approach. The prior IHR only applied to a short list of infectious diseases (e.g. cholera, plague and yellow fever), whose spread was historically associated with travel and trade. Article 1 of the new IHR defines "disease" as "an illness or medical condition, irrespective of origin or source, that prevents or could present significant harm to humans", which will include 1) naturally occurring infectious disease, whether of known or unknown illogical origin; 1) the potential international spread of non-communicable diseases caused by chemical or radiological agents in products moving in international commerce and 3) suspected intentional or accidental releases of biological, chemical or radiological substances. In other words, public health risks caused by bioterrorism or nuclear radiation are also covered by the new IHR. This "all-risks" approach demonstrates an important shift in the purpose of global health governance. The prior IHR were driven by prioritised trade interests, but the IHR (2005) instead focus on human health. The result is a set of more flexible and adaptable rules with more public health legitimacy. The principle to expand the domain of public health is found throughout the IHR (2005). Response to public health crises is now standardised into the following stages: reporting health events, handling epidemiological data, making WHO recommendations and limiting national health measures across the spectrum of health events. The expanded scope creates a more demanding framework than anything that ever appeared in the traditional approach.

Third, the IHR (2005) incorporate human rights principles. With the emergence of international human rights regimes, people have gradually realised the impact of public health interventions on civil and political rights, including basic safety and freedom of movement. Human rights issues therefore have also become an important consideration in the IHR (2005).

To start, the IHR (2005) embodies general human rights principles. Article 3.1 of the IHR (2005) stipulates that "the implementation of these Regulations shall be with full respect for the dignity, human rights and fundamental freedoms of persons". The human rights considerations in the IHR (2005) can be traced back to the definition of human rights in the preamble to the Constitution of WHO ratified in 1948. "The enjoyment of the highest attainable standard of health is one of the fundamental rights of every human being without distinction of race, religion, political belief, economic or social condition" (Constitution of WHO, 1946, p. 1). This article also raises the question whether the IHR (2005) conform to existing international human rights principles. For a public health policy to legitimately impose restrictions on civil and political rights, it must respond to a pressing public or social need, pursue a legitimate aim, be proportionate to the legitimate aim, and be no more restrictive than is required to achieve the purpose sought

WHO and global health governance 71

by restricting the right (UN Economic and Social Council, 1985). Such rights-restricting measures must also be implemented in a non-discriminating manner,[10] and individuals whose rights and freedom are affected by these policies must be treated with a humanitarian spirit, respectfully and in a dignified manner.[11] The IHR (2005) as a whole reflect the requirements of international human rights conventions. Articles 23, 31 and 43 require states parties to clarify public health risks to justify public health measures imposed on individuals and to use appropriate health response measures, which shall be no more "intrusive and invasive than other measures taken to achieve adequate protection of health". These provisions also apply to recommendations made by WHO under the new IHR. Article 42 states that "all health measures shall be implemented in a transparent and non-discriminatory manner". In addition, Article 32 stipulates that

> States Parties shall treat travellers with respect for their dignity, human rights and fundamental freedoms and minimise any discomfort or distress associated with such measures, including by: (a) treating all travellers with courtesy and respect; (b) taking into consideration the gender, sociocultural, ethnic or religious concerns of travellers; and (c) providing or arranging for adequate food and water, appropriate accommodation and clothing, protection for baggage and other possessions, appropriate medical treatment, means of necessary communication if possible in a language that they can understand and other appropriate assistance for travellers who are quarantined, isolated, or subject to medical examinations or other procedures for public health purposes.

The extent to which the IHR (2005) incorporate human rights principles has significant implications with respect to their interpretation and implementation through international human rights conventions. If states parties do not integrate human rights considerations into the operation of their respective public health systems, such incorporation will be irrelevant. As human rights problems with HIV/AIDS outbreaks and other public health concerns suggest, the effectiveness of human rights components in the IHR (2005) relies on political commitment and compliance from member states.

The IHR (2005) also contain provisions on informed consent and privacy. Articles 23 and 31 stipulate that "State Parties cannot apply health measures to travellers without their prior express informed consent, except in situations that warrant compulsory measures." Article 45 further stipulates that

> health information collected or received by a State Party from another State Party or from WHO which refers to an identified or identifiable person shall be kept confidential. State Parties may disclose and process personal data where essential for assessing and managing a public health risk but must ensure that the personal data are kept confidential. . . .Upon request, WHO shall as far as practicable provide an individual with his or her personal data.

72 WHO and global health governance

By recognising the importance of the right to informed consent and privacy, the new IHR have improved traditional methods of health governance, but some problems remain. For example, compulsory measures implemented without informed consent are not conducive to human rights principles. In addition, there is no requirement in the IHR (2005) for states parties to take necessary and appropriate procedural protections when implementing such compulsory measures. Regarding the right to privacy, the provisions of Article 45 entrust the obligations of protecting personal health data to the state party through national law. Similarly, when coping with public health crises, requirements for constituents to protect privacy ought to abide by national rules. These provisions have thus subjected privacy protections to disparate levels of national privacy protection rather than to internationally recognised privacy standards.

Fourthly, the IHR (2005) to some extent have transcended traditional concepts of national sovereignty under which the public health system within a country is an internal affair and not open to foreign interference of various channels.

The IHR (2005) highlight the importance of national capacity for upholding global health governance. "It is clear that strengthening a weak health system is necessary, which will not only enable the people of the country to enjoy the best health services, but also ensure global health security" (WHO, 2007, p. 63). Articles 5 and 13 of the IHR (2005) require state parties to develop, strengthen and maintain core surveillance and response capabilities, requirements involving public health sovereignty in state parties. The prior IHR mandated countries to strengthen the relevant public health capabilities only at points of entry and exit, a methodology still based on the old concept formed in the 19th century when prevention of cross-border transmission of diseases was achieved only through precautionary measures in border areas of various countries. In other words, the prior IHR focused on how to block disease outside the country rather than on building up internal disease management and public health systems within the country. In the context of frequent flow of trade and human mobility, such strategy can in no way adequately address global epidemics. The focus of the IHR (2005) on constructing internal public health mechanisms is a more proactive strategy in global health governance, one that seeks to control and govern the spread of infectious disease from its source. The revised provision has addressed the weakness in global health governance arising from insufficiencies in national monitoring and the lack of emergency response mechanisms. Since the internal public health system is an issue of national sovereignty, the provision that governs internal public health response mechanisms transcends the traditional concept of national sovereignty. Of course, the IHR (2005) also confer some degree of flexibility to the public health system capacity building of member states. For example, Article 5 stipulates that

> Each State Party shall develop, strengthen, and maintain, as soon as possible but no later than five years from the entry into force of these Regulations, the capacity to detect, access, notify, and report events; A State Party may report to WHO on the basis of a justified need and an implemented plan and,

in so doing, obtain an extension of two years; the State Party may request a further extension not exceeding two years from the Director-General, who shall make a decision.

Although the provisions of the IHR (2005) on surveillance and response capacities recognise the critical need for capacity building, questions remain with respect to realising this goal. The most pressing question concerns the availability of financial and technical resources needed to improve national core capacities. This is especially true in developing countries, where inadequate investment, paralysis in the health infrastructure for lack of trained health workers, and damage to health infrastructure brought by armed conflicts as well as natural disasters have often led to a dire shortage of necessary resources. Some developing countries find it particularly difficult to respond effectively to public health crises. Adding to their misfortunes, public health events of international concern tend to take place in developing countries with poor public health infrastructures. WHO's goal to help developing nations establish public health capacities is beyond the reach of its arm. Nor does the new IHR stipulate obligations on state parties to provide financial and technical resources to support capacity building for other countries. Although Article 44 of the IHR (2005) urges state parties to provide financial and technical resources, these provisions are not binding. Given the funding needed to address global health issues, for example, to increase access to AIDS treatment and to achieve the health-related UN MDGs, the IHR (2005) neither specify on how to meet the core competencies nor provide a clear solution and strategy.

The IHR (2005) oblige state parties to report public health emergencies of international concern. Article 6 requires each state party to notify WHO of all events in its territory that may constitute a public health emergency of international concern. But whether a state party has or can develop surveillance capabilities sufficient to fulfil these obligations remains a serious question. There is another problem in requiring notification. Some state parties may choose not to report diseases governed by the IHR because they fear other countries will implement excessive trade and travel restrictions. Although broader and more stringent notification requirements can weaken the incentives for state parties not to comply, it is not fool proof against the havoc wrought by non-compliance, for WHO itself is a "toothless health regulator" (Ho, 2006). It simply does not have a penalty or an enforcement mechanism to deal with a breach of obligation.

The IHR (2005) formally identifies non-governmental actors as one of their sources of information. One of the main reasons why the prior IHR did not work effectively is that it limited the information sources for WHO to state parties only. Wary of massive economic losses in the event of embargoes and quarantines, some governments refused to notify WHO of incidents, supply needed information or to cooperate. Some were unable to monitor relevant outbreak information due to technical restraints. This limitation on information sources handicapped WHO's ability to respond to disease outbreaks. The IHR (2005) clearly specify that unofficial information may sometimes be prioritised over official information, thus expanding WHO's information channels. "In the context of infectious

74 *WHO and global health governance*

disease control, a key feature of global health governance that emerged in the 1990s was the direct involvement of non-state actors in surveillance for outbreaks and disease events" (Fidler, 2004, pp. 132–133). This practice is now formally included in the IHR (2005). Articles 9 and 10 allow WHO to take into account reports from sources other than notifications or consultations from or with governments and to seek states parties in whose territories the events are allegedly occurring.

In fact, ever since the beginning of the IHR's revision process, WHO has recognised that access to non-governmental sources of information is critical to constructing an effective global surveillance system. The use of telecommunications in disease verification and testing has increasingly become a new phenomenon in global health governance. WHO's Global Outbreak Alert and Response Network (GOARN) has harnessed new information technologies, including the World Wide Web, to form a collaborative network of institutions and experts that pools human and technical resources. GOARN can identify, confirm and respond to outbreaks of international significance; it can also send response teams to the world within 24 hours to provide direct support to the relevant departments of the country. This network can bridge huge gaps due to insufficient national capacity and protect global health in the event a country delays reporting an outbreak out of political considerations or other reasons. It plays an important role in the effective implementation of the functions of the new IHR. During the SARS outbreak, WHO demonstrated its ability to obtain information from non-governmental sources. NGOs under WHO possess information channels that grant WHO the right to require member states to verify information from such channels. These provisions incentivise member states to comply with the notification requirements. Therefore confronted with a public health threat and wishing to minimise negative economic impact, a member state would fare best to keep its cooperation with WHO and other countries. "This source of information and verification rules places global health governance above national sovereignty" (Fidler & Gostin, 2006, p. 90).

The IHR (2005) grant WHO two important and unprecedented powers. First, it authorises WHO to decide whether a disease outbreak constitutes a public health emergency of international concern. Article 12 states that

> the Director-General shall determine, on the basis of the information received, in particular from the State Party within whose territory an event is occurring, whether an event constitutes a public health emergency of international concern. Although the Director-General must consult with the State Party in which the disease occurred, he or she is not bound by the views of State Parties.

In other words, WHO's right to take action overrides a state party's refusal to cooperate. Articles 2, 15 and 16 stipulate that if the director-general determines that a public health emergency of international concern is occurring, then he or she shall issue non-binding, temporary recommendations to state parties on the most appropriate ways to respond. The director-general may also issue non-binding, standing recommendations on routine, periodic application of health measures for specific, ongoing public health risks. The new IHR contain criteria for issuing temporary or standing recommendations and examples of the kinds of measures recommended by WHO. These powers allow WHO to provide leadership in adopting scientific measures that appropriately balance health protection with respect for human rights and acknowledgement for trade concerns.

Although state parties have no legal obligation to comply with the temporary or long-term recommendations issued by WHO, the IHR (2005) contain binding limits on the types of health measures that state parties may take to address public health hazards. The purpose of these restrictions is to ensure maximum safety of health with minimal interference with traffic and human rights. Article 31 stipulates that "Invasive medical examination, vaccination or other prophylaxis shall not be required as a condition of entry of any traveller to the territory of a State Party." Article 35 further stipulates that "no health documents, other than those provided for under these Regulations or in recommendations issued by WHO, shall be required in international traffic". Articles 37 to 39 of the new IHR also adjusted the sanitary measures states parties may take on ships, aircraft, cargo and containers, and standardised the types of sanitary documents required for ships and aircraft. It allows states parties to implement health measures in response to specific public health hazards or public health emergencies of international concern in accordance with their national law and international obligations. But Article 43 also stipulates that

> such measures shall be based on scientific principles, available scientific evidence and available information from WHO and other relevant intergovernmental organisations and international bodies. Such measures shall not be more restrictive of international traffic and not more invasive or intrusive to persons than reasonably available alternatives that would achieve the appropriate level of health protection.

These provisions map out a path similar to the one taken by WTO regarding health protection measures, such as the Agreement on the Application of Sanitary and Phytosanitary Measures. However, the IHR (2005) depart from the Agreement in that they do not have a strong enforcement mechanism should the state party not comply with its health obligations according to mandates. The implementation of the Agreement is facilitated by the mandatory dispute settlement procedures in WTO, while the dispute settlement mechanism in the IHR (2005) is voluntary in nature. The lack of enforcement mechanisms in the IHR (2005) suggests that it unclear whether state parties will comply with its provisions.

3.3.3 Political conflicts exposed by the IHR (2005)

Three political conflicts collectively bearing on the efficiency of the IHR (2005) were brought to the fore during the revision of the IHR. As state parties failed to reach a consensus, WHO eventually chose to be intentionally vague regarding these points, a vagueness underpinning the eventual insufficiency of WHO in its desired future roles.

76 WHO and global health governance

3.3.3.1 Conflicts between the IHR (2005) and other international regimes

The expanded list of diseases exposes the IHR (2005) to conflicting jurisdiction with other international mechanisms also entrusted to manage transnational health hazards. These organisations include the International Atomic Energy Agency (in charge of nuclear accidents), WTO (which can issue health measures to restrict international trade), and the Codex Alimentarious Commission, which sets food standards and guidelines to protect consumer health and promote safe trade. Despite efforts by WHO to coordinate with various other international organisations, discrepancies with respect to goal and function make it hard to reconcile the IHR (2005) with competing policies from these organisations. Because so many international organisations share legislative power on health-related issues, efforts to issue directives and impose obligations are easily dispersed and become ineffective. The conflicts between the IHR (2005) and other international regimes have resulted in an "institutional overload" in global health governance.

3.3.3.2 Conflicts in the relationship between WHO and BWC

Regarding the relationship between WHO and the BWC, one conflict concerns whether the scope of notification stipulated in the IHR (2005) would include public health risks associated with biological, chemical and radioactive weapons. It is highly controversial to make provisions that apply to the deliberate release of such agents. The IHR (2005) only requires state parties to share information with WHO if they have evidence of a deliberate release of these agents in their territories. The spirit of this provision is that responses in public health policies should be commensurate with the gravity of the public health crisis, be it naturally occurring or deliberately introduced. But the provision is politically controversial because it relates to national and international security issues regarding weapons of mass destruction. Precedents and guidelines for WHO to respond to incidents involving weapons of mass destruction have been made. For example, WHO published the first edition of *Health aspects of biological and chemical weapons* in 1970. After the anthrax terrorist attacks in the United States, the WHO Secretariat prepared a report titled *The deliberate use of biological and chemical agents to cause harm: public health response* in the spring of 2002 in preparation for the 55th World Health Assembly. This report suggested that "the Organization's basic activity in this area is to strengthen public health disease alert and response systems at all levels, as such as a system will detect and respond to diseases that may be deliberately caused" (WHO, 2002, p. 2). In response to potential biological attacks, WHO issued a new publication in 2004 titled *Public health response to biological and chemical weapons: WHO guidance*. However, to include the deliberate release of infectious diseases in the scope of the IHR (2005) is to potentially implicate WHO in highly sensitive political areas, including putting it in the position of having to determine whether a state party has violated the BWC. Some claim that entangling WHO in national and international security politics is detrimental to its core public health functions. WHO is slipping into a "dangerous position" where

WHO and global health governance 77

its "political neutrality" would be undermined (Pearson, 2005, p. 16). The United States and its allies strongly support WHO's role in the investigation of suspicious biological terrorism incidents, whereas some developing countries, including Pakistan and Iran, oppose the practice, partly because they fear being asked by WHO to hand in highly sensitive security information and partly because they believe that WHO is at risk of being politicised, which could lead to the collapse of the organisation's surveillance system (Check, 2005, p. 686).

Another conflict has to do with whether WHO should help enforce compliance with the BWC. The BWC, adopted in 1975, is the first multilateral disarmament treaty banning an entire category of weapons of mass destruction. Ratified by a total of 151 countries, it also forms an essential part of the international disarmament system and an international collective security framework anchored by the United Nations. Compliance with the BWC is of critical importance to prevent bioterrorism because terrorists are most likely to acquire biological weapons from within one of the member states. Fortunately, there is no evidence that terrorists have or will soon be able to independently develop such weapons. No country would risk its own security to furnish biological weapons to terrorists. Terrorists would sooner buy, steal or invade a national biological project than replicate the costly and time-consuming development process of biological weapons (Rosenberg, 2007, p. 7). Some contend the virus spores used in the anthrax attacks almost certainly originated from a defence laboratory in the United States (Rissanen, 2002, p. 710). A corollary to this conjecture is that the BWC will determine to a large extent its odds in successfully combating biological terrorism. If WHO is to play a role in the prevention of biological terrorism, should it play a role in compelling countries to comply with the BWC, which is closely associated with controlling biological terrorism?

Since 2002, eight review conferences of the BWC have been held. There have been debates concerning surveillance and inspection of the use of biological weapons and suspected outbreaks of infectious diseases on the conferences. WHO has been a participant in each review conference. If WHO were to verify and investigate "any outbreak of an infectious disease" as stipulated in the IHR (2005), it would enforce compliance with the BWC. Strengthening WHO's global disease surveillance capabilities will help improve the effectiveness of the BWC. If WHO performs the inspection function, it will help to monitor compliance with the BWC by member states. However, there is considerable disagreement among WHO member countries regarding the relationship between WHO and the BWC. The United States believes WHO should play an important role in facilitating compliance with the BWC, but Brazil and some other countries strongly oppose WHO's involvement. Their view is the same as what some scholars have argued elsewhere:

> If countries perceived WHO staff or consultants as intelligence agents with a dual responsibility to investigate treaty violations as well as health matters, they may consequently be unwilling to report outbreaks at their onset and reluctant to request the help of WHO or permit its entry.
>
> (Woodall, 2005, p. 651)

78 *WHO and global health governance*

There are also concerns that WHO's public health mission may lose momentum if it is obligated to investigate whether a state party has violated the BWC or a resolution of the UN Security Council (Pearson, 2005). At any rate, WHO has also tried to steer away from participating in surveillance activities going beyond its health mandate. In its programme of work for the biennium 2004–2005, WHO used the following statement to declare its attempt to distance itself from BWC:

> The disarmament and non-proliferation dimensions of the BWC are clearly outside the public health mandate of WHO. This explains why the primary emphasis of WHO's work on deliberately caused diseases is on the public health preparedness and response to the deliberate use of biological agents that affect health.
>
> (WHO, 2004)

In view of the member states' divergent views regarding the relationship between WHO's public health notification obligations and the BWC, WHO treats this issue with a fair degree of obscurity. The new IHR's delineation of WHO's degree of involvement in bioterrorism investigation is murky. They do not address explicitly how information about suspicious deliberate releases of nuclear, biological or chemical events is to be shared, nor do they specify how WHO should play its role in compliance with the BWC. There are only two obscure provisions in the IHR that touch on the issue. One is in Article 7, which says, "If a State Party has evidence of an unexpected or unusual public health event in its territory, irrespective of origin or source, which may constitute a public health emergency of international concern, it shall provide WHO with all relevant public health information". The other is in Article 14: "WHO shall cooperate and coordinate its activities, as appropriate, with other competent intergovernmental organisations or international bodies in the implementation of these Regulations, including through the conclusion of agreements and other similar arrangements" (WHO, 2005). Fidler (2005) also pointed out such "obscurity" (p. 335) in his research on international health law. In fact, although the information WHO collected and analysed can be used to prevent bioterrorism and to assess whether a country has breached an arms control treaty or a Security Council resolution, the IHR (2005) does not entrust to WHO this function to assess such information, nor does it explicitly prohibit it from doing so. By allowing for a certain degree of flexibility for WHO to play a role, the IHR (2005) also sows the seeds of conflict among the member states on these issues.

Despite the failings and controversies analysed previously, the IHR (2005) are still an unprecedented global health governance mechanism that defines the relationship between international mechanisms and public health. It epitomises the trend to securitise global health issues and may well become the central mechanism for global health governance in the 21st century. The contribution they make to global health governance is of epoch-making significance. They have provided a framework for countries to build closer international health cooperation and better national health capabilities. They have injected fresh vitality into cross-border horizontal public health governance as well as vertical public health governance endeavours within a national border. Of course, IHR is no magic shot or a cure-all. For decades, maintaining member states' compliance with IHR has always been a challenge. Controversies surrounding WHO's aggressive action during the SARS epidemic may prevent the organisation from taking similar actions specified in the IHR (2005). In addition, the weakening global and local public health capacity also suggest that WHO's efforts to improve health conditions in developing countries have not been very effective over time. The implementation of the new IHR will not change the situation soon, especially because they do not require developed countries to provide emergency assistance to another country afflicted by a public health emergency. Without financial backing from developed countries, WHO's own assistance programs rest upon on shaky foundations. In the past, to avoid the implementation of health measures that could restrict trade or violate human rights, member states were compelled to comply with relevant international restrictions; violations were nevertheless common, even in these circumstances. Compliance with the IHR (2005), despite their strengths over the old version, will not necessarily fare better. There are still gaps in their coverage of urgent global health issues, such as worsening access to AIDS treatment in developing countries and the brain drain of health workers from developing to developed countries.

3.4 The limitations of WHO in global health governance

WHO plays an indispensable role in today's global health governance. Some scholars even thought that "WHO has moved closer to becoming a ministry of health for the world" (Cooper et al., 2007, p. 19). However, being an intergovernmental organisation, it is confronted with impasse arising from collective action and political factors from major countries. WHO governance efficiency, particularly with respect to its member states' compliance with the IHR (2005), is varied. Overall, the efficiency of WHO's global health governance efforts is contingent upon the following factors.

3.4.1 Politicisation of WHO

Politicisation refers to the practice of introducing political agendas to a non-political institution by its member states, thereby causing dysfunction when the introduced agenda exceeds the institution's scope of mandate. International organisations are designed to provide a communication channel for political units (member states) in both cooperation and disputes, thus subjecting organisations to political rivalries among party states. They are subject to the power struggle of nation-states (Verbeek, 1998, p. 17). WHO is no exception to the trend. It is not safe from politicisation despite its consistent efforts to maintain its functional neutrality through disassociating itself with international regimes involved with traditional political affairs, blocking political issues that lie beyond its mandate and focusing on cross-border medical and health technological cooperation to

80 WHO and global health governance

"attain the highest possible level of health by all people". At the World Health Assembly in 1983, Dr Halfdan Mahler, then director-general of WHO, voiced his strong opposition to engaging political issues at the World Health Assembly: "If we move to areas outside the Constitution's mandate, we will find ourselves in a minefield which we have been trying to avoid all along" (Williams, 1987, p. 63). In fact, politicisation in WHO has been evident throughout its history and is found all the way back to 1850 when the international health cooperation first started. Dr Henry Kissinger criticised the trend in the mid-1970s, noting the tendency for specialised agencies to be preoccupied with political considerations (Nerfin, 1976, p. 86). In the 1980s, some scholars also raised their concerns about the trend of politicisation in the specialised agencies of the United Nations (Cox, 1994, pp. 99–113). "Politicisation of WHO is nothing new" (Siddiqi, 1995, p. 30). It finds full expression in the following aspects.

First, WHO's institutional structure and arrangement are politicised. The main bodies of WHO are the World Health Assembly, the Executive Board and the Secretariat. The World Health Assembly is composed of delegates from member states. Each member can send no more than three delegates. Although delegates are chosen for their technical or managerial competence in the field of health, they also represent the interests of their respective governments. They therefore naturally assume a diplomatic role in the event of a conflict of interest for their country. Some members have taken advantage of the platform provided by WHO to promote their political position. During the Cold War, the World Health Assembly descended into a political arena between Israel with its support from the United States and Arab countries backed by the Soviet Union. Additionally, the Executive Board is equally prone to political influence. The Board is expected to represent all member states of the organisation as opposed to only countries from which the Board members are selected. Board members are referred to by the Constitution as "individuals", meaning they are selected due to their expertise in the field rather than their political affiliation. Therefore, they shall speak for their viewpoints independent from the positions of their respective governments. The principle behind this provision holds that health is inherently apolitical. Yet whether the Board can in practice transcend politics is altogether a different question. It might be able to when discussing technical issues but certainly not when international politics, the election of the director-general and a budget proposal are among agenda items. Therefore, "the independence of the Executive Board is a myth" (Beigbeder, 1997, p. 32).

Second, WHO's normative functions are politicised. As a specialised international agency, WHO indeed "is rarely involved in political issues such as international and regional security" (Slaughter, 2004, p. 22). But it is also true that it has shown an interest in security policies outside its traditional milieu in recent years, thus triggering normative changes. The stance WHO takes on nuclear weapons, for instance, is clearly the result of the political tug-of-war between nuclear and non-nuclear states. In 1993, based on Resolution WHA46.40, adopted in May 1993, the then director-general of WHO asked the International Court of Justice (ICJ) to provide an advisory opinion on whether a country's use of nuclear weapons would violate its obligations under international law, including the Constitution of the WHO, due to adverse health consequences that would result from such

WHO and global health governance 81

use.[12] The ICJ refused to rule on the matter in 1996, citing that there were many causes for human health to deteriorate; whether the reasons were legal or not "is no excuse for WHO to take measures to prevent these consequences." "The use of nuclear weapons always produces health and environmental consequences. But this does not mean that the discussion of its legality falls within the purview of WHO" (Shao, 2006, pp. 518–537). The ICJ's opinion suggests it does not support the politicised motion submitted by WHO, but the matter itself is a testament to WHO's politicised leanings. In addition, WHO's participation in each review conference of the BWC and its connection with traditional international security mechanisms, such as the UN Security Council, are further illustrations.

Such politicisation has introduced controversy among its member states, acted against member states to reach consensus and drained WHO's resources, altogether impeding WHO from taking its proper role in global health governance. The nature of WHO as an intergovernmental organisation makes it predestined for internal politicisation. As US scholar Christopher Osakwe emphasised,

> A study on the discussions on the specialised agencies of the United Nations will bring us to a more realistic conclusion: compared with the efforts to maintain international peace and security, issues in international education, cultural or scientific cooperation, and even international postal and telecommunications exchanges, are no less political, not to mention those more sensitive issues on international labour or on health legislation.
>
> (Ameri, 1982, p. 106)

Yet, though we consider the politicisation of WHO inevitable, the consequences of politicisation may not be all deleterious. If initiatives prompted by political motivations meet the needs of the time and can garner consensus from the international community, they may present an opportunity for member states to place more commitment in global health governance. WHO's engagement in the verification of the use of bioterrorism and of members' compliance with the BWC, for instance, will benefit global health governance.

3.4.2 WHO's lack of compulsory dispute settlement mechanism

Despite the achievement made by WHO in global health governance, the absence of an effective compulsory dispute settlement mechanism in the IHR (2005) leaves much to be desired. This absence is illustrated in two aspects: First, although the IHR (2005) have clearly improved on the prior versions by introducing an arbitration mechanism to resolve disputes between members, Article 56 covering this area still lacks an effective penalty clause. Second, on the verification of outbreaks, Article 9 stipulates that

> WHO may take into account reports from sources other than notifications or consultations and shall assess these reports according to established epidemiological principle and then communicate information on the event to the State Party in whose territory the event is allegedly occurring.

82 *WHO and global health governance*

The question remains whether WHO still has the power to send its staff to investigate an outbreak without the nation's explicit request if its government fails to perform its verification obligations. In particular, Article 9 is vague on procedures in the event a member state opposes any on-sight investigations by WHO. Such murkiness is bound to undercut WHO's surveillance efficiency. In a way, these two deficiencies will put a dent in the role the IHR plays in global health governance. In light of this problem, the United Nation secretary-general's High-level Panel on Threats, Challenges and Change issued a report in 2004, recommending that

> The Director-General of WHO may, at any time, report to the Security Council cases of suspicious or mass outbreak of infectious disease; If confronted by States that have the capacity to undertake their obligations but repeatedly fail to do so, the Security Council should be prepared to support WHO investigators or directly deploy experts that can report to the Security Council. If the International Health Regulations could not aid investigation and response coordination efforts, the Security Council may need to take additional measures to ensure compliance.
>
> (2004, p. 47)

However, such recommendations have never been implemented. Overall, three reasons lead to the absence of a compulsory resolution mechanism in the IHR (2005).

3.4.2.1 *WHO's functionalism orientation*

A powerful theory underpinning all specialised agencies of the United Nations, functionalism holds that human affairs are divided into political and non-political—in other words technical—categories. The former is a field full of controversy and conflicts; the latter is one in which international consensus is more easily achieved. Functionalists want to use non-political international organisations as platforms to help strengthen international cooperation and are committed to solving health, cultural, scientific, technological and economic issues with its end goal of maintaining world peace and reducing international conflict. As "functional" organisations, the activities of international organisations are directly related to "economic, social, technical, and humanitarian affairs and these activities have a direct bearing on values such as prosperity, welfare, social justice, but not with war prevention or eliminating national insecurity" (Claude, 1971, p. 378). In Mitrany's words, "functional arrangements have the patent virtue of technical self-determination" (1975, p. 68). This "technical self-determination" excludes political participation. In reality, though, it is extremely difficult to set up a compulsory dispute settlement mechanism in an international organisation without political commitment and participation from its member states. Today's global health issues are rarely purely technical; they often impinge on the international social development and global security. Restricting WHO to the field of medical technological cooperation will only result in a loss of function in its global health governance. In short, in the case of WHO, the technical self-determination is a false proposition. The politicisation of WHO's activities has shown that "realism trumps functionalism" (Hazelzet, 1998, p. 29).

3.4.2.2 WHO's sensitivity to sovereignty

As a neutral organisation focusing on technical health issues, WHO has always been careful to avoid sovereignty issues in its operation. During the SARS epidemic, it issued warnings urging international travellers not to visit Toronto or Beijing. This prompted heavy criticism from the Canadian government, who contended that it was an issue of national sovereignty and that WHO had no authority to publish such travel alerts. WHO soon retracted these warnings against travelling to Toronto. This is the only time WHO embroiled itself in a sovereignty controversy. Unlike the International Atomic Energy Agency, WHO does not have a verification mechanism. If a member government chooses not to report a domestic outbreak or not to allow WHO's intervention, WHO lacks the authority to sanction such a breach. A deeper reason for the new IHR's lack of binding force and verification mechanism is that WHO is overly cautious with respect to issues relating to sovereignty. For example, the IHR (2005) have an article that authorises WHO to carry out "field investigations". Many countries find the practice controversial; they consider this article an infringement on their sovereignty (Trucker, 2005, pp. 338–347). A spokesman for WHO once commented: "A member state has the final decision on whether to allow WHO staff to enter its territory for verification; If a government does not allow this to happen, there is no other way" (Alaman, 2003). Another reason behind WHO's particular sensitivity to sovereignty is that "health issues have to be balanced with many complex and difficult policies under the concept of sovereignty" (Jackson, 2006, p. 248).

3.4.2.3 WHO's neglect for international law

The status of international law has given it unique function in contemporary international society.

> The place of international law in our present international society gives it a distinctive stamp. Because the central rules of this society are considered to have the status of law, and not merely of morality, the sense of their binding force is an especially strong one.
>
> (Bull, 2012, p. 137)

However, in the field of global public health, WHO has not fully tapped into the functions of international law. International health jurists L'hirondel and Yach (1998) argue that, among the responsibilities of WHO, global health issues—such as international control of infectious diseases, tobacco use, abuse of antibiotics, international trade of blood and human organs, setting biological and chemical product standards and allogeneic organ transplants—all require the intervention

84 *WHO and global health governance*

of international law (p. 79). "Global health should be a major area for attention in international law, but the reality is quite the opposite" (Gostin, 2007, p. 993). In global health governance, member states are reluctant to develop international legal mechanisms to create obligations and incentives that are binding to them. Such reluctance is particularly apparent in WHO's case. As a core international regime for global health governance, WHO has regarded international law as a no-go area since its founding in 1948. Compared with other specialised agencies of the UN, such as WTO and the International Atomic Energy Agency, WHO appears far less adept at using international legal mechanisms or treaties to govern global public health. Although WHO's Constitution has given the organisation legislative power and the World Health Assembly the authority to adopt conventions or agreements within its competence, the conventions or agreements adopted still have to reach a two-thirds majority in the World Health Assembly and is subject to being approved by the constitutional processes of each member before it is effective.[13] In short, WHO has never fully exercised the extensive normative powers granted by its Constitution. As Tomasevski (1995), an expert on international law, noted, "WHO has made so few international laws that people are led to believe health protection is not affected by international law" (p. 859). Such neglect has reduced the IHR (2005) to a toothless sleeping treaty. A majority of international law scholars also agree that the history of global health governance since 1948 onwards demonstrates international health legal mechanisms have been systematically marginalised.[14]

There are many reasons that lead WHO to adopt a "non-legal approach" to global health governance. One has to do with the personnel make-up of the organisation consisting primarily of public health professionals rather than experts in international law, thereby making the organisation heavily functionalist. WHO evades the "higher politics" of international law because it considers itself essentially a science and technology institution. Wilson Jameson (1948), president of the first World Health Assembly, once observed: "Let's face the facts and refrain from a discussion of legal technicalities into which we, as an assembly of public health experts, are perhaps hardly competent to enter" (p. 77). As Fidler and Gostin (2008) aptly described,

> The common argument used to explain WHO's antipathy toward international law is that WHO is dominated almost exclusively by people trained in public health and medicines, introducing an ethos prone to reduce global health problems as medical-technical issues. The medical-technical approach does not need international law because the approach mandates application of the medical or technical resource or answer directly at the national or local level.
>
> (p. 1099)

Similarly, Taylor (1992) also believes that

> The WHO's reluctance to use laws and legal mechanism to advance its health strategy is largely due to the organisation's own internal dynamics and

WHO and global health governance 85

political activities. In particular, this reluctance is largely due to organisational culture established by the conservative medical community that dominates this mechanism.

(p. 303)

3.4.3 Weaknesses of the IHR (2005)

The IHR (2005) is the first international treaty adopted by WHO within the framework of international law. The way it is designed will, to a large extent, determine the efficiency of WHO in global health governance. Although the IHR (2005) have vastly improved on their prior versions, for example, by expanding the scope of notifiable diseases and by increasing information channels to enhance its global health surveillance, problems remain concerning its strict adherence. Compliance with an international treaty depends on the one hand on the "compliance pull" of the treaty and on the other on the compliance capacity of its member states. Unfortunately, the IHR (2005) did not take institutional measures to amend these flaws. Therefore, "it is a frustrating task to translate IHR into a global health surveillance regime" (Baker & Fidler, 2006, p. 1064).

3.4.3.1 Insufficient "compliance pull" of the IHR (2005)

Theoretically speaking, international cooperation with a goal to provide global public goods involves, on the one hand, compulsory intervention by an international regime to regulate and restrain free actions of the member states and, on the other hand, continuous design and innovation of such regimes to provide selective incentives to induce member states to take actions that safeguard, or at least do not harm, the public interest. Yaqing Qin (1999) argued that as a process determinant, the influence of an international regime derives from its authority and relevance, its reward and punishment mechanisms and its service. An international regime is a set of rules widely acknowledged or agreed upon by state members of the international community. Rational members will use the regime to achieve its own self-interest. The regime in turn rewards members that play by the rules and punishes those that do otherwise. Members, therefore, must learn to define or redefine their national interests in alignment with the regime (pp. 279–280). In other words, the "compliance pull" of an international regime depends on whether it has an in-built punishment and reward function. Regrettably, the IHR (2005) does not have these two functions, so member states are insufficiently incentivised to comply. Member states who choose to follow the IHR (2005) in reporting outbreaks might suffer heavy losses brought by excessive reactions from other countries. For example, a plague broke out in India in 1994. The outbreak triggered measures that went far beyond acceptable levels, including food import bans, flight cancellations and travel warnings. Some countries even started to repatriate Indian workers even as many of them had left India years before the outbreak. WHO was powerless to respond to these reactions. There are also member states who may not notify the organisation of the outbreaks due to fears of

86 *WHO and global health governance*

overreaction from other countries. These countries get away with such choices since the IHR (2005) have no means of imposing penalties, nor do they stipulate rewards for those who comply with relevant clauses.

As a result, members are poorly incentivised to comply with the regulations. WHO must design adequate incentive structures to ensure better compliance. It is essential to turn the negative rewards, including trade, travel and economic restrictions, into positive rewards exemplified by human, financial and technical support to help countries who lack public health capabilities cope with an outbreak. These incentives, once in place, will much increase the "compliance pull" of the IHR (2005). In addition, during an outbreak, WHO must monitor the ground closely to make sure trade embargos and travel restrictions enforced by member countries shall not exceed the limits set by the organisation. It is regrettable that WHO has been dragging its feet in taking up such practice or proactive strategies. Its challenge on the European Union's ban on fresh fish imports from cholera-stricken East African countries is a rare exception to its general action in this regard.[15]

3.4.3.2 Failure of the IHR (2005) to address the incapability of developing countries to comply

As noted by Lawrence Gostin, "Capacity building must be at the heart of effective global health governance" (Gostin, 2008, p. 384). However, the IHR (2005) does not address the incapacity of developing countries to comply. As the most important norm in global health governance, its compliance is in the interest of all countries. Some countries, especially developing countries, fail to comply with the IHR not due to intent but rather due to their incapability—or a lack of capability. Many developed countries are in areas at low risk for public health emergencies (e.g. bird flu). It is in these countries' interest if high-risk member states comply with the regulations, so an early warning can enable them to take appropriate measures to protect their own citizens. For the developing countries unable to control disease outbreaks, early detection and notification of public health emergencies may in fact be thoroughly counterproductive. Early notifications may lead to overreaction by other countries and in turn incur significant economic losses. In addition, to ask resource-strapped developing countries to invest in the infectious disease surveillance infrastructure may divert funds away from investing in more pressing public health issues, such as the treatment and control of tuberculosis, malaria and HIV/AIDS. As a result, these countries often find it difficult to comply with the regulations due to their limited ability to manage public health crises, giving rise to the observation that "the countries least likely to comply are those that have the least ability to comply" (Dry, 2008, p. 17). Failure to comply on the part of developing countries due to their insufficient public health capacity will make it less likely to effectively respond to global health crises. Furthermore, the IHR (2005) require all member states to assess their core competence two years after the document goes into effect to better detect and respond to public health emergencies, and it additionally requires member states to achieve the core

WHO and global health governance 87

competencies within the ensuing three years. For many underdeveloped countries, this expectation is unrealistic. At the same time, the IHR (2005) do not specify the obligations WHO and developed countries ought to take in assisting developing countries to build their public health capacity, which will ultimately affect the effectiveness of WHO's global health governance efforts.

3.5 World Health Organization reforms

An important specialised agency of the United Nations, WHO has also faced pressure to reform due to allegations of its poor governance. Since the 1990s, the agency increasingly came under widespread criticism from many sides for its failure to assume its proper role as the leader in global health governance.[16] WHO "is suffering a crisis of trust both internally and internationally" (Godlee, 1994a, p. 1427). As a matter of fact, calls for reform were heard as early as 1993 (WHO, 1993). In 1998, Gro Harlem Brundtland, then WHO director-general, promised to usher in major changes to the organisation to revitalise its role in global health affairs. "Dr. Brundtland's (reform) is the first serious attempt to rethink a complex agency within the UN-system and make it work in a world vastly different from 1948, the year when the UN was founded" (Robbins, 1999, p. 32). She indicated her resolve by saying, "We cannot point to the *Constitution of WHO* and say we have the power to be a governing body; We must earn leadership" (WHO, 1998b, p. 4). By launching the Roll Back Malaria initiative and subsequently leading negotiations on the conclusion of the Framework Convention on Tobacco Control, WHO is brought back to the centre stage of international political economy. But Brundtland's in-house structural reform did not achieve much. As Gavin Yamey (2002a) observed, "Dr. Brundtland is far more successful in advancing WHO's international status than it is in reforming it internally" (p. 1173). Margaret Chan, who took over the agency since 2007, wanted to carry through the reform. On May 5, 2011, she released *WTO Reforms for a Healthy Future*, a report receiving wide support from the World Health Assembly. At the special meeting of the Executive Board on November 1, 2011, Chan once again addressed the need for WHO reform (WHO Director-General Address Need for WHO Reform, n.d.). The World Health Assembly officially adopted her reform agenda on May 26, 2012, kicking off "the most extensive administrative, governance, and fiscal reform ever" (Chan, 2011a). However, considering the severe challenges posed by WTO's institutional difficulties, democratic deficit and financial distress, the prospects of the reforms remain dim.

3.5.1 Background for reform

It is believed that WHO was already at a moment of crisis in the early1990s (Smith, 1995). On top of its agenda was how WHO could effectively address emerging global health challenges through reforms. As Barry Bloom (2011) put it, "WHO needs a big change" (p. 143). There are many reasons behind this need.

88 WHO and global health governance

3.5.1.1 WHO's weakening capacity to lead and coordinate

WHO has been increasingly marginalised in global health governance in recent years, coinciding with a surge in the number and influence of other actors in the field (see Table 3.2). First, international organisations such as WTO and the World Bank have boosted their presence in global health governance. "The World Trade Organization is becoming the most important international regime in global health governance" (Williams, 2005, p. 73). The World Bank has also increased its investment in global health and become the largest funder of health governance activities in low-income countries. It has listed infectious disease control as one of the five global public goods it focuses on (World Bank Development Committee, n.d., p. 6). Some global health experts even believe that the World Bank has, in lieu of WHO, assumed the de facto leadership role in global health governance (Godlee, 1994b). Second, many more global public private partnerships and private foundations are now devoted to this cause. Notable examples include Stop TB Partnership; Global Fund to Fight AIDS, Tuberculosis and Malaria and the Bill & Melinda Gates Foundation. While these non-state actors have helped to fill the governance vacuum left by WHO, they have also brought two types of risks for global health governance to bear: One is that such partnerships often focus much more on specific disease projects than on the project for capacity building that many developing countries urgently need in their basic health systems; the other is that, with so many non-communicating actors in the scene, global health governance has become more "fragmented" than ever. The United States, for instance, through the President's Emergency Plan for AIDS Relief (PEPFAR) and the Global Health Initiative (GHI) initiatives, has risen to be the largest state actor in global health governance. In 2009, it spent US$10.2 billion on global health, far higher than WHO's total budget of the year (US$3.5 billion). In this light, WHO has simply been dwarfed by the stupendous investment of member states. To restore its diminishing influence, Brundtland tasked WHO's Commission on Macroeconomics and Health to release *Macroeconomics and Health: Investing in Health for Economic Development* (Commission on Macroeconomics and Health, 2001), a report that incorporated health issues into the global development agenda and sought to improve the leadership and coordination role of the WHO by

Table 3.2 Actors in Global Health Governance

Category	Examples
State Actors	OECD countries (e.g. The President's Emergency Plan for AIDS Relief and Global Health Initiative in the United States), emerging powers (e.g. China's health assistance to Africa)
Multilateral Lenders	World Bank, WTO, UN Development Program
NGOs	International NGOs (e.g. Oxfam, International Red Cross), NGOs in donor countries
Private Charities	Bloomberg Family Foundation, Bill & Melinda Gates Foundation, Rockefeller Foundation
Global Funds and Alliances	Global Fund to Fight AIDS, Tuberculosis and Malaria; Global Alliance for Vaccines and Immunization; Roll Back Malaria

leading the global health development. Brundtland also initiated negotiations on the Framework Convention on Tobacco Control. By engaging foreign affairs, finance and health ministers and policymakers of various countries in the negotiations, the organisation's image as a leader in global health governance had improved, but its waning capacity in organisation and leadership was not reversed.

3.5.1.2 WHO's entrenched financial crisis

As globalisation deepens, global health agenda has garnered increasing international attention, attracting many actors to the cause. Investment in the global health sector grew exponentially from US$5.7 billion in 1990 to US$26.7 billion in 2010 (Butler, 2011). This bourgeoning trend stands in stark contrast with the financial situation of WHO, which, despite being a leader by default in global health governance, was woefully under-resourced and sometimes mired in budget crises. The budget proposed for its 2012–2013 fiscal year was US$4.8 billion, of which US$3.96 billion was approved (ibid.), meaning almost US$90 million would be added to its deficit in the next two years. One reason for this trend is that many donor countries have simply cut their contributions amidst the current global economic crisis. Compounding this difficulty, another reason is that WHO settles its expenditure in Swiss francs, but its income is in US dollars. The weakening US dollar against the Swiss franc has resulted in a decline in the purchasing power of the agency. With no cut in its global operations and programs, a financial crisis has become all but inevitable. As a matter of fact, the Helms-Biden Reauthorization Act (i.e. the United Nations Reform Act), which was passed in the United States in 1999, foreshadowed WHO's financial plight. The Act put in place several conditions for the reform of the UN system, one of which is a ceiling imposed on member contributions. Ever since this "zero-growth policy" went into effect, membership dues have not been raised a single cent. After Brundtland came to office, she once proposed to raise member contributions to ease the budget pressure, but she ran into strong resistance from big donor countries. United States, Japan and Germany, for example, argued that no UN organisation should violate the zero-growth policy. If countries contributed more than their due to WHO, it would set a precedent for other UN agencies as well. As a result, Brundtland's push for more funding proved futile.

3.5.1.3 WHO's excessive reliance on extra-budgetary funding

Centralisation and independence are important for the efficiency of international organisations (Abbott & Snidal, 1998). WHO is no exception to this rule. In the absence of a centralised structure, WHO has tried to strengthen its role to better help enhance global health governance by maintaining its independence. Unfortunately, and yet irrefutably, "such independence has also been threatened" (Hoffman, 2010, p. 514). The organisation is financed through two main sources. First, member states pledge a set amount based on their wealth and population. The second is through voluntary contributions, which come mainly from developed countries, multinational pharmaceutical companies and private foundations, often with pre-specified conditions. With member states' contributions vis-à-vis voluntary contributions in grave disproportion, WHO's organisational independence in decision-making is in doubt. Hamstrung by the zero-growth policy on member contributions, WHO has become more reliant on voluntary contributions (see Figure 3.1), thus compromising its independence. During the swine flu epidemic in 2010, WHO was accused of being too closely tied to multinational pharmaceutical manufacturers in exaggerating the effects of the H1N1 virus (Stein, 2010; Cohen & Carter, 2010). This might be taken as a sign that the agency's decision-making process has been unduly influenced by private interests. In fact, under Brundtland's watch, WHO had already sought to redress the problem through

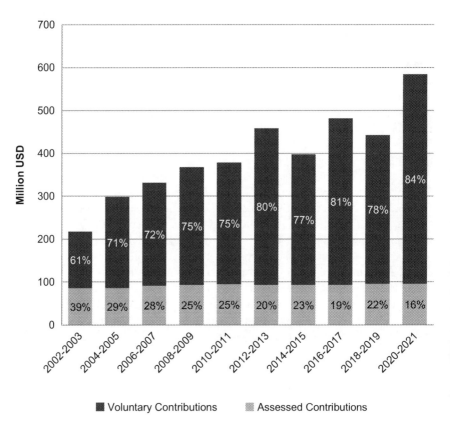

Figure 3.1 Proportion of Assessed Contributions and Voluntary Contributions in the WHO Budget

Sources: Data about WHO's Assessed Contributions,

Retrieved from www.who.int/about/finances-accountability/funding/assessed-contributions/en/

Data about WHO's Voluntary Contributions,
Retrieved from www.who.int/about/finances-accountability/funding/voluntary-contributions/en/

reforms. The first measure Brundtland took in office was to introduce a fiscal disclosure policy, which asked all senior WHO officials to declare the economic interests, patents and positions they hold in the private sector (Dove, 1998). But the reform accomplished little. Unable to raise membership dues, Brundtland then turned to voluntary contributions for more funding. In the first annual (2000–2001) budget of her first term, voluntary contributions had increased by 19% over the previous year (Andresen, 2002, p. 35). As a result, WHO has allowed itself to grow more reliant on pre-specified voluntary contributions. This not only makes funding less sustainable and predictable but also seriously jeopardises its independence and impartiality in decision-making.

3.5.1.4 WHO's inherent structural defect

WHO adopts a decentralised "Byzantine" structure. Its six regional offices are highly autonomous and independent from each other within the UN system. WHO has no personnel rights at the regional level. Employees of regional offices are individually elected. Although representatives to each member state represent the WHO Secretariat at the state level, they are appointed by and accountable to only to their respective regional directors-general. This has resulted in poor communication between regional offices and the WHO headquarters. In addition, the headquarters has no control in the decisions and budget of the regional offices. Each regional office thus monopolises their own health governance agenda, undermining WHO's efforts at global health coordination. As some WHO experts observed, "there is not one WHO, but seven" (Butler, 2011, p. 430). Brundtland tried to overcome this by improving communication among headquarters departments as well as between headquarters offices and regional offices. She first removed the position of assistant director-general at the headquarters and then reduced, merged and transformed the previous 50 programmes into 35 departments grouped into eight clusters, each with a technical budget expert appointed as its executive director. The reform resulted in a more balanced internal governance structure and helped restore the professional and technical authority of WHO. Second, Brundtland started a cabinet system into the headquarters' decision-making procedure. She held regular weekly consultations with her cabinet ministers to discuss and make decisions on major WHO issues. This in some ways has changed the indecisive image of WHO. By developing a more holistic approach to decision-making, Brundtland reduced the degree of compartmentalisation of WHO under which "the right hand never knows what the left hand is doing" (Godlee, 1994a, p. 1426). Finally, to increase WHO's control over the regional offices, Brundtland asked the regional offices to help her find vacant regional or country positions that will be filled by professionals previously working in headquarters in Geneva. This was the first time the headquarters had asked to be involved with regional personnel decisions. Unfortunately, these efforts received only lukewarm responses from regional offices. Brundtland's reform to make WHO a better coordinated organisation did not gather much traction in the end.

92 *WHO and global health governance*

3.5.2 *WHO's reform agenda*

On December 15, 2010, Dr Margaret Chan released a report titled *The future of financing for WHO*, in which she argued, "for WHO to play a more effective role in global health leadership, fundamental changes are needed in the way the organisation works" (WHO, 2010, p. 1). In another report, *WTO Reforms for a Healthy Future*, released in May 2011, Chan (2011a) identified the goals and expected outcomes of the reform (WHO, 2011). In summary, the reform proposals fall into three areas:

3.5.2.1 *Stronger leadership and coordination capacity*

First, there is a strong need to build WHO's internal governance capacity. The lack of policy coordination between the headquarter, regional and country levels leads to overlapping responsibilities and wasted resources, making it difficult for WHO to effectively implement collective global health actions. It is of essential importance to unify functions and units across the three levels of the agency to have a better coordinated task force. As Chan (2011b) argued, "WHO must become a more integrated and better networked organisation. . . . Through reforms, the work of the headquarters and the activities of the six regional offices will be coordinated to increase efficiency and improve performance". But this is the most difficult goal to achieve because it targets squarely at the inherent structural weakness of the organisation. "Unless deep-seated structural problems are solved, reforms will only scratch the surface" (Butler, 2011, p. 431). WHO must clarify the division of functions on the three levels and exercise more oversight and control over regional and country offices to ensure coherence of its policies.

Second, WHO should make the organisation more inclusive and improve its interaction mechanisms with other global health governance actors. WHO is no longer the only actor in global health governance. In *The future of financing for WHO*, Chan (2010) pointed out that

> Global health policy is shaped by a wide range of stakeholders from the public, private, and voluntary sectors. It has become increasingly important that these voices are also heard in WHO. Better inclusivity leads to more public support, in turn contributing to a stronger leadership role for WHO.

WHO must work with other stakeholders in global health governance to address global health issues. This requires WHO to become more inclusive and allow more voice and representation from stakeholders in designing global health governance norms and standards. As the legislative body of WHO, the World Health Assembly can involve more actors in the discussion of global health issues. These changes will help make the assembly more democratic and science-driven, thereby reducing the "democratic deficit" of the process.

3.5.2.2 *More predictable, sustainable financing*

Fiscal pressure has become a bottleneck restricting WHO's functioning. Budget reforms are therefore a focal point to strengthening WHO's efficiency. As some experts have observed, "it is never too much to emphasise the link between the WHO budget and its reform agenda" (Daulaire, 2011). While it is almost impossible to increase member contributions, WHO can adopt the following two approaches to address its financial constraints in addition to simplifying and making more efficient its institutional structure.

First, WHO needs to identify strategic priorities in global health governance. "In a landscape crowded with global health initiatives and partnerships, leadership must be achieved through strategic and selective engagement; WHO is unable to direct and coordinate all activities and policies in the many sectors affecting public health today" (WHO, 2010, p. 6). Therefore, WHO needs to avoid over-extending itself; instead, it should set strategic priorities, maximise its resource efficiency, and be more selective in choosing priority programs. As opposed to undermining its prominence in global health governance, this strategic de-scaling will only strengthen the organisation's traditional comparative advantage rather than undermine the prominent role it plays in global health governance. But setting strategic priorities among so many global health issues is not easy. As Chan conceded, "improving the way this Organization sets its priorities is the hardest part of the reform process, and likely the most critical" (2012).

Secondly, WHO needs to reform its financing mechanism. According to Chan, "flexible financing remains an important part of the reform, which will enable WHO to adapt more quickly to changing challenges" (WHO, 2011, p. 3). In recent years, investment in global health by state actors, non-state actors, and various public-private partnerships has grown explosively. In comparison, funding for WHO remains dimly insufficient. Therefore, "WHO will work to attract new donors and widen its resource base, for example, drawing on Member States with emerging economies, foundations and the private and commercial sector, without compromising independence or adding to organisational fragmentation" (Chan, 2010). If funding of other actors is incorporated into WHO's Global Health Governance Program, the organisation's funding resources will be greatly boosted. This is conditioned on WHO's willingness to join hands with private foundations, NGOs, existing partnerships and the private sector in general. Moreover, such cooperation must be predicated on the condition that WHO shall not be unduly influenced by vested interests in decision-making.

3.5.2.3 More flexibility in coping with global health crises

An important purpose of the reforms is to ensure that WHO can keep pace with the changing times and effectively respond to emerging global health challenges. Chan claimed that WHO "is aiming to build an excellent, flexible, and efficient organisation" (WHO, 2011, p. 3). Currently, it appears that WHO is too slow and rigid in its response to public health emergencies. For example, in October 2010, a massive cholera struck Haiti and resulted in over a thousand deaths. Three days after the epidemic was declared, a riot broke out in the hardest-hit area; local people claimed the disease was spread by UN peacekeepers from Nepal. Despite extensive media coverage, WHO had remained consistently silent on the issue (McNeil, 2010). The lack of action in the crisis signals the organisation's

94 *WHO and global health governance*

lack of flexibility in handling health emergencies. What's more, WHO's sluggish response to the Ebola crisis in West Africa in 2014 attracted even stronger criticism from many quarters. The problems exposed during the crisis underscore the urgency of the reform. According to a response evaluation report written by an independent expert team commissioned by WHO, "WHO does not have the capacity or culture to respond to public health emergencies". WHO must improve its emergency capacity through immediate reforms. As Chan indicated, "At WHO, we learned how rigid and unresponsive our management systems have become. This has to change. This Organization needs to sail, streamlined, swift on course, and quick to shift as new threats to health emerge" (2011b). To cope with the growing public health crisis, WHO needs to improve its crisis management mechanisms. Increasing the flexibility in crisis response should feature prominently on its reform agenda.

3.5.3 *Hurdles to WHO reforms*

International organisations seek reforms when they become dysfunctional. Theories on international organisations usually attribute causes of dysfunction to the organisation's own governance structure, external pressure, as well as its material (financial) constraints (Barnett & Finnemore, 1999, p. 716). Similarly, in WHO's case, the reasons have to do with its own internal governance structure, external political interference and budget crisis. As an effort to incorporate reform, WHO developed a High-Level Implementation and Monitoring Framework in May 2012, which specified the reform goals, priority activities and a roadmap for the next one to three years (WHO, 2012). However, there are still many hurdles to cross as WHO seeks to overcome its dysfunction.

First, WHO is stuck in an institutional dilemma. Its Constitution stipulates that

> The regional committee shall be composed by representatives of the Member States and Associate Members in the region concerned. Regional committees shall adopt their own rules of procedure; the functions of the regional committee shall be to formulate policies governing matters of an exclusively regional character".[17]

This makes WHO's governance structure highly decentralised. Each of the six regional offices has its own separate personnel, administrative and financial arrangements. The leadership of the regional offices is elected by the member states of the region. This structure is a double-edged sword: If directors of the regional offices could serve the area in a transparent and accountable manner, such a decentralised arrangement would boost WHO's efficiency. In reality, regional offices are not held accountable to the people they represent but rather to the Ministries of Health in the region. There is hence a chance that regional offices may succumb to geopolitical pressures from regional powers, thereby making it hard for WHO to effectively coordinate the communication between headquarters and regional offices. In the end, WHO suffers from overlapping functions and lack of clarity in divisions of responsibility. To achieve better communication between the headquarters and the regional offices, to overcome the separation and disconnection of authority and to effectively improve the efficiency of its internal governance, WHO must transform its "decentralised" system, as stipulated in the Constitution, into a "centralised" system with greater control over various regional offices. However, overcoming this institutional hurdle is not easy. In fact, Brundtland's frustration in her structural reform was also an important reason for her decision not to run for a second term (Yamey, 2002b).

Second, WHO suffers from a democratic deficit. What WHO provides is a global public good. According to the Triangle of Publicness theory proposed by the UN Development Programme experts Inge Kaul et al., the effective provision of global public goods depends on achieving publicness in both decision-making and the distribution of benefits (1999). Barnett and Finnemore (2004) also believed the authority of international organisations stems from their unbiased stance, the pursuit and protection of the interests of a wide range of international communities and their own expertise. These views all demonstrate that achieving democratic decision-making and income balance is essential to restoring an international organisation's authority and crucial to its efficiency in providing global public goods. Whether WHO can revive its authority through reforms and whether it can provide global public goods for health more effectively depend, in large measure, on its ability to achieve the democracy of decision-making and the publicity of benefit distribution. However, given the entrenched democratic deficit in WHO, achieving such goals can be difficult. Two factors contribute to this deficit.

One is that power politics has always troubled WHO. "Any convincing view of global governance cannot ignore the power inequalities between nations" (Held, 2002, p. 12). International regimes represent the interests and policies of big powers (Krasner, 1999). By the same token, being a functional international organisation, WHO is unable to shake off the power politics that often shackle international relations and therefore may denigrate into an arena of power struggle among big nations, resulting in the democratic deficit in its decision-making. Some experts even hold that, in the global health governance process, political interest of big powers exerts more influence on WHO than do its internal reforms (Huang, 2012). Decisions made in WHO, from policy decisions taken by its governing body to action resolutions adopted by its regional offices, are virtually all the result of compromise between the member states. Such compromises are emblematic of a broader pattern in global power structure. As some scholars suggested, "the work of international mechanisms such as WHO depends very much on the distribution of power in the world" (Navarro, 2008, p. 152). For instance, the five permanent members of the UN Security Council are implicitly members of WHO's Executive Board. WHO is driven by member states, but these members may prioritise their own interests. The drive for self-interest from member states makes it difficult for WHO to focus on global health issues due to conflicting interests between individual member states and global welfare. As a result, big powers may often abuse platforms provided by international organisations to

96 WHO and global health governance

pursue their own interests in the name of global public welfare. For example, led by developed countries including the United States, WHO has prioritised global infectious disease surveillance over basic health capacity building in developing countries. If an infectious disease breaks out in a developing country, alarms trigged would help developed countries put up a "Machino Line of Defence" (Jin & Karackattu, 2011, p. 185) well in advance. In short, democratic deficit due to power politics is the most entrenched obstacle in the way of WHO's reforms.

The second has to do with money politics. WHO must have an inclusive global health governance structure for many global health governance actors to work effectively. If WHO could involve non-state actors in its governance process, it would create more representation and motivation (Tang, 2011). But this integration is tricky. As WHO broadened its funding base from voluntary contributions and from "public private partnerships" with the private sector, it implicitly granted legitimacy to non-state actors to demand their share in decision-making, thus placing an influence on WHO's impartiality, fairness and accountability. In response, Chan proposed to set up a World Health Forum, an informal scheme made up of government representatives, civil society organisations, the private sector, and other relevant stakeholders to increase WHO's inclusiveness (WHO, 2011, pp. 14–15). However, the proposal was rejected by many countries, who believed this would change WHO's intergovernmental nature and lead to an even larger democratic deficit. After all, they argue, the World Health Assembly still operates on the basis of one-country/one-vote. Besides, some NGOs are also concerned that if such a forum were to be set up, it would allow the private sector, especially multinational pharmaceutical companies, to tamper with WHO's decisions, thereby undermining WHO's legitimacy as a neutral and democratic institution (NGOs Call on Member States to Stop the World Health Forum, 2011).

Finally, financial distress. This current round of reform was triggered by the WHO fiscal crisis, which was long in the making. In the early days of WHO, developed and developing countries had already diverged over the amount of "assessed contributions" (Chisholm, 2008). The current world economic recession has only exacerbated WHO's fiscal plight. A research report released by the Institute for Health Metrics and Evaluation of the University of Washington shows that, since the outbreak of the European debt crisis, Western developed countries have already cut or slowed down funding to WHO to rein in their own deficit (Institute for Health Metrics and Evaluation, 2011). In her report to the Executive Board in May 2011, Chan said that to increase predictability and flexibility of WHO's financing to effectively respond to emerging health challenges, "Member states shall consider increasing 'Assessed Contributions' and re-examine its national policy on limiting the growth of contributions" (WHO, 2011, p. 13). However, most member states were unenthusiastic about such a proposal. Furthermore, low- and middle-income countries had no intention to pressure developed countries to increase their "assessed contributions" either.

With the hope of raising more "assessed contributions" dashed, WHO's Geneva headquarters was forced to cut more than 300 of its staff in 2011.[18] But this does not fundamentally cure the pain. At the same time, WHO allowed itself to increasingly rely on voluntary contributions from the private sector or developed countries. In her report, Chan argued that WHO should expand the funding by bringing various foundations and private business sectors into its fold (WHO, 2010). But the real problem, however, is that there is always an irreconcilable conflict of interest between the independence of WHO and its reliance on the private sector. The tendency to rely on voluntary pre-specified contributions would further worsen the agency's transparency and accountability. Thailand is among countries who believe that WHO has become a donor-driven organisation rather than an organisation for public interest and that current discussions will not yield any substantive result (Faid & Gleicher, 2011, p. 8). Some scholars even contend that attracting more funds from for-profit or neoliberal ideology-driven actors might ultimately result in trading-off WHO's decision-making processes that prioritise the public interest, the "soul" (Richter, 2012, p. 141) of the organisation.

Summary

As the core international regime in global health governance, WHO has played a vital role in the provision of global public goods for health by formulating and implementing public health policies at the global level. The wide representation of its member states has strengthened its legitimacy. However, like other international mechanisms, the politicisation and unequitable distribution of benefits have hindered its global health governance function. For example, the revised IHR were originally not intended to improve public health security in developing countries, but rather to prevent the spread of disease from developing to developed countries. Developing countries with poor public health capabilities will find neither the strength nor motivation to comply with the new IHR. As public health and security become more reliant on each other in today's world, this will create a global "black hole in epidemic prevention". In addition, the absence of a dispute settlement mechanism in WHO has made full compliance with the IHR a distant reality. Only by strengthening the public health capacity and improving the compliance capacity of developing countries as well as strengthening the binding force of relevant norms can WHO overcome problems of collective action in its efforts to provide more global public goods for health and in turn truly serve as "the directing and coordinating authority on international health work".

WHO was once widely acclaimed for its leadership role in global health. However, with the rise of other actors in the scene, with its own internal governance problems, "WHO is becoming irrelevant" (Chow, 2010). Under Brundtland's stewardship, the agency carried out a series of reforms, though not particularly effective in the end. The current round of reforms Chan promoted will present another opportunity in that it will not only help WHO keep up with the times and adapt to the changing global health landscape, thereby "guiding the global health governance system forward" (Gostin & Mok, 2009, p. 10), but it will also reinvigorate its leadership position. However, given the mounting challenges posed by its institutional structure, democratic deficits and fiscal difficulties, the reform prospects are far from rosy. "The legitimacy of

98 *WHO and global health governance*

a governance system depends not only on its effectiveness, but also on how agents who are subject to its authority perceive its impartiality and legitimate social purpose" (Stevenson & Cooper, 2009, p. 1381). This rule also applies to WHO. Therefore, whether the organisation can re-establish its authority in the field of global health governance through reforms depends not only on whether it can improve governance efficiency but also on whether it can truly commit itself to improving the health and well-being of all human beings, especially to strengthening basic health capacity building in the least-developed countries. As Chinese Ambassador He Yafei (2011) said at the briefing on WHO's governance reform, the reform should be driven by the health needs of developing countries, especially those of the least developed countries, to shore up the weak links in the global health system. In short, the reform shall not only aim to promote governance efficiency but also tackle global health justice issues to achieve "the attainment by all peoples of the highest possible health".[19] At the 69th World Health Assembly held in May 2017, Dr Tedros Adhanom Ghebreyesus from Ethiopia was elected as the new director-general of WHO. He is the first African picked to lead the organisation since its establishment in 1948. After taking office, Ghebreyesus has made WHO reform one of his five main priorities.[20] It remains to be seen whether he can coordinate different member states and other stakeholders, be brave enough to tackle the structural and institutional challenges of WHO and eventually bring the organisation back to the centre of authority to promote global health governance.

Notes

1 Goodman believes that "quarantine" derives from "quaranta" implemented in Venice in the year of 1403, a period that equals the length of time Jesus and Moses stayed in the desert in the Bible. See Goodman (1971). For details on the history of "quarantine", see Mafart and Perret (1998), Sehdev (2002).

2 For example, in Shakespeare's (2013) famous tragedy *Romeo and Juliet*, Father John was caught in an outbreak of plague on the way to Mantua and was isolated, so he could not give Father Lawrence's letter (which tells Romeo that his lover Juliet is not dead) to Romeo. Had Father John not been isolated, the tragic deaths of Romeo and Juliet would have been prevented.

3 At this meeting, Austria, Britain, France and the Kingdom of Sardinia claimed that isolation measures were invalid and opposed the isolation of ships; the other three Italian city-states, the Russia Empire, Spain, Greece and Italy support the isolation policy; Portugal did not want to undertake any obligations.

4 In view of the limited coverage of the disease and the outbreak of other epidemics, yellow fever was added to the 1912 International Sanitary Conference; typhus, relapsing fever and smallpox were included in 1926.

5 See Article 23 (6) of the Covenant of the League of Nations. Retrieved from www. camlawblog.com/articles/caribbean/league-of-nations-charter/.

6 According to Siddiqi (1995, p. 20), even Howard-Jones, an expert in this field, was baffled by OIHP's refusal to make any concessions. According to Howard-Jones (1978, p. 73), many countries are both members of the OIHP and the HOLN. It was unbelievable that the recommendations made by member states in Geneva were rejected by the same member states in Paris.

WHO and global health governance 99

7 Other regional offices include the Regional Office for Africa (AFRO), the Regional Office for South East Asia (SEARO), the Regional Office for Europe (EURO), the Regional Office for the Eastern Mediterranean (EMRO) and the Regional Office for the Western Pacific (WPRO).

8 The 1946 Charter of the International Labour Organization stipulates that the labour conventions that have been adopted by a two-thirds majority of the member states and signed by the President of the Congress or the director-general of the International Labour Organization, should be approved after the decision is notified to all member states. Similar conventions are also adopted by the FAO. See Li (1987).

9 The articles or annexes cited in this section all come from the revised articles or annexes of the IHR by WHO on May 23rd, 2005. For details, see *International Health Regulations (2005)*, Retrieved from www.who.int/ihr/publications/9789241580496/en/.

10 See Articles 21 and 26 of the International Covenant on Civil and Political Rights. Retrieved from www.ohchr.org/en/professionalinterest/pages/ccpr.aspx.

11 Ibid., Article 10 (1).

12 Article 76 of the Constitution of the World Health Organization stipulates that "Upon authorization by the General Assembly of the United Nations or upon authorization in accordance with any agreement between the Organization and the United Nations the Organization may request the International Court of Justice for an advisory opinion on any legal question arising within the competence of the Organization."

13 See Articles 2 and 19 of the Constitution of the World Health Organization.

14 For example, Taylor believes that "WHO's success in promoting the implementation of universal health services in member states is extremely limited, in part because WHO does not focus on the role of legislation in the "Health for All" Strategy. See Taylor (1992). Fidler believes that "WHO is facing a 'tsunami' of international law. WHO needs to change its attitude towards international law. Although WHO is accused of paying too little attention to international law, international relations before World War II were flooded with too much international health law", see Bezuhly et al. (1997), Fidler (1998), Plotkin (1996), Sturtevant et al. (2007) and Taylor (1997).

15 During the period when the European Union banned imports of fresh fish from three East African countries due to cholera outbreaks, WHO exercised its governance function by issuing a statement condemning the sanctions and claimed that such sanctions were not based on reliable principles of epidemiology. WHO's statement forced the European Union to lift this restriction and resolved the issue through WHO's Dispute Resolution Panel. See WHO. (1998, February). *Director-General Says Food Import Bans Are Inappropriate for Fighting Cholera*. WHO Press Release WHO/24. Retrieved from http://who.int/inf-pr-1998/en/pr98-24.html.

16 For more criticism on WHO, see Chow (2010), Gostin and Mok (2009), Horton (2002), Huang (2016), McColl (2008) and Sridhar (2009).

17 See Article 50 of the Constitution of the World Health Organization.

18 To restore some of the functions lost at the headquarters due to layoffs, WHO has established 43 positions in the World Health Organization Administration and Information Technology Center in Kuala Lumpur, Malaysia, a move designed to reduce WHO's long-term financial pressures.

19 See Article 1 of the Constitution of the World Health Organization.

20 The other four priorities include universal health coverage; health emergencies; the health of women, children and adolescents and the impact of climate and environmental changes on health. See www.who.int/dg/biography.

References

Abbott, K. W., & Snidal, D. (1998). Why States Act through Formal International Organizations. *Journal of Conflict Resolution*, 42(3), 9.

100 *WHO and global health governance*

Alaman, L. K. (2003, May 28). World Health Organization: Expected to Gain Broader Powers. *New York Times*. Retrieved from www.nytimes.com/2003/05/28/science/sciencespecial/28INFE.html

Ameri, H. (1982). *Politics and Process in the Specialized Agencies of the UN*. Hants: Gower House.

Andresen, S. (2002, August). *Leadership Change in the World Health Organization: Potential for Increased Effectiveness?* Retrieved from www.fni.no/doc&pdf/FNI-R0802.pdf

Baker, M. G., & Fidler, D. P. (2006). Global Health Surveillance under New International Health Regulations. *Emerging Infectious Diseases*, 12(7), 1064.

Barnett, M., & Finnemore, M. (1999). The Politics, Power, and Pathologies of International Organizations. *International Organization*, 53(4), 716.

Barnett, M., & Finnemore, M. (2004). *Rules for the World: International Organizations in Global Politics*. Ithaca, NY: Cornell University Press.

Beck, A. (1970). *A History of the British Medical Administration of East Africa, 1900–1950*. Cambridge, MA: Harvard University Press.

Beigbeder, Y. (1997). *L'Organisation Mondial de la Santé*. Paris: Presses Universitaires de France.

Bezuhly, M., Wojick, M. E., & Fidler, D. P. (1997). International Health Law. *The International Lawyer* (31), 645.

Bloom, B. (2011, May 12). WHO Needs Change. *Nature*, 473, 143.

Bull, H. (2012). *The Anarchical Society: A Study of Order in World Politics*. New York: Columbia University Press.

Butler, D. (2011, May 26). Revamp for WHO. *Nature*, 473(7348), 430–431.

Carvalho, S., & Zacher, M. (2001). The International Health Regulations in Historical Perspective. In A. T. Price-Smith (Ed.), *Plagues and Politics: Infectious Disease and International Policy*. Basingstoke, Hampshire: Palgrave Macmillan.

Chan, M. (2010, December 15). *The Future of Financing for WHO*. Retrieved from http://apps.who.int/gb/ebwha/pdf_files/EB128/B128_21-en.pdf

Chan, M. (2011a, May 16). *WHO Director-General Reminds Health Officials: Never Forget the People*. Retrieved from www.who.int/dg/speeches/2011/wha_20110516/en/index.html. Accessed September 11, 2012.

Chan, M. (2011b, November 1). *WHO Director-General Addresses Need for WHO Reform*. Opening Address at the Executive Board Special Session on WHO Reform. Geneva, Switzerland. Retrieved from www.who.int/dg/speeches/2011/who_reform_01_11/en/index.html

Chan, M. (2012). *Reform of Priority Setting at WHO*. Geneva, Switzerland. Retrieved from www.who.int/dg/speeches/2012/reform_priorities_20120227/en/index.html

Check, E. (2005). Global Health Agency Split over Potential Anti-Terrorism Duties. *Nature*, 434, 686.

Chisholm, B. (2008). *WHO and the Cold War*. Vancouver: University of British Columbia Press.

Chow, J. (2010, December 8). Is the WHO Becoming Irrelevant? *Foreign Policy*.

Claude Jr., I. L. (1971). *Swords Into Plowshares* (4th ed.). New York: Random House.

Cohen, D., & Carter, P. (2010, June 12). WHO and the Pandemic Flu Conspiracies. *British Medical Journal*, 340.

Commission on Macroeconomics and Health. (2001). *Macroeconomics and Health: Investing in Health for Economic Development*. Geneva: WHO.

Constitution of WHO. (1946). Retrieved from https://apps.who.int/gb/bd/pdf_files/BD_49th-en.pdf#page=7

WHO and global health governance 101

Cooper, A. F., Kirton, J., & Schrecker, T. (2007). *Governing Global Health: Challenge, Response, Innovation.* Hampshire: Ashgate Publishing Ltd.

Cox, R. W. (1994). The Crisis of World Order and the Problem of International Organization in the 1980s. *Cooperation and Conflict,* 29(2), 99–113.

Daulaire, N. (2011, May 17). *World Health Organization Reform Agenda Must Address Budget Issue While Not Reducing WHO's Impact.* Statement by U.S Representative on the Executive Board of the World Health Organization. Retrieved from http://geneva.usmission.gov/2011/05/18/who-reform/

Dorelle, P. (1969). Old Plagues in the Jet Age: International Aspects of Present and Future Control of Communicable Disease. *Chronicle of the World Health Organization* (23), 103–111.

Dove, A. (1998). Brundtland Takes Charge and Restructures the WHO. *Nature Medicine,* 4(9), 992.

Dry, S. (2008). *Epidemic for All? Governing Health in a Global Age.* STEPS Working Paper 9. Brighton: STEPS Centre, p. 17.

Faid, M., & Gleicher, D. (2011). World Health Assembly Discusses Reforms of the WHO. *Health Diplomacy Monitor,* 2(3), 8.

Fidler, D. P. (1998). The Future of the WHO: What Role for International Law. *Vanderbilt Journal of International Law* (31), 1079–1998.

Fidler, D. P. (1999). *International Law and Infectious Diseases.* Oxford: Clarendon Press, pp. 19–28.

Fidler, D. P. (2004). *SARS, Governance and the Globalization of Disease.* London: Palgrave Macmillan.

Fidler, D. P. (2005). From International Sanitary Conventions to Global Health Security: The New International Health Regulations. *Chinese Journal of International Law,* 4(2), 335–344.

Fidler, D. P., & Gostin, L. O. (2006). The New International Health Regulations: An Historic Development for International Law and Public Health. *Journal of Law, Medicine & Ethics,* 34(1), 90.

Fidler, D. P., & Gostin, L. O. (2008). *Biosecurity in the Global Age: Biological Weapons, Public Health, and the Rule of Law.* Redwood City, CA: Stanford University Press.

Foreman-Peck, J. (1983). *A History of the World Economy: International Economic Relations since 1850.* London: FT Prentice Hall.

Godlee, F. (1994a). WHO in Crisis. *British Medical Journal,* 309(6966), 1426–1427.

Godlee, F. (1994b). WHO in Retreat: Is It Losing Its Influence? *British Medical Journal,* 309(6967), 1494.

Goodman, N. M. (1971). *International Health Organizations and Their Work.* Edinburgh: Churchill Livingstone.

Gostin, L. O. (2007). A Proposal for a Framework Convention on Global Health. *Journal of International Economic Law,* 10(4), 4.

Gostin, L. O. (2008). Meeting Basic Survival Needs of the World's Least Healthy People: Towards a Framework Convention on Global Health. *The Georgetown Law Journal,* 96, 378.

Gostin, L. O., & Mok, E. (2009). Grand Challenges in Global Health Governance. *British Medical Bulletin* (90), 7–18.

Grein, T. W., Kamara, K. B., & Rodier, G. et al. (2000). Rumours of Diseases in the Global Village: Outbreak Verification. *Emerging Infectious Disease,* 6(2), 97–102.

Hammond, T. H. (1986). Agenda Control, Organization Structure and Bureaucratic Politics. *American Journal of Political Science,* 30(379), 379–420.

102 WHO and global health governance

Hazelzet, H. (1998). The Decision-Making Approach to International Organizations. In B. Reinalda & B. Verbeek (Eds.), *Autonomous Policy Making by International Organizations*. New York: Routledge.

He, Y. (2011, April 11). Ambassador of China in United Nations Office at Geneva He Yafei Attends the World Health Organization's Briefing on Its Governance Reforms. *China's Ministry of Foreign Affairs*. Retrieved from www.china-un.ch/chn/hyyfy/t816973.htm

Headrick, D. R. (1981). *The Tools of Empire: Technology and European Imperialism in the Nineteenth Century*. Oxford: Oxford University Press.

Headrick, D. R. (1988). *The Tentacles of Progress: Technology Transfer in the Age of Imperialism, 1850–1940*. Oxford: Oxford University Press.

Held, D., & McGrew, A. (2002). *Governing Globalization*. Cambridge: Polity Press.

Ho, A. (2006). WHO: A Health Watchdog without Legal Teeth, in reference of X. Gong (2006) Infectious Disease Control from the Perspective of International Law (Unpublished PhD dissertation). Wuhan University, Wuhan.

Hoffman, S. J. (2010). The Evolution, Etiology and Eventualities of the Global Health Security Regime. *Health Policy and Planning*, 25(6), 514.

Horton, R. (2002). WHO: The Causalities and Compromises of Renewal. *The Lancet*, 359(9317), 1605–1611.

Howard-Jones, N. (1975). *The Scientific Background of the International Sanitary Conferences, 1851–1938*. Geneva: WHO.

Howard-Jones, N. (1978). *International Public Health Between the Two World Wars: The Organizational Problems*. Geneva: WHO.

Huang, Y. (2012). *World Health Organization Reform*. New York: Council on Foreign Relations.

Huang, Y. (2016). *How to Reform the Ailing World Health Organization?* New York: Council on Foreign Relations.

Institute for Health Metrics and Evaluation. (2011). *Financing Global Health 2011: Continued Growth as MDG Deadline Approaches*. Seattle: University of Washington.

Jackson, J. H. (2006). *Sovereignty, the WTO, and Changing Fundamentals of International Law*. Cambridge: Cambridge University Press.

Jameson, W. (n.d.). *Official Records of the World Health Organization*, No. 13, First World Health Assembly, Geneva, 24 June to 24 July 1948. Geneva: WHO, p. 77. Retrieved from http://whqlibdoc.who.int/hist/official_records/13e.pdf

Jin, J., & Karackattu, J. T. (2011). Infectious Diseases and Securitization: WHO's Dilemma. *Biosecurity and Bioterrorism: Biodefense Strategy, Practice and Science*, 9(2), 185.

Kaul, I., Grunberg, I., & Stern, M. A. (1999). *Global Public Goods: International Cooperation in the 21st Century*. Oxford: Oxford University Press.

Krasner, S. (1999). *Sovereignty: Organized Hypocrisy*. Princeton: Princeton University Press.

Lee, K. (1998). *Historical Dictionary of the World Health Organization*. Lanham, MD and London: The Scarecrow Press, Inc.

L'hirondel, A., & Yach, D. (1998). Develop and Strengthen Public Health Law. *World Health Statistics Quarterly*, 51(1), 79.

Li, H. (1987). *Introduction to the Law of Treaties*. Beijing: Law Press·China.

Mafart, B., & Perret, J. L. (1998). History of the Concept of Quarantine. *Med Trop* (58), 14–20.

McColl, K. (2008). Europe Told to Deliver More Aid for Health. *The Lancet*, 371(9630), 2072–2073.

McNeil Jr., D. G. (2010, November 21). Cholera's Second Fever: An Urge to Blame. *New York Times*.

Mitrany, D. (1975). The Prospect of Integration: Federal or Functional? In A. J. R Groom & Taylor (Eds.), *Functionalism*. London: University of London Press.

Navarro, V. (2008). Neoliberalism and Its Consequences: The World Health Situation since Alma Ata. *Global Social Policy* (8), 152.

Nerfin, M. (1976). Is a Democratic United Nations Possible? *Development Dialogue*, 2, 86.

NGOs Call on Member States to Stop the World Health Forum. (2011, May 17). Retrieved from www.evb.ch/en/p25019347.html

Pearson, G. S. (2005, May). *The UN Secretary-General's High-Level Panel: Biological Weapons Related Issues*. Strengthening the Biological Weapons Convention Review Conference Paper No. 14. Bradford: Department of Peace Securities, University of Bradford.

Plotkin, B. J. (1996). Mission Possible: The Future of the International Health Regulations. *Temple International and Comparative Law Journal* (10), 503.

Qin, Y. (1999). *Hegemonic System and International Conflict: The US' Supporting Behaviours in International Armed Conflicts (1945–1988)*. Shanghai: Shanghai People's Publishing House, pp. 279–280.

Rao, G. (1996). *The Law of International Organizations*. Beijing: Beijing University Press.

Richter, J. (2012). WHO Reform and Public Interest Safeguards: An Historical Perspective. *Social Medicine*, 6(3), 141.

Rissanen, J. (2002). Left in Limbo: Review Conference Suspended on Edge of Collapse. *Disarmament and Diplomacy*, 62, 710.

Robbins, A. (1999). Brundtland's World Health. *Public Health Reports*, 114, 32.

Roelsgaard, E. (1974). Health Regulations and International Travel. *Chronicle of the World Health Organization* (28), 265–268.

Rosenberg, B. H. (2007). A Counter-Bioterrorism Strategy for the New UN Secretary-General. *Disarmament and Diplomacy*, 84, 7.

Secretary-General's High-Level Panel on Threats, Challenges and Change. (2004). *A Safer World: Our Shared Responsibility*. New York: United Nations.

Sehdev, P. S. (2002). The Origin of Quarantine. *Clinical Infectious Diseases* (35), 1071–1072.

Shakespeare, W. (2013). *Romeo and Juliet*. Act 5 Scene 2. (S. Zhu, Trans.). Beijing: World Book Publishing Company.

Siddiqi, J. (1995). *World Health and World Politics*. Columbus: University of South Carolina Press.

Siegfried, A. (1965). *Routes of Contagion*. New York: Harcourt Press.

Shao, S. (2006). *Newest Cases of the International Court of Justice*. Beijing: The Commercial Press.

Slaughter, A. (2004). *A New World Order*. Princeton: Princeton University Press.

Smith, R. (1995). The WHO: Change or die. *British Medical Journal*, 310, 543.

Sridhar, D. (2009). *Global Health: Who Can Lead?* London: Chatham House Publishing.

Stein, R. (2010, June 4). Reports Accuse WHO of Exaggerating H1N1 Threat, Possible Ties to Drug Makers. *Washington Post*.

Stern, A. M., & Markel, H. (2004). International Efforts to Control Infectious Diseases, 1851 to the Present. *Journal of the American Medical Association*, 292(12), 1476.

Stevenson, M. A., & Cooper, A. F. (2009). Overcoming Constraints of State Sovereignty: Global Health Governance in Asia. *Third World Quarterly*, 30(7), 1381.

104 *WHO and global health governance*

Sturtevant, J. L., Anema, A., & Brownstein, J. S. (2007). The New International Health Regulations: Considerations for Global Health Surveillance. *Disaster Medicine Public Health Preparedness* (1), 117–121.

Tang, B. (2011). Partnership and the Expansion of the Autonomy of International Organizations: Taking the World Health Organization's Experience in Global Malaria Control as an Example. *Foreign Affairs Review*, 2, 132.

Taylor, A. L. (1997). Controlling the Global Spread of Infectious Diseases: Toward a Reinforced Role for the International Health Regulations. *Houston Law Review* (33), 1327.

Trucker, J. B. (2005). Updating the International Health Regulations. *Biosecurity and Bioterrorism: Biodefense Strategy, Practice, and Science*, 3, 338–347.

Tomasevski, K. (1995). Health. In O. Schachter & C. Joyner (Eds.), *United Nations Legal Order*. Cambridge: American Society of International Law and Cambridge University Press.

Taylor, A. L. (1992). Making WHO Work. *American Journal of Law & Medicine*, 18(4), 303.

UN Economic and Social Council, UN Sub-Commission on Prevention of Discrimination and Protection of Minorities. (1985). *Siracusa Principles on the Limitation and Derogation of Provisions in the International Covenant on Civil and Political Rights*. UN Doc. E/CN.4/1985/4, Annex. New York: United Nations Plaza.

Velimirovic, B. (1976). Do We still Need International Health Regulations? *Journal of Infectious Diseases* (133), 478–482.

Verbeek, B. (1998). International Organizations: The Ugly Duckling of International Relations Theory. In B. Reinalda & B. Verbeek (Eds.), *Autonomous Policy Making by International Organizations*. New York: Routledge.

WHO. (1946). *The Constitution of World Health Organization*. Geneva: WHO.

WHO. (1970). *Health Aspects of Chemical and Biological Weapons: Report of a WHO Group of Consultants*. Geneva: WHO.

WHO. (1993). *Report of the Executive Board Working Group on the WHO Response to Global Change: Executive Board 92nd Session*. Geneva: WHO.

WHO. (1998a, January). *Provisional Draft of the International Health Regulations*. Geneva: WHO.

WHO. (1998b, May 16). *Dr Gro Harlem Brundtland Speech to the Fifty-First World Health Assembly*. Geneva, p. 4. Retrieved from http://apps.who.int/gb/archive/pdf_files/WHA51/eadiv6.pdf

WHO. (2004). *Preparedness for Deliberate Epidemics: Programme of Work for the Biennium 2004–2005*. WHO/CDS/CSR/LYO/2004.8, p. 4. Retrieved from www.who.int/csr/resources/publications/deliberate/WHO_CDS_CSR_LYO_2004_8.pdf

WHO. (2005). *The International Health Regulations (2005)*. Geneva: WHO.

WHO. (2007). *World Health Report 2007: A Safer Future: Global Health Security in the 21st Century*. Geneva: WHO.

WHO. (2010, December 15). *The Future of Financing for WHO*. Geneva: WHO.

WHO. (2011, May 5). *World Health Organization: Reform for a Healthy Future*. Geneva: WHO.

WHO. (2012, May 16). *WHO Reform: High-Level Implementation and Monitoring Framework*. A65/INF.DOC./6. Geneva: WHO.

WHO Director-General Address Need for WHO Reform. (n.d.). Retrieved from www.who.int/dg/speeches/2011/who_reform_01_11/en/index.html

WHO, & WTO. (2002). *WTO Agreements & Public Health: A Joint Study by the WHO and the WTO Secretariat*. Geneva: WHO.

Williams, D. (1987). *The Specialized Agencies and the United Nations*. London: C. Hurst & Company.

Williams, O. (2005). The WTO, Trade Rules and Global Health Security. In A. Ingram (Ed.), *Health, Foreign Policy & Security*. London: The Nuffield Trust.

Woodall, J. P. (2005). WHO and Biological Weapons Investigations. *The Lancet*, 365, 651.

World Bank Development Committee. (n.d.). *Poverty Reduction and Global Public Goods: Issues for the World Bank in Supporting Global Collective Action*, p. 6. Retrieved from http://siteresources.worldbank.org/DEVCOMMINT/Documentation/90015245/DC-2000-16(E)-GPG.pdf

World Health Assembly. (1995, May 12). *Revision and Updating of the International Health Regulations*. WHA48.7. Geneva: WHO.

Yamey, G. (2002a). Have the Latest Reforms Reversed WHO's Decline. *British Medical Journal*, 325, 1107–1112.

Yamey, G. (2002b). WHO's Management: Struggling to Transform a Fossilised Bureaucracy. *British Medical Journal*, 325, 1173.

4 World Trade Organization and global health governance

Human welfare depends on both free trade and public health security. Efforts to balance the relationship between trade and public health have persisted throughout the entire history of global trade. This chapter mainly analyses the impact of global trade on public health through the lens of international regimes and studies the relationship between global trade and public health from the perspective of global health security. WTO is a main international regime that formulates global trade norms, and its various agreements inevitably exert a significant influence on global health governance. D. T. Jamison, an American public health expert, believes WTO is the most influential international regime in the field of public health (Jamison et al., 1998, p. 514). Exaggeration in his point of view aside, his view reflects the non-trivial role WTO plays in global health security. Because the various agreements under WTO concerns trade and production stipulate policies that affect health of people in member countries, they have posed limitations on these countries' autonomy in managing their public health. In short, "these agreements have the potential to change the architecture of global health governance significantly and have direct implications on various public health communities and national health systems" (Williams, 2005, p. 73). Therefore, "the connections among global trade, international trade agreements, and public health deserve more attention" (Shaffer, 2005, p. 23).

4.1 Links between WTO and global public health

Trade accompanied human society throughout history, and ever-expanding trade has become a catalyst for increasing global interdependence. This deepening global interdependence has gradually extended to the field of public health security. Early cooperation in international public health was primarily driven by commercial interests. "If, in the old colonial days, it was true that 'trade follows the flag', it was equally true that the first faltering steps towards international health cooperation followed trade" (Howard-Jones, 1975, p. 12). In other words, issues of international health and international trade have been tied to, and interacted with, each other since the colonial days. The ever-expanding international trade has resulted in globalisation, "which is changing the landscape of global public health" (Drager & Beaglehole, 2001, p. 803). Globalisation is mainly manifested in economic aspects. "Although economic globalization has attracted wide attention, its implications for public health remain poorly understood" (Shaffer, 2005, p. 23). Therefore, it is necessary to discuss the influence and roles of WTO as a major organisation that formulates economic and trade norms on global health governance.

4.1.1 Background, purposes and principles of WTO

The idea of establishing WTO was proposed at the Bretton Woods conference held in July 1944. At the time, the vision for it was that an international trade organisation should be established along with the World Bank and the International Monetary Fund so these three could form a "currency-finance-trade" trinity that would shape the world economy after World War II. An agreement to establish WTO was reached in the Havana Charter signed at the International Conference on Trade and Employment in 1947. Nonetheless, the agreement was soon shelved due to opposition from the United States. In the same year, the United States proposed to formulate the General Agreement on Tariffs and Trade (GATT) as a temporary contract to promote trade liberalisation. The GATT hosted a total of eight rounds of multilateral negotiations on tariff and trade from 1947 to 1993. After the Uruguay Round initiated in 1986, the European Community and Canada formally proposed to set up WTO in 1990. The GATT Ministerial Conference held in Marrakesh, Morocco, in April 1994 formally decided to establish WTO as a replacement for the GATT of 1947. WTO, IMF and the World Bank have since been regarded as the three pillars of world economic development.

All international organisations have their purposes; however, WTO is unique because in addition to the principles stipulated in the preamble to the Agreement Establishing the World Trade Organization, the preambles to the GATT, the Havana Charter, and the General Agreement on Trade in Services also constitute main parts of WTO's principles. The main purposes of WTO in summary are as follows: 1) improve people's living standards. In its preamble, *WTO Agreement* clearly states that WTO member countries "recognise that they aim to improve people's living standards when handling various relations in the trade and economic fields". 2) Fully guarantee the continuing growth of employment, real income and effective demand. The purpose of formulating rules, regulations and systems for WTO is to create a loose yet orderly international trading environment to increase employment opportunities around the globe, boost general income and expand the international market for products and services. 3) Expand production and trade of goods as well as trade in services. Since members "recognised the growing importance of trade in services to the development of the world economy", the preamble to the WTO Charter clearly states that "expanding trade in services" is one of the main goals of WTO. To achieve this purpose, the Uruguay Round reached a General Agreement on Trade in Services and other documents. 4) Make appropriate use of world resources. WTO agreement stipulates that "efforts should be made to make rational use of world resources based on the Sustainable Development Goals." 5) Ensure the developing countries' share in international trade growth

108 *WTO and global health governance*

and their economic development. In its preamble, the WTO Charter states that "there is need for positive efforts designed to ensure that developing countries, and especially the least developed among them, secure a share in the growth in international trade commensurate with the needs of their economic development"; 6) Establish an integrated multilateral trading regime—that is, "develop an integrated, more viable and durable multilateral trading system".[1]

As an important international trade regime, WTO operates by certain principles. It formulated a series of trade principles and rules to ensure and promote equal, fair and mutually beneficial trade among members, avoid trade discrimination and trade friction and achieve liberal trade worldwide. In general, WTO has the following basic principles: 1) The most-favoured-nation (MFN) treatment principle. The preambles to the General Agreement on Tariffs and Trade in 1994 and the Agreement Establishing WTO clearly stipulate that all parties should "eliminate discriminatory treatment from international trade relations" and that all members should give each other MFN treatment. It is required that members should not discriminate against each other when they trade with each other; all members are equal regardless of their size. Any benefits, preferences, privileges or immunities provided by one member to another shall be immediately and unconditionally available to all other members. 2) The principle of national treatment. When one member's goods or services enter the territory of another member, they should enjoy the same treatment as those enjoyed by the import country's own domestic goods or services. In the field of trade for services, specific national treatment can be negotiated; that is, agreements can be reached through negotiation of members on an equal basis, and national treatment can be granted to different degrees in different industries according to the agreement. 3) The principle of market access. Members are required to gradually open their markets, reduce tariffs and lift restrictions on imports, so that foreign goods can enter their markets and compete with their domestic products. These commitments to the gradual opening of their markets are binding and implemented under the principle of non-discriminatory trade. 4) The principle of promoting fair competition and trade. Members are not to engage in unfair trade competition; in particular they should not dump or unduly subsidise their exported products. When any member enhances exports of its own products through dumping or subsidising, which would cause substantial damage to the importing country, the importing country can follow certain procedures to collect anti-dumping and countervailing duties. Nonetheless, these measures should not be abused for protectionist purposes. 5) Principle of transparency. Members of WTO shall publish the trade-related laws, regulations, policies and practices that they formulated and implemented, and the related changes thereof, including amendments, additions or abolitions. Those unpublished should not come into force. Meanwhile, they shall also inform WTO of these laws, regulations, policies and practices and the changes thereof. The purpose of this principle is to effectively guarantee the stability and predictability of the international trading environment.

From this analysis, it is clear that the main goal of WTO is to coordinate and promote global free trade. In WTO's regime, global trade takes precedence over everything else. Under the free trade doctrine, WTO is bound to overlook public health issues. In some ways, WTO has even become the very reason that leads to public health crises in a vast number of developing countries. Given the close relationship between trade and public health, how to balance the interests between the two within the framework of WTO has become an urgent issue in global health governance.

4.1.2 Connection between WTO and public health issues

4.1.2.1 Trade and public health: an old but relevant topic

Trade has existed since the very beginning of humankind, in its inception in the form of bartering. Throughout the thousands of years of human civilisation, public health issues such as infectious diseases have had a profound impact on human history. Both trade and public health pose familiar challenges. Nevertheless, it was only in recent years that a connection has been forged between the two. The long history behind the two concepts does not rule out their relevance to today's world. For thousands of years, merchants, invaders, and natural forces have spread diseases and changed history. In fact, quarantine practice established to combat infectious diseases was directly developed from trading activities. In as early as 1377, the first quarantine in human history was used in Ragusa (Dubrovnik, part of modern-day Croatia), a port city on the Dalmatia coast. Since the first day of the quarantine, the city isolated travellers from areas affected by the epidemic for 30 days (*trentini giorni*) or 40 days (*quaranti giorni*). From this was born the modern concept of "quarantine" and the entry-exit inspection and quarantine system widely in use today. During the Italian city-state period in the 15th century, to avoid the spread of the infectious disease, merchant ships from areas suffering from the Black Death were required to moor in a secluded port for 40 days before they reached the bustling Venice port. In the early 19th century, European countries implemented different or sometimes counter-productive quarantine policies, which impeded commercial trade. To protect their business interest, major European countries started to cooperate on international public health. The international spread of infectious diseases was portrayed as a threat to countries' economic interests. This mode dominated international health cooperation in the 19th century. Many subsequent international public health conferences were held, based on which came the IHR, which fully reflected the close link between trade and public health. Its purpose is "to limit the international spread of infectious disease to maximised global security at minimum interference with international business". This purpose demonstrates the importance of coordination between global trade interests and global health interests.

4.1.2.2 WTO and public health issues

WTO has broader jurisdiction and greater power than its predecessor GATT. Since WTO's establishment, its impact on world trade has become increasingly

110 *WTO and global health governance*

prominent, and its concerns have also extended to all aspects of society. The free trade that it advocates has brought a wide range of goods to people and promoted the cross-border movement of people but also spread potential infectious pathogens that might follow those goods. WTO agreements, such as the Trade-Related Aspects of Intellectual Property Rights (the TRIPS Agreement) and the liberalisation of trade in services, have had a significant impact on public health governance in countries around the world, especially that of developing ones. "Those concerned with health and security worldwide cannot afford to ignore the profound changes generated by global trade" (Shaffer, 2005, p. 33). On August 22, 2002, WHO and the Secretariat of WTO published a joint study on the relationship between trade rules and public health. This 171-page study shows that WTO agreements and public health are in many aspects closely connected. In the preface, Gro Harlem Brundtland, former director-general of WHO, and Mike Moore, former director-general of WTO, pointed out that, "There is much common ground between trade and health. Another important message is that health and trade policymakers can benefit from closer cooperation to ensure coherence between their different areas of responsibilities" (WHO & WTO, 2002, p. 1).

From the initial fight against infectious diseases all the way to the establishment and improvement of the multilateral trade regime led by the GATT and WTO in the 20th century, trade liberalisation has affected public health in many ways. Trans-boundary outbreaks of diseases have directly disrupted trade and transportation. International trade policies can also have an indirect influence on public health. For example, reducing barriers to trade can lower prices for medical equipment and health-related products, such as medicines and blood products; changes to international rules on patent protection can affect accessibility to essential medicines and the transfer of diagnostic devices and technology; in terms of health services, trade policies will affect the construction of a country's public health system. Conversely, national and international health standards and rules, such as *Codex Alimentarius*, food trade guidelines and recommendations, the IHR and the Framework Convention on Tobacco Control, can also exert a significant influence on trade. The free movement of goods and population driven by economic globalisation represented by WTO and environmental protection issues have made it increasingly difficult for sovereign states to prevent and control the spread of infectious diseases on their own (Feng, 2005, p. 61). In particular, due to the deepening economic globalisation in the second half of the 20th century, infectious diseases have spread around the world at an unprecedented rate, inflicting public health problems that develop from purely internal affairs to global health crises. Admittedly, many reasons lead to public health crises, including the spread of infectious diseases, food safety issues, the inaccessibility to medicines and the transfer of health technologies. The four main WTO agreements have had an important impact on certain aspects of public health. They include the Agreement on Trade-Related Aspects of Intellectual Property Rights (TRIPS), the General Agreement on Trade in Services (GATS), the Agreement on the Application of Sanitary and Phytosanitary Measures (SPS), and the Agreement on Technical Barriers to Trade (TBT) (see Table 4.1).

Table 4.1 Specific Health Issues and Most Relevant WTO Agreements

Public health issues	The Agreement on the Application of Sanitary and Phytosanitary Measures (SPS)	The Agreement on Technical Barriers to Trade (TBT)	The Agreement on Trade-Related Aspects of Intellectual Property Rights (TRIPS)	The General Agreement on Trade in Services (GATS)
Infectious disease control	X	X		
Food safety	X			
Tobacco control		X	X	X
Environment	X	X		
Accessibility to medicines			X	
Health service	X			X
Emerging issues				
Biotechnology	X	X	X	
Information technology			X	
Traditional knowledge			X	

Source: WHO & WTO, *WTO Agreement & Public Health: A Joint Study by the WHO and WTO Secretariat*, 2002, p. 59.

Undoubtedly, some WTO regulations involve considerations of public health. For example, the Marrakesh Agreement Establishing WTO states in its preamble that

> The Parties to this Agreement, Recognizing that their relations in the field of trade and economic endeavour should be conducted with a view to raising standards of living, ensuring full employment and a large and steadily growing volume of real income and effective demand, and expanding the production of and trade in goods and services, while allowing for the optimal use of the world's resources in accordance with the objective of sustainable development, seeking both to protect and preserve the environment and to enhance the means for doing so in a manner consistent with their respective needs and concerns at different levels of economic development.

Clearly, the phrases "raising standards of living" and "in accordance with the objective of sustainable development" in the preamble consider both individual health and national public health. Article 20 of the GATT stipulates that as long as measures are not applied in a manner constituting a means of arbitrary or unjustifiable discrimination between countries where the same conditions prevail, or a disguised restriction on international trade, nothing in this Agreement shall be construed as preventing the adoption or enforcement by any contracting party of

112   *WTO and global health governance*

measures necessary to protect human, animal or plant life or health. Given WTO's free trade orientation, even though the aforementioned provisions can contribute to global health security, it is still not WTO's main goal.

4.1.3 Negative impact of WTO norms on global health governance

Economists believe "there is a positive correlation between human health and per capita income and education level. Environmental degradation, such as poor sanitation and unclean drinking water, happen to the worst in the poorest countries" (Samuelson & Nordhaus, 2003, p. 296). In other words, health is directly proportional to economic development. Therefore, many supporters of WTO believe that free trade promoted by WTO will bring a win-win situation to all participants. In fact, although WTO is not a welfare-oriented international mechanism, it also relates to global welfare since the idea behind its establishment is that expanded trade can have a positive impact on global welfare. The preamble to the Agreement Establishing WTO includes objectives to support development and raise living standards, objectives beneficial to global health. For example, the growing wealth generated from international free trade can be used to purchase and build public health facilities, which can enhance the overall health level. Through international trade, the best health products (such as medicines and medical services) are made available internationally.

Although WTO has strengthened the development of the global economy, such development does not naturally lead to the improvement of countries' public health security, especially those of developing ones. "Much of this health crisis reflects the underlying economic reality of globalization. The greatest gains from trade liberalization have gone to the wealthiest nations" (Hilary, 2001, p. 7). In other words, public health security in most developing countries has not improved in the tide of economic growth promoted by WTO. On the contrary, it is getting even worse. Consequently, the gap between developed and developing countries in public health has further widened. Leaving the problems of poverty and diseases unsolved in developing countries will lead to potentially serious consequences for all members of the international community. In view of the global interdependence in the field of public health security, it is necessary to examine the negative impact of various WTO agreements on global health security. WTO has four major agreements that can negatively affect public health security in developing countries. To start with, the TRIPS Agreement affects the price of and accessibility to essential medicines. The GATS agreement directly hinders the cross-border movement of patients and health professionals as well as the foreign ownership of medical equipment.

The SPS inhibits food safety and the spread of infections across countries. The TBT also puts a check on relevant health norms and standards. All these agreements are related to public health and entail corresponding obligations of members. Based on different obligations members have to fulfil under each agreement, these agreements present challenges to global health security in the following two ways: First, many agreements require members to deregulate those areas of public health that restrict trade or require members to conform national public health regulations to internationally harmonised standards. As a result, members may lose their freedom to decide how they achieve public health goals. For example, the TRIPS Agreement stipulates that all countries, rich or poor, must provide patent protection for new medicines for at least 20 years. As a result, developing countries lost their freedom in patent protection, thus delaying the production of low-cost generic medicines which public health institutions in developing countries and poor people in these countries depend on for survival. The highly undifferentiated provisions of the TRIPS Agreement protect the high prices of patented medicines, and many poor people infected with otherwise curable diseases lost their lives because they could not afford expensive medicines or vaccines. The prevalence of HIV/AIDS is just one example. This is not to say that the intellectual property system is of no use at all but that some flexibility should be allowed in the implementation of this system. As the American economist Lester C. Thurow (1997) argued,

> In a global economy, a global system of intellectual property rights is needed. This system must reflect the needs both of countries that are developing and of those that have developed. The problem is similar to the one concerning which types of knowledge should be in the public domain in the developed world. But the Third World's need to get low-cost pharmaceuticals is not equivalent to its need for low-cost CDs. Any system that treats such needs equally, as our current system does, is neither a good nor a viable system.
>
> (p. 103)

As another example, *Codex Alimentarious* of the Food and Agriculture Organization, adopted voluntarily by countries around the world, provides scientific and non-binding standards for food safety. This codex is also used by the Agreement on the Application of Sanitary and Phytosanitary Measures to judge the legitimacy of food standards and health measures of the member countries. The TBT and the TRIPS Agreement have also adopted similar standards and regulatory norms. The aforementioned WTO agreements have greatly restricted the freedom of members in their public health governance, making it impossible for members to enforce corresponding public health policies in accordance with their specific domestic public health situations. In 2001, the UN Economic and Social Council passed a resolution acknowledging the negative influence of such agreements as the TRIPS Agreement on the right to health, the right to food, and the right to self-determination. The Council required member countries to take note of the fact that they should prioritise their international obligations to protect human rights mandated by international law over enforcing their own economic and trade policies and international trade agreements (UN Committee on Economic, Social and Cultural Rights, 2000). Be that as it may, the resolution is essentially non-binding in comparison to the force of WTO agreements.

Second, the obligations of the members enshrined in WTO agreements have facilitated the privatisation of knowledge or products that are necessary to promote human health, as well as that of the previously public national health system.

114 *WTO and global health governance*

Taking the TRIPS Agreement as an example: Medical knowledge, biological resources and pharmaceuticals are subject to a whole new balance of interest between patent holders and the wider public. The promotion of private ownership of such products as essential medicines has had a profound influence on public health security. In 1968, British biologist Garrett Hardin coined the term "the tragedy of the commons" in his published paper to describe a situation where public resources are often inappropriately used due to a lack of corresponding rules (1968, pp. 1243–1248). The global promotion of intellectual property rights, especially in such areas as biomedical research, is now implying "an 'anti-commons' in which people underuse scarce resources because too many owners can block each other . . . More intellectual property rights may lead paradoxically to fewer useful products for improving human health" (Heller & Eisenberg, 1998, p. 698). Similarly, the GATS has almost transformed WTO from an anti-protectionist body to a global institution promoting privatisation. It views essential services, such as public health, as areas that can be regulated by market-oriented policies rather than as public goods. "Whilst the WTO's health-related rules are detailed and highly complex, when taken together they suggest a new and emerging global political economy of health which is privately orientated" (Williams, 2005, p. 77). The privatisation tendency of WTO agreements has exacerbated market failures in global public health. In particular, in the vast number of developing countries, the privatisation of public health has made the already inadequate public health system more fragile. Such privatisation runs counter to the nature of global public goods for health. An unrestricted and fully adjustable private market is the most powerful driving force of globalisation that leads to inequality in health. In short, by representing forces of globalisation, WTO has promoted trade liberalisation and privatisation at national and even global levels through its various agreements, but it also leads to serious shortages of global public goods for health, thereby having a negative effect on global health governance.

4.2 WTO agreements and global health governance: a case study of the conflict between TRIPS and accessibility to medicines

Although WTO is mainly viewed as an organisation committed to facilitating free trade, the complex interactions of many principles in WTO's various agreements suggest that WTO itself is also a regime for development. Since health protection is a development issue, WTO thus becomes an important player in global health governance, whose function is manifested in the four agreements under its framework. As Gong (2006) observed,

> In a sense, WTO has become the central horizontal regime for international law on infectious diseases after its creation in 1995. The Agreement on Trade-Related Aspects of Intellectual Property Rights, the Agreement on the Application of Sanitary and Phytosanitary Measures, and the WTO's powerful dispute settlement mechanism made WTO more important for infectious disease control policy than the discredited IHR. The trade regime's

ascendancy over the classical regime is apparent in the contrast between the public health attention and controversy generated by WTO agreements and the IHR's obscurity in global health discourse.

(p. 65)

In other words, WTO plays a different role from those of other international regimes in global health governance. This section examines the role of WTO agreements in global health governance through the conflict between the TRIPS Agreement and accessibility to medicines.

The TRIPS Agreement is one of the final results achieved in the Uruguay Round of the GATT. It was signed on April 15, 1994, and became effective on January 1, 1995. It is to date the most comprehensive multilateral agreement on intellectual property. It is also a global multilateral agreement that has had the greatest influence on the intellectual property and legal systems of countries and regions around the world. It also forms one of the three pillars of WTO together with the Agreement on Trade in Goods and the Agreement on Trade in Services. The purpose of the TRIPS Agreement is to promote more adequate and effective protection of intellectual property rights in international trade so that holders of intellectual property rights can benefit from their technological inventions. In so doing, holders of intellectual property rights can be motivated to continue working on more inventions and creations, thereby making the material and spiritual results of technology and arts as widely available to the public as possible. The TRIPS Agreement also aims to reduce the distortion and obstruction of international trade by intellectual property protection and ensure that the implementation and procedures of the TRIPS Agreement do not hinder legal trade. However, since 2001, given the grave threats to people's health by HIV/AIDS, tuberculosis and malaria, public health problems in developing countries have received increasing attention from the international community. In 2002 alone, 15 million people worldwide had reportedly died of infectious diseases, and tens of millions were battling death after contracting HIV/AIDS. In Africa and Latin America, deadly infectious diseases such as malaria, tuberculosis and HIV/AIDS were fast spreading, putting people's health and the economy in serious jeopardy. Reasons for public health crises in these areas are manifold, but the critical one is the lack of access to effective and affordable medicines. Oxfam, an international charity, published a 2001 report titled "Patent Injustice: How World Trade Rules Threaten the Health of Poor People", which examined the prohibitive drug prices inflated by WTO's patent system and its catastrophic impact on poor countries (Oxfam, 2001). The report took efavirenz and nelfinavir, two Western patented medicines for AIDS, under scrutiny. According to statistics in October 2001, under patent protection Stonathan could sell for as much as US$4,730, as opposed to US$485 of similar generic medicines, while nelfinavir could fetch US$3,508 under patent protection, compared to only US$201 of generic medicines. Developing countries estimated that they could save 80–90% of their expenses if they were allowed to produce generic medicines (Cheng, 2001). But the TRIPS Agreement has prevented them from producing these patent-protected medicines at the same time

116　WTO and global health governance

depriving them of the ability to afford expensive patent medicines. It thus contributes to serious public health crises in developing countries.

4.2.1　Public health-related articles in the TRIPS Agreement

The close connection between trade and public health means the TRIPS Agreement also affects public health issues. Specifically, the TRIPS Agreement seeks to strike a balance between patent rights (private interest) and access to medicines (public interest). Clashes between the two existed long before the TRIPS Agreement was signed and were the main contention of the Uruguay Round. The TRIPS Agreement attempts to reconcile such conflict through the following articles:

1　The preamble to the TRIPS Agreement stipulates that each member shall establish minimum standards for the protection and enforcement of intellectual property rights, thereby promoting technological innovation, technology transfer and social development. There is no doubt that public health is an important aspect of social development. The purpose of intellectual property protection of medicines should not be to obtain monopolised profits but rather to facilitate the transfer of technologies and the improvement of public health and contribute to public health security.

2　Article 7 of the TRIPS Agreement sets out the objectives of intellectual property protection. The protection and enforcement of intellectual property rights should contribute to the promotion of technological innovation and to the transfer and dissemination of technology, to the mutual advantage of producers and users of technological knowledge and in a manner conducive to social and economic welfare and to a balance of rights and obligations. In other words, the TRIPS Agreement must effectively protect intellectual property rights of those who create such technologies while ensuring potential users of such technologies may enjoy the benefits they bring. The intellectual property protection mechanism must be oriented not only towards self-interest but also towards social welfare.

3　Article 8(1) of the TRIPS Agreement concerning this principle states that members may in formulating or amending their laws and regulations adopt measures necessary to protect public health and nutrition and promote the public interest in sectors of vital importance to their socio-economic and technological development, provided that such measures are consistent with the provisions of this agreement. In other words, members may take necessary measures to enhance public health security on the condition that these measures do not breach the agreement.

4　Article 27(2) of the TRIPS Agreement provides that members may exclude from patentability inventions, the prevention within their territory of the commercial exploitation of which is necessary to protect public order and social norms, including the protection of human, animal and plant lives and health as well as the prevention of serious harm to the environment, provided that such exclusion is not made merely because the exploitation is prohibited by their law. In other words, members may refuse to recognize it.

5 Article 27(3) of the TRIPS Agreement provides that members may exclude from patentability diagnostic, therapeutic and surgical methods for the treatment of humans or animals. In other words, members may refuse to acknowledge patent protection that can affect the treatment of diseases.

6 Article 31 of the TRIPS Agreement stipulates that if any member is in the event of a national emergency or other circumstances of extreme urgency or in cases of public non-commercial use, a compulsory license for the patent right can be granted. People can apply for the use of some subject matter of a patent through the administrative application process. If these conditions are met, the national authority can issue a compulsory license for the patent and directly allow the applicant to use the subject matter of the patent without authorisation of the patent holder. The provision indicates that in case of a public health crisis, the country can enforce a compulsory license for the use of the patent medicine. This provision represents one of the most important ways in which the TRIPS Agreement seeks to strike a balance between promoting accessibility to medicines and enhancing the development of new medicines.

7 Article 65 of the TRIPS Agreement on transitional arrangements stipulates the following: If a member state is a developing nation, if the member state is either transitioning from a centrally planned economy to a free-market economy or if it is undertaking transformation of its intellectual property system and facing challenges with implementing relevant regulations, then this member state is entitled to delay the implementation date by five years. That is, the member state has until 2000 to implement the TRIPS Agreement.

8 Article 66 of the agreement states that, in view of the special needs and requirements of least-developed country members, their economic, financial and administrative constraints and their need for flexibility to create a viable technological base, such members shall not be required to apply the provisions of this agreement for a period of ten years from the date of application. In other words, these least developed countries (LDCs) may enjoy a ten-year transition period in their implementation of patent rights on medicines.

These articles demonstrate WTO's endeavour to balance patent rights for medicines and the access to essential medicines. For developing countries and LDCs in particular, a transition period of five to ten years will temporarily ease the pressure on their implementation of patent rights for essential medicines. But on the whole, the TRIPS Agreement is still a victory scored by developed countries because it forces the international community to accept the international intellectual property protection system they have long championed. WTO's effort to balance patent rights for medicines and access to essential medicines is just a fraction of what is needed to solve public health crises. For countries with backwards pharmaceutical technology, the compulsory licensing for pharmaceutical patent rights stipulated in the TRIPS Agreement is purely for show. For developing

118 *WTO and global health governance*

countries that do have technologies to produce medicines, the lack of clarity in how to implement compulsory licensing has also filled actual implementation with controversy.

4.2.2 *Declaration on the TRIPS Agreement and public health issues*

Given the TRIPS Agreement's failure to resolve global health issues, especially its failure to improve the accessibility of essential medicines in developing countries, WTO members held the Fourth Ministerial Conference in Doha, Qatar, on November 14, 2001. Developing countries pushed to make public health and intellectual property rights a focal point of the Conference. After three days of negotiations on patent rights and public health, delegates finally passed The Doha Declaration on the TRIPS and Public Health (referred to as the Doha Declaration), an unprecedented agreement in WTO's history. At the opening ceremony of the conference, then director-general of WTO Mike Moore acknowledged the significance of the moment, noting that any consensus reached between public health and the TRIPS Agreement could become a "deal-breaker" of this new round of negotiations (WTO, 2001). The implications of the Doha Declaration in addressing global health issues include first, the Doha Declaration recognised the gravity of the public health problems afflicting many developing countries, especially those resulting from HIV/AIDS, tuberculosis, malaria and other epidemics. All parties agreed that the TRIPS Agreement should not prevent members from taking measures to protect public health. Accordingly, while reiterating their commitment to the TRIPS Agreement, they affirmed that the agreement should be interpreted and implemented in a manner supportive of WTO members' right to protect public health.

> We agree that the TRIPS Agreement does not and should not prevent Members from taking measures to protect public health. Accordingly, while reiterating our commitment to the TRIPS Agreement, we affirm that the Agreement can and should be interpreted and implemented in a manner supportive of WTO Members' right to protect public health and, in particular, to promote access to medicines for all.
>
> (WTO, n.d.a)

Members have full rights to make use of the flexibility articles provided in the TRIPS Agreement. Flexibility articles stipulate that the interpretation of specific articles of the TRIPS Agreement should be in line with its objectives and purposes; each member has the right to grant compulsory licensing and may independently decide the reasons for granting such licenses; each member has the right to decide what may constitute a public health crisis, including but not limited to national emergencies or other circumstances of extreme urgency, such as those related to HIV/AIDS, tuberculosis, malaria and other infectious diseases; members have freedom on the question of the exhaustion of intellectual property rights as long as most-favoured-nation principle and national treatment principle provisions are not violated. To a certain extent, this helps developing countries solve the public health crises they face.

Second, the Doha Declaration further clarifies the flexibility on pharmaceutical patents provided in the TRIPS Agreement. Article 31 stipulates that although members can issue compulsory licensing for patent rights on medicines, the flexible measures are still conditioned by various prerequisites. These prerequisites are often used by developed countries to thwart developing countries' efforts to issue compulsory licenses for patent medicines. As a result, developing countries must battle various constraints when trying to do so. It is for this reason that, in practice, a member state will rarely use "compulsory license" unless there is an absolute reason to do so. South Africa and Brazil, who faced very high infection rates of HIV/AIDS, were the first two countries to issue compulsory licenses for patents on HIV/AIDS medicines. Both countries have since drawn lawsuits, condemnations and accusations from Western developed countries, particularly the United States. The Doha Declaration later addresses this by stipulating that "every member has the right to grant compulsory licenses and also has the right to independently determine the reasons for granting such compulsory licenses".[2] There is another prerequisite built into the TRIPS Agreement—a compulsory license must be issued predominantly for the supply of the domestic market of the member granting the license. This provision may not present an obstacle for developing countries with strong capabilities to produce generic drugs, such as India, Brazil and China. However, it renders LTDs who are unable to produce generic medicines powerless to grant compulsory licenses. Moreover, when facing severe public health crises, these LTDs are unable to import medicines at low prices from countries that can issue compulsory licenses. The Doha Declaration acknowledges that WTO members with insufficient or no manufacturing capacities in the pharmaceutical sector could face difficulties in making effective use of compulsory licensing under the TRIPS Agreement. Article 6 of the Doha Declaration states that

> We recognise that WTO members with insufficient or no manufacturing capacities in the pharmaceutical sector could face difficulties in making effective use of compulsory licensing under the TRIPS Agreement. We instruct the Council for the TRIPS Agreement to find an expeditious solution to this problem and to report to the General Council before the end of 2002.
>
> (WTO, n.d.b)

This provision became the famous "Paragraph 6" of the Declaration. In addition, the Doha Declaration sets two specific tasks. First, it instructs the Council for the TRIPS Agreement to find an expeditious solution to the problem faced by countries with insufficient or inadequate pharmaceutical production capacity in making effective use of the compulsory licensing provisions of the TRIPS Agreement and to report to the General Council before the end of 2002. Second, it extended the deadline for least-developed countries to apply provisions on pharmaceutical patents to January 1, 2016. The TRIPS Council was mandated by the Ministerial Conference to take necessary action to perform these tasks.

120 *WTO and global health governance*

In short, the legitimacy of the WTO pharmaceutical patent rights has been constantly challenged by public health crises arising from infectious diseases in developing countries every year. The choice concerns whether the organisation should maintain its protection of pharmaceutical patents at the expense of right to life or instead amend the TRIPS Agreement and protect public health and uphold human rights. Fortunately, WTO chose the second option (He, 2004, p. 107). The Doha Declaration has positive implications for public health governance. It confirms public health's precedence over private property rights. It affirms member states' right to make full use of the flexibility articles under the TRIPS Agreement and their sovereign right to take steps to safeguard public health. It advances WTO's role in global health governance. Nevertheless, in spite of its clarification on the TRIPS Agreement's relevant provisions, the extension of the transition period for LDCs to implement the TRIPS Agreement, and the freedom given to member states to independently determine public health emergencies and issue compulsory licenses, the Doha Declaration has not addressed the fundamental conflict between the TRIPS Agreement and health promotion.

4.2.3 *The protocol amending the TRIPS*

Although the Doha Declaration has further confirmed and specified the flexibility articles concerning pharmaceutical patent rights under the TRIPS Agreement and raised the issues unresolved by "Paragraph 6", it has not legally provided new rights for developing members. Issues of this kind may only be resolved through consultations among members. On August 30, 2003, after one year and eight months of arduous negotiations, the General Council of WTO finally passed the Protocol on the Implementation of Paragraph 6 of the Doha Ministerial Declaration on the TRIPS and Public Health. Subsequently in December 2005, the WTO General Council incorporated amendments to the Doha Declaration and the Protocol into the TRIPS Agreement. This signalled the success of WTO members to be able to reach consensus on the solutions to public health issues. As Dr Supachai Panitchpakdi, former WTO director-general, described,

> This is a historic agreement for the WTO. It allows poorer countries to make full use of the flexibilities in the WTO's intellectual property rules in order to deal with the diseases that ravage their people. It proves once and for all that the organisation can handle humanitarian as well as trade concerns. This particular question has been especially difficult. The fact that WTO members have managed to find a compromise in such a complex issue bears testimony to their goodwill, and it provides opportunities for poor countries to 'access essential medicines' in a way that does not violate intellectual property laws.
>
> (Supachai Panitchpakdi, 2003)

The revisions to the TRIPS Agreement in the Protocol are mainly manifested in the following aspects:

1 According to the Protocol, the revised TRIPS will enable WTO members to grant their domestic companies compulsory licenses for producing and even exporting specific patent medicines as long as they meet certain conditions. This is a breakthrough in the TRIPS Agreement because the patented medicines that are compulsorily licensed are no longer restricted to their domestic markets. This revision allows underdeveloped countries that are unable to grant compulsory licenses due to their less-developed pharmaceutical producing capacities to import low-priced medicines from other developing countries that can issue compulsory licenses. For example, currently, two-thirds of the 40 million people in the world infected with HIV/AIDS are from Africa. To give treatment to people who have to buy prohibitively expensive patented medicines, this agreement allows that African countries that are unable to issue compulsory licenses for the patent rights of related medicines may now import generic HIV/AIDS medicines from India or Brazil at far lower prices.

2 The TRIPS Agreement provides in principle that WTO members must pay adequate remuneration to patent holders which grant compulsory licenses for their patents. The Protocol further confirms that in the case where both an exporting member and an importing member grant a compulsory license for the same product, the patent licenses fee should only be paid by the exporting member. This reduces the cost of issuing compulsory licenses in developing countries.

In short, the Protocol allows WTO members to grant compulsory licenses for the purpose of exporting medicines to "qualified import members", a breakthrough in the TRIPS Agreement which stipulated that compulsory licenses "can only be granted to those products mainly supplied to the domestic market". The Protocol empowers developing and least developed members who are facing public health crises due to HIV/AIDS, malaria, tuberculosis and other epidemic diseases by lending authority to issue compulsory licenses for patents without patent holders' authorisation. These countries can produce, use and sell patented medicines for the aforementioned diseases, or they can import these medicines from other members that can enforce compulsory licenses. In so doing, the market price of patented medicines can be greatly reduced, which will help control and alleviate public health crises more quickly and effectively.

Although WTO members have made many efforts to balance patent rights and the access of medicines in developing countries, as well as patent rights and the right to human health, developed countries have not changed their stance on the use of intellectual property rights to monopolise profits. In fact, some Western developed countries still cling to unilateralism and double standards regarding issuing compulsory licenses for producing patented medicines. For instance, following the anthrax attack that took place after the September 11 terrorist attack, the United States decided to stockpile Cipro. However, seeing that Bayer's patent rights on Cipro were not due to expire until 2003, the United States threatened to override Bayer's patent using "emergency" provisions unless the German

122 *WTO and global health governance*

company lowered the price of the drug. Bayer eventually assented to sell Cipro at one-fifth of its market price. The Cipro story was reported by the *Financial Times*, which, ironically, on the same day also ran a report on how the US-led group, including Canada, had blocked Brazil and India's proposal to issue a ministerial declaration at the Doha Round, who wanted to declare to the world that nothing in the agreement shall prevent member states from taking measures to protect their public health. Meanwhile, the United States has accused developing countries, for instance, South Africa and Brazil, of granting compulsory licenses to HIV/AIDS medicines and has filed lawsuits against these countries for their violation of the TRIPS Agreement. The United States is thus often accused of judging pharmaceutical patents by a double standard. It is true that intellectual property protection regimes can promote technological innovation to a certain extent, but the contributions of inventions are meaningful only if we can manage to make them affordable and accessible to the poor. In fact,

> The privileges granted to inventors by patent laws are prohibitions on other men, and the history of inventions accordingly teems with accounts of trifling improvements patented, that have put a stop, for a long period, to other similar and much greater improvements. . . . The privileges have stifled more inventions than they have promoted. . . . Every patent is a prohibition against improvements in a particular direction, except by the patentee, for a certain number of years; and, however, beneficial that may be to him who receives the privilege, the community cannot be benefited by it. . . . On all inventors it is especially a prohibition to exercise their faculties; and in proportion as they are more numerous than one, it is an impediment to the general advancement. . . .
>
> (Machlup & Penrose, 1950, p. 24)

Similarly, the patent rights on medicines also hinder the development of the global community so that "IPRs have been regarded as food for the rich countries and poison for poor countries" (Commission on Intellectual Property Rights, n.d.). As Indira Gandhi once contended, "The idea of a better-ordered world is one in which medical discoveries will be free of patents and there will be no profiteering from life and death" (Zhuang & Du, 2003).

The TRIPS Agreement is only one example of WTO's influence on global health governance to have restricted access to medicines in developing countries. The other reason has to do with the "10/90 gap", meaning as little as 10% of global funding for research is spent on as many as 90% of global health issues. Given the low purchasing power of developing countries, Western pharmaceutical companies tend to avoid developing medicines for prevalent tropical diseases that ravage developing countries, such as malaria and dengue fever. Instead, they focus on medicines for public health problems in developed countries, resulting in a huge public health investment gap between developing and developed countries. For example, in 2001, developed countries spent an estimated US$101.6 billion in national health research, accounting for 96% of the global total, while developing countries only spent an estimated US\$4.3 billion, only 4% of the global total (Global Forum for Health Research, 2004, p. 15). This huge investment gap is also an important reason for public health crises in developing countries. In addition to the TRIPS Agreement, the other WTO agreements have also affected global public health. Take GATS, which is committed to the liberalisation and privatisation of global trade in services, for example.[3] It has inevitably affected health services as they are part of global trade in services. The GATS resulted in a significant migration of health professionals from developing to developed countries, further weakening the already inadequate public health systems of these developing countries. Many critics of GATS consider it an important cause for the disastrous consequences of public health. As WTO expert Owain Williams warned, "The *General Agreement on Trade in Services* is playing a role in what has been described as a 'collapse' in global public health" (Williams, 2004, p. 78). The SPS Agreement and the TBT Agreement have affected public health security at national and global levels in similar ways. SPS, for instance, allows member governments to take measures to protect public health, but at the same time subject these measures to stringent sanitary standards and risk assessment procedures (WHO & WTO, 2002). Balancing the two proves challenging. Moreover, by claiming agricultural products in developing countries do not meet health standards, some developed countries have taken the opportunity to implement trade protection measures. If members cannot resolve such disputes and lodge an appeal to the "General Council", the dispute settlement body of WTO, the final decision will be made by senior trade officials rather than public health experts. In fact, WTO has neither the ability nor the authority to set health standards for food and products because it does not have scientific credibility nor does it possess medical and public health technologies (Koivusalo, 2002, p. 175). Therefore, the health and quarantine measures in the SPS may become "green barriers" in disguise.

4.3 WTO's role in global health governance: some limitations

"WTO is becoming the single most important international institution in the architecture of global health governance" (Williams, 2005, p. 73). As a main symbol of current globalisation, WTO exerts much influence on global health governance with its unparalleled regulatory authority. "WTO has become more important than WHO in formulating infectious disease policies" (Fidler, 2003, p. 285). In particular, the TRIPS Agreement plays an irreplaceable role in enhancing access to essential medicines in developing countries. Nonetheless, since WTO is not a regime oriented towards public health security, protecting global health security is thus not the primary goal in its operation. Some scholars comment, "It would thus be Pollyanna-ish to expect WTO policies and jurisprudence to align perfectly with the goal of promoting health" (Bloche & Jungman, 2007, p. 253). In some aspect, WTO has even worked to the detriment of global health security. Specifically, there are several factors restricting WTO's role in global health governance.

124 *WTO and global health governance*

4.3.1 WTO's free trade doctrine

The philosophical tenet behind WTO is that a non-discriminatory and competitive open market for international trade can promote the welfare of all countries. Free trade boosts economic growth, which can help reduce poverty and strengthen public health security. This inspiration has been fully manifested in the principles and purposes of WTO and is reflected from many recent analyses of the relationship between globalisation and public health (e.g. Dollar, 2001; Feachem, 2001). For these reasons, the main goal of WTO is to promote free trade and the trade-related interests of member states rather than to ensure public health security. Although WTO clearly stipulates that trade measures should not hinder members' endeavours to protect public health security, when a conflict arises between protecting trade-related interests and maintaining public health security, WTO leans strongly towards the former. For example, WTO requires members to demonstrate the scientific efficacy of health policies that come at a cost to trade, but business practices that hinder public health policies are given free passes. "This unfair application of scientific evidence undermines WTO's claim that it would always represent the interests of the general public" (Gong, 2006, p. 77). "This puts the WTO in the indefensible position of refusing to tolerate irrational government policy in matters of public health while continuing to tolerate irrational government trade policies such as tariffs and quotas" (Charnovitz, 2000, p. 13). In other words, WTO adheres to a strict view of "market fundamentalism",[4] which has led to "market failure" in global health governance. As Orbinski and Burciul (2006) pointed out, the lack of medicines for "neglected diseases" is not due to a lack of knowledge or lack of ability of scientists, but due to "market failure" (p. 117). In other words, under the current system, major pharmaceutical companies have no vested interest to develop medicines that people need the most.

Taking the TRIPS Agreement as an example, WTO believes it helps promote technological innovation and free trade. However, many studies have shown that patent protection will not necessarily stimulate research and development.[5] In fact, the TRIPS Agreement is not in complete alignment with WTO's purpose to promote free trade. Its patent rights protection hinders free competition. In this sense, WTO's protection of intellectual property rights is a tax levied on the developing countries using patented products of developed countries. American scholar Panagariya pointed out that the geographical expansion of patents will increase monopolised rights, present an adverse impact on product distribution and transactions and impede growth in research and development of developing countries. In his view,

> The extension of North's patent law to South will lead to both efficiency loss and transfer of benefits from Southern consumers to innovators. Since innovators are mainly located in North, South will lose on both counts: monopoly distortion and the transfer from its consumers to innovators in North. Global welfare will also decline.
>
> (Quotation from Kaul et al., 2003, p.414)

WTO and global health governance 125

Stephen Lewis, the United Nations' special envoy for HIV/AIDS in Africa, named the practice of prioritising intellectual property and free trade over the right to human health as a "mass murder by complacency" (Lewis, 2003). American economist John Jewkes is even sharper in his criticism by saying, "It is almost impossible to conceive of any existing social institution so faulty in so many ways. It survives only because there seems to be nothing better" (Jewkes et al., 1971, p. 255).

In summary, WTO's free trade framework demonstrates the tension between intellectual property rights driven by economic globalisation and public health security as a global public good. The solution to this tension lies not in the removal of global trade rules but in achieving an appropriate balance between public health security and global trade. Moreover, human development and public health should be a priority characterising this balance. As Georg Merck, founder of the multinational pharmaceutical company Merck & Company (MSD) (2003), said, "We try never to forget that medicine is for the people; It is not for the profits" (p. 42).

4.3.2 *WTO regulations have broadened the public health divide between developed and developing countries*

> While globalization offers great opportunities, its benefits are very unevenly shared and its costs are unevenly distributed. The gap resulting from this uneven distribution is strinkingly pronounced in the field of public health. Among many phenomena that threaten the important balance of the world, the North-South 'public health gap' may be one of the most worrisome.
>
> (United Nations, n.d. pp. 1-2)

Far from filling this gap, WTO's rules have somehow managed to exacerbate the inequity. In formulating global health policies, the broad representation of member countries in WTO may lead us to believe that inequality is not an issue for WTO. This is far from the truth. Many poor countries are simply not eligible to be represented at WTO meetings. In particular, informal meetings convened by the chairman of a committee or the director-general of WTO and attended by a few stakeholder delegations as well as the so-called "Green Room" meetings are all dominated by developed countries. The TRIPS Agreement of WTO has worsened the divide between developed and developing countries in public health arena. Developing countries are generally net importers of technologies, most of which are provided by developed countries that hold most of the patents in the world. Therefore, developed countries have spared no efforts to formulate policies that can protect their intellectual property rights in the framework of TRIPS. For developing countries, the introduction of the patent system cannot solve public health problems (Wilson, 2005). Developed countries remain coldly indifferent to public health crises of developing countries in setting the agenda of WTO. The Group of Eight (G8), in particular, has been playing an important role in WTO's decision-making process. However, judging by WTO's agenda, G8's

126 *WTO and global health governance*

response to globalisation's effect on human health and development disasters can be described as cruelly indifferent (Labonte & Schrecker, 2004, pp. 1661–1676). Were the United States to endure a prevalence of AIDS infections comparable to that in Africa, it would be hard to imagine the country would persist to be as fervent an advocate for intellectual property protection for drugs. WTO looks like a rules-based system, but it is obvious that there is always one set of rules for rich countries and another set for poor ones (Chen, 2003). It is this double-standard nature of rules that has created or widened the North–South Divide in public health.

4.3.3 *Privatisation of global public goods for health*

Health security is a typical global public good. An important reason for the under-supply of public goods has to do with "market failure". Since there is no "world government" in the international community, "market failure" in the supply of global public goods for health becomes even more serious. Only through adequate international cooperation can the negative effects of "market failure" be mitigated and the supply of global public goods for health improved. The private market is neither incentivised nor empowered to address the problems in the supply of public goods for global health. However, WTO agreements have gone the contrary direction by advocating privatisation in areas of health security. Dominated by developed countries, WTO attempts to facilitate the supply of global public goods for health by "privatizing the market". In terms of the provision of global public goods for health, such privatisation of WTO has been particularly reflected in the system of intellectual property rights of medicines. The TRIPS Agreement explicitly declares intellectual property rights are private rights. That is to say, intellectual property rights of pharmaceutical products are also private rights. At present, most of the intellectual property rights for pharmaceuticals are held by multinational corporations in developed countries. These for-profit companies make research plans based on the market needs of the developed countries rather than the needs of impoverished people in developing countries. Accordingly, the focus of their research is mainly on non-communicable diseases rather than infectious diseases such as malaria, cholera, AIDS, dengue fever and others prevalent in developing countries. It is estimated that less than 5% of the global funding for pharmaceutical research and development is spent on diseases that primarily affect developing countries (Commission on Macroeconomics and Health, 2001, p. 79). This has also widened the gap between developed and developing countries in their access to health products. Consequently, shares of the world medicine market vary tremendously from one region to another (see Table 4.2). Of the 1,393 medicines approved for development between 1975 and 1999, as few as 13 were for the treatment of tropical diseases (Trouiller & Olliaro, 2002, p. 2189). On the other hand, along with globalisation and the increase in population movements around the world, infectious diseases can no longer be geographically contained. Transnational population movements and economic trends have made the world, both developed and developing countries alike, more vulnerable to infectious diseases such as SARS, tuberculosis and avian influenza. Failure to address the public health issues of developing countries will have potentially serious consequences for all members of the international community. Therefore, medicine development must be viewed as a global problem to be addressed through global cooperation, rather than as a problem reserved for multinational pharmaceutical corporations. Globalisation, promoted by multinational corporations and advocated by WTO, is not the path to the future. Similarly, medicine research and development led by multinational pharmaceutical companies is not the right path towards global health governance. Such privatisation will only exacerbate the market failure in the supply of global public goods for health.

4.3.4 Power politics and double standards in WTO

Although WTO is a functional organisation, it is still gripped by the power politics. This power politics is manifested in their decision-making power and in issue linkage power. "In contemporary WTO practice, weak governments are often marginalized in WTO decision-making" (Charnovitz, 2005, p. 950). Under the WTO framework, developed countries led by the United States first use strong decision-making power to fix their intellectual property rights for pharmaceutical products and then apply issue linkage power to threaten any country that might resort to such flexibilities as compulsory licensing or parallel import for promoting accessibility and affordability of medicines. As it is pointed out, "compulsory licensing under the TRIPS Agreement was intended as a lifeline. But, in practice, any country reaching for this lifeline has been handcuffed by United States trade negotiators" (Vick, 1999, p. A1). Robert Keohane believed that international regimes would be of effect only when the needs of those countries that

Table 4.2 World Pharmaceutical Market by Region or Country (Unit: US$1 billion)

Region/country	2004	2005	Global sales share in 2005 (%)
North America	249	268.8	44.4
Europe	169.2	180.4	29.8
Japan	66.1	69.3	11.4
Oceania	7.1	7.7	1.3
CIS	4.2	5.0	0.8
Southeast Asia	25.3	28.8	4.6
Latin America	24.4	26.6	4.4
Indian subcontinent	6.6	7.2	1.2
Africa	6.3	6.7	1.1
The Middle East	4.7	4.9	0.8
World total sales	562.9	605.4	100.0

Source: WHO, Public Health, Innovation and Intellectual Property Rights, *Report of the Commission on Intellectual Property Rights, Innovation and Public Health*, Geneva, WHO, 2006, p. 28.

128 *WTO and global health governance*

are both willing and able to provide international regulations and decision-making processes are met (Keohane, 1982). Similarly, when these regulations are not in line with their interests, compliance issues are quickly cast aside. As an international regime, WTO is designed to protect the interests and meet the needs of the major players that have formulated its norms in the first place. There is no doubt that Western developed countries have a dominant influence on WTO. It is common for them to apply double standards in their compliance with WTO norms. Nowhere are such double standards more apparent than in the practice of the compulsory licensing of pharmaceutical patents in the TRIPS Agreement. But such practice will in no way help the implementation of loopholes intended to improve the accessibility of medicines, thereby negatively affecting global health governance.

In view of WTO's structural flaws and contradictions in global health governance, "it would thus be Pollyanna-ish to expect WTO policies and jurisprudence to align perfectly with the goal of promoting health" (Bloche & Jungman, 2007, p. 253). This also has important implications for China's health governance. China has the world's largest number of hepatitis B patients. Infectious diseases such as tuberculosis and HIV/AIDS are also on the rise. As a large country accounting for one-fifth of the world's population, China's effective health governance is a huge contribution the country makes to global health governance.

First, China should speed up relevant legislation to provide a more solid legal foundation for the enforcement of "compulsory licensing". Article 50 of the new Patent Law of the People's Republic of China formally implemented on October 1, 2009, stipulates that to enhance public health, the Patent Administration Department of the State Council may enforce compulsory license for patent rights on foreign patented medicines. However, this law does not specify the circumstances under which compulsory licenses should be issued. China should, through proper legislation, set a quantifiable implementation standard for using compulsory license and use patented medicines of the broadest impact to China as a benchmark. In the event of an epidemic, China should not hesitate to enforce compulsory license for foreign patented medicines to break the drug monopoly of foreign pharmaceutical companies, thereby lowering the price of these medicines and promoting the accessibility of such medicines. Taking hepatitis B as an example, as many as 120 million people are living with hepatitis B in China, making the disease as much a medical issue as a social one. A key medicine to treat hepatitis B is lamivudine produced by the pharmaceutical giant GlaxoSmithKline. Although China is the largest exporter of the active pharmaceutical ingredients for lamivudine, due to patent protection that restricts domestic companies from producing lamivudine-finished medicines, Chinese hepatitis B patients still have to bear prohibitive treatment expenses. A grant in China for a compulsory license for lamivudine would vastly increase accessibility to this drug.

Second, China should use issue linkage power and be more proactive in using flexibility measures such as compulsory license and parallel import. Despite the severity of the public health burden caused by infectious diseases such as hepatitis B and tuberculosis, China to date has never issued any compulsory license for related medicines, probably due to fears of potential trade retaliation and the subsequent impact on international relations. Given the interdependence between China and developed countries in economy and its own strong economic strength, China should be brave to tap into its issue linkage power and grant compulsory licenses when necessary.

Finally, public health is at its core a public good, of which government should be the main supplier. The privatisation approach advocated by WTO is bound to cause market failure in public health, making organisations and agents engaged in public health more profit-driven rather than service-driven and leading to a serious undersupply of public goods. Therefore, any reform of China's public health system should steer clear of the privatisation approach. In terms of supply of necessary medicines, China might consider setting up a national fund to incentivise research on medicine for diseases that may be of wide influence. In return, pharmaceutical companies should shorten the duration of patent protection or supply the market with lower-priced patented medicines.

Summary

World trade issues and global health have been intimately connected with each other for decades. As the most important international trade regime, WTO inevitably has a significant impact on global health governance. Under the influence of its free trade doctrine, WTO has not put the solution to global health issues on the top of its agenda. Moreover, WTO agreements have aggravated global health situations to a certain extent. Dominated by developed countries, WTO has been designed first to satisfy the economic interests of developed countries instead of serving the global public interest. The effective supply of public goods is determined by the publicness in decision-making and in the distribution of benefits. In terms of WTO's decision-making on public health, most developing countries are at a disadvantage and therefore cannot make their demand for public health benefits heard. In other words, WTO is unable to achieve publicness in decision-making and in the distribution of benefits. Due to the lack of such publicness, WTO can only provide club goods for developed countries, not public goods for the whole world. Led by the United States, developed countries want to solidify their economic interests in the form of international law under the WTO framework while at the same time marginalise the public health interests of developing countries. Given the interdependence in global health security, both developed and developing countries are stakeholders in global health security, and public health crises in developing countries will inevitably generate negative externalities in the global dimension. Therefore, WTO can only play its due role in global health governance if it both takes developing countries' public health interests into account when making relevant norms and manages to provide global public goods for health rather than the club goods for developed countries. Every piece of legislation is a tool to realise public interest. Therefore, China should be more proactive to use WTO's flexibility provisions to promote access to medicines. This in itself is a contribution to global health governance.

130 *WTO and global health governance*

Notes

1 See the World Trade Organization website. Retrieved from www.wto.org/.
2 World Trade Organization, *Declaration on the TRIPS Agreement and Public Health*, November 9–14, 2001. Retrieved from www.who.int/medicines/areas/policy/tripshealth.pdf.
3 World trade services are classified into 12 categories with more than 160 pieces of content. These service categories include 1) commercial services, 2) communication services, 3) construction services, 4) sales services, 5) education services, 6) environmental services, 7) financial services, 8) health and social services, 9) tourism and related services, 10) culture, entertainment and sports services, 11) transportation services and 12) other services. See the *General Agreement on Trade in Services*. Retrieved from www.wto.org/english/docs_e/legal_e/26-gats.pdf.
4 The term "market fundamentalism" originally appeared in the book *The Crisis of Global Capitalism* by American financial tycoon George Soros, and it means faith in free markets and free trade.
5 For example, American economists Levin and Nelson found in a classic study that companies from 130 industries all pointed out in a report that patent rights are the least important means of protecting the competitive advantage of new products. See also Levin et al. (1987), Levin (1986).

References

Bloche, M. G., & Jungman, E. R. (2007). Health Policy and the World Trade Organization. In I. Kawachi & S. Wamala (Eds.), *Globalization and Health*. Oxford: Oxford University Press.

Charnovitz, S. (2000). The Supervision of Health and Bio-Safety Regulation by World Trade Rules. *Tulane Environmental Law Journal* (271), 13.

Charnovitz, S. (2005). Transparency and Participation in the World Trade Organization. *Rutgers Law Review*, 56(4), 950.

Chen, J. (2003). *The Role of International Institutional Institutions in Globalization*. Northampton: Edward Elgar Publishing, Inc.

Cheng, D. (2001, November 22). Drug Disputes between Brazil and the United States: Concerns over Intellectual Property Rights and Public Health. *Economic Daily*.

Commission on Intellectual Property Rights. (n.d.). *Integrating Intellectual Property Rights and Development Policy*, p. v. Retrieved from www.iprcommission.org/papers/pdfs/final_report/CIPRfullfinal.pdf

Commission on Macroeconomics and Health. (2001). *Macroeconomics and Health: Investing in Health for Economic Development*. Geneva: WHO.

Drager, N., & Beaglehole, R. (2001). Globalization: Changing the Public Health Landscape. *Bulletin of the World Health Organization*, 79(9), 803.

Dollar, D. (2001). Is Globalization Good for Your Health? *Bulletin of the World Health Organization*, 79(9), 827–833.

Feachem, R. (2001). Globalization Is Good for Your Health, Mostly. *British Medical Journal* (323), 504–506.

Feng, J. (2005). *Public Health Crisis and Reform of WTO Intellectual Property System-Focusing on the TRIPS Agreement*. Wuhan: Wuhan University Press.

Fidler, D. P. (2003). Emerging Trends in International Law Concerning Global Infectious Disease Control. *Emerging Infectious Diseases*, 9(3), 285.

Global Forum for Health Research. (2004). *Monitoring Financial Flows for Health Research*. Geneva: WHO.

WTO and global health governance 131

Gong, X. (2006). Infectious Disease Control from the Perspective of International Law (Unpublished doctoral dissertation). Wuhan: Wuhan University.

Hardin, G. (1968). The Tragedy of the Commons. *Science* (162), 1243–1248.

He, X. (2004). Analysis of the "Paragraph 6" of the WTO Doha Declaration. *Law Review* (6), 107.

Heller, M. A., & Eisenberg, R. S. (1998). Can Patents Deter Innovation? The Anticommons in Biomedical Research. *Science*, 280, 698.

Hilary, J. (2001). *The Wrong Model: GATS, Trade Liberalization and Children's Rights to Health*. London, England: Save the Children.

Howard-Jones, N. (1975). *The Scientific Background of the International Sanitary Conferences 1851–1938*. Geneva: WHO.

Jamison, D. T., Frenk, J., & Knaul, F. (1998). International Collective Action in Health: Functions, and Rationale. *The Lancet* (351), 514.

Jewkes, J., Sawyers, D., & Stillerman, R. (1971). *The Source of Invention*. New York: Norton & Company.

Kaul, I., et al. (Eds.). (2003). *Providing Global Public Goods: Managing Globalization*. Oxford: Oxford University Press.

Keohane, R. (1982). The Demand for International Regimes. *International Organization*, 36(2), 332–355.

Koivusalo, M. (2002). Assessing the Health Policy Implications of WTO Trade and Investment Agreements. In Kelley Lee (Ed.), *Health Impacts of Globalization: Towards Global Governance*, London: Palgrave Macmillan.

Labonte, R., & Schrecker, T. (2004). Committed to Health for All? How the G7/G8 Rate. *Social Science and Medicine*, 59(8), 1661–1676.

Levin, R. C. (1986). A New Look at the Patent System. *American Economic Review*, 199(76).

Levin, R. C., Klevorick, A. K., Nelson, R., & Winter, S. (1987). Appropriating the Returns from Industrial R&D. *Brookings Papers on Economic Activity*, 783.

Lewis, S. (2003). *Mass Murder by Complacency*. Retrieved from https://cicd-volunteerin-africa.org/fighting-with-the-poor/mass-murder-by-complacency

Machlup, F., & Penrose, E. (1950). The Patent Controversy in the Nineteenth Century. *The Journal of Economic History*, 10(1), 24.

Merck. (2003). Supporting China's AIDS Control. *China WTO Tribune*, 2003(2), 42.

Meri, K. (2002). Assessing the Health Policy Implications of WTO Trade and Investment Agreements. In K. Lee (Ed.), *Health Impacts of Globalization: Towards Global Governance*. New York: Palgrave Macmillan, p. 175.

Orbinski, J., & Burciul, B. (2006). Moving beyond Charity for R&D for Neglected Diseases. In J. Clare, P. Illingworth, U. Schuklenk, & A. Arbor (Eds.), *The Power of Pills: Social, Ethical, and Legal Issues in Drug Development, Marketing & Pricing*. London: Pluto Press.

Oxfam. (2001, February). *Patent Injustice: How World Trade Rules Threaten the Health of Poor People*. Retrieved from www.oxfam.org.uk/cutthecost/patent.pdf

Panitchpakdi, S. (2003). *Speech on the Fifth Session Ministerial Conference*. Retrieved from www.wto.org/english/news_e/pres03_e/pr350_e.htm

Samuelson, P., & Nordhaus, W. (2003). *Economics* (X. Chen, Trans.). Beijing: Posts & Telecom Press.

Sexton, S. (n.d.). *GATS, Privatization and Health*. Retrieved from www.thecornerhouse.org.uk/itemshtml?x=52188

Shaffer, E. R. (2005). Global Trade and Public Health. *American Journal of Public Health*, 95(1), 23–33.

132 *WTO and global health governance*

Thurow, L. C. (1997, September–October). Needed: A New System of Intellectual Property Rights. *Harvard Business Review*, 103.

Trouiller, P., & Olliaro, P. (2002). Drug Development for Neglected Diseases: A Deficient Market and a Public Health Policy Failure. *The Lancet*, 359, 2189.

UN Committee on Economic, Social and Cultural Rights. (2000, August 11). *CESCR General Comment 14, the Right to the Highest Attainable Standard of Health.* Retrieved from www.refworld.org/docid/4538838d0.html

United Nations. (n.d.). *United Nations Millennium Declaration.* Retrieved from https://www.un.org/en/ga/president/55/pdf/priorities/millenniumsummit.pdf

Vick, K. (1999, December 4). African AIDS Victims Losers of a Drug War: US Policy Keeps Prices Prohibitive. *Washington Post*, p. A1.

WHO. (2006). *Public Health, Innovation and Intellectual Property Rights, Report of the Commission on Intellectual Property Rights, Innovation and Public Health.* Geneva: WHO.

WHO & WTO. (2002). *WTO Agreement & Public Health: A Joint Study by the WHO and WTO Secretariat.* Geneva: WHO.

Williams, O. (2004). The WTO, Trade Rules and Global Health Security. In A. Ingram (Ed.), *Health, Foreign Policy & Security.* London: The Nuffield Trust.

Wilson, C. A. D. (2005). The TRIPS Agreement: Is It Beneficial to the Developing World, or Simply a Tool Used to Protect Pharmaceutical Profits for Developed World Manufactures? *Journal of Technology Law & Policy*, 10, 248.

WTO. (2001, November 14). Declaration on the TRIPS Agreement and Public Health. WT/MIN(01)DEC/2. Retrieved from www.who.int/medicines/areas/policy/tripshealth.pdf

WTO. (n.d.a). *Declaration on the TRIPS Agreement and Public Health.* Retrieved from www.who.int/medicines/areas/policy/tripshealth.pdf

WTO. (n.d.b). *Para. 6 of Declaration on the TRIPS Agreement and Public Health.* Retrieved from www.who.int/medicines/areas/policy/tripshealth.pdf

WTO and WHO, WTO Agreements & Public Health: A Joint Study by the WHO and the WTO Secretariat, Geneva: WHO, 2002.

Zhuang, Z., & Du, J. (2003). *Theoretical and Empirical Analysis of Intellectual Property Protection in Developing Countries.* Wuhan: Wuhan University (Social Science Edition), No. 4.

5 International human rights regimes and global health governance

> It is my aspiration that health will finally be seen not as a blessing to be wished for, but as a human right to be fought for.
>
> —Kofi Annan[1]

As Louis Henkin put it: "Ours is the age of rights; Human rights is the idea of our time, the only political-moral idea that has received universal acceptance" (Henkin, 1990, p. v). Notwithstanding the exaggeration, this quote illustrates how deeply ingrained human rights are in our minds. The universal acknowledgement of human rights means they have not only been accepted by all societies and governments in principle as well as in rhetoric but also incorporated in national constitution and legislation. But human rights should not be enshrined by domestic political and legal systems only. The international community should also shoulder the obligation to internationalise and institutionalise human rights. Since the end of World War II, the international community has adopted a series of international instruments, such as the Universal Declaration of Human Rights and the International Covenant on Civil and Political Right. Together they constitute international human rights regimes. These human rights regimes have been playing an increasingly important role in the field of international relations and in turn have received more attention from the international community. The reorganisation of the UN Commission on Human Rights into the Human Rights Council at the 60th session of the General Assembly in 2006 is just one example of their growing prominence.[2]

Human rights provide a basis for addressing societal and global problems through active participation, increased transparency and accountability. Therefore, it is not only feasible but also necessary to solve global health issues from the perspective of human rights. Many of the current international human rights regimes, including the Universal Declaration of Human Rights, the International Covenant on Economic, Social and Cultural Rights and the United Nations Convention on the Rights of the Child, have all directly or indirectly addressed public health issues. Moreover, the introduction of the right to health into international human rights regimes has not only obliged governments to provide health services and protect the health of their citizens, but also clarified their responsibilities to

134 *International human rights regimes*

promote the health of their citizens. Examining global health issues from the perspective of human rights marks the return to human-centred thinking. The human rights-based approach for global health governance also illustrates a human-based worldview. In short, human rights protection and health promotion complement and mutually reinforce each other.

5.1 Development of international human rights regimes and their links with public health

Despite its long historical presence, not until the end of World War II was "human rights" adopted as a term in International Relations Studies. Moreover, it was not until the founding of the United Nations that the international community started to pay attention to human rights. Although human rights cannot "unify the world" or shift policy directions in contemporary international relations, it nevertheless affects a country's foreign policy and international relations. As a nascent field in International Relations Studies, global health governance is also subject to this influence. As J. M. Mann, a public health expert from Harvard University, once put it, "we are creating, participating in and witnessing an extraordinary moment in social history—the emergence of a health and human rights movement—at the intersection and at the time of two enormous paradigm shifts" (1997, p. 113).

5.1.1 *Historical background to the development of international human rights regimes*

In the 17th century, the "rights of man" was understood as the rights of individuals to confront each other or the government in whose jurisdiction they lived. In 1776, the 13 colonies in North America jointly adopted the United States Declaration of Independence, a document Karl Marx referred to as the first declaration of human rights. The Declaration explicitly states that "all men are created equal" and are "endowed by their Creator with certain unalienable Rights, that among these are Life, Liberty and the Pursuit of Happiness". However, it was not until the appearance of the 1789 French Declaration of the Rights of Man and of the Citizen that "human rights" was explicitly proposed in an institutional instrument in the modern history. Nevertheless, in those days, human rights issues were treated as domestic concerns and rarely captured international attention.

Before World War II, "human rights were rarely discussed in international politics" (Donnelly, 1997, p. 3). As Davidson (1993) observed:

> The International concern with human rights is a phenomenon or comparatively recent origin. Although it is possible to point to a number of treaties or international agreements affecting humanitarian issues before the Second World War, it is only with the entry into force of the United Nations Charter in 1945, that it is possible to speak of the advent of systematic human rights protection within the international system.

(p. 1)

Notwithstanding the truth of this observation, some human rights issues had already found their way into international agreements and regimes in the early 20th century. For example, the 1926 Convention to Suppress the Slave Trade and Slavery addressed the slave trade, the International Labour Organization began to concern itself with workers' rights after World War I and the protection of ethnic minorities in certain regions became a focus of the League of Nations. The Declaration by United Nations, signed in Washington, DC, on January 1, 1942, is the first international instrument that brought human rights issues to the fore. It proclaimed that "being convinced that complete victory over their enemies is essential to defend life, liberty, independence and religious freedom, and to preserve human rights and justice in their own lands as well as in other lands" (Li & Wan, 1992, p. 177). After World War II, although national governments had different political stances on human rights, avocation for human rights in the international community was so popular that the construction of international human rights regimes had become an irresistible historical trend. By legalising and institutionalising human rights issues on a global scale, the UN played an indispensable role in constructing international human rights regimes. From the beginning, the UN was destined to be a human rights institution. The UN Charter, signed on June 26, 1945, states in its preamble that "we the peoples of the United nations are determined to reaffirm faith in fundamental human rights, in the dignity and worth of the human person, in the equal rights of men and women and of nations large and small". Two of the purposes of the UN are directly related to human rights: One is to "develop friendly relations among nations based on respect for the principle of equal rights and self-determination of peoples". The other is to "promote and encourage respect for human rights and for fundamental freedoms for all".

5.1.2 Development phases of international human rights regimes

As for the historical development of human rights, the best known—albeit rather contentious—theory is "three generations of human rights", presented by Karel Vasak, a former legal adviser to the United Nations Educational, Scientific and Cultural Organization (UNESCO). It consists of the following views: 1) The first generation of human rights was formed during the American War of Independence and the French revolution. This view sought to uphold people's freedoms and protect people from intrusions by their states. It fundamentally reflected citizens' civil and political rights as those enshrined in the International Bill of Rights. Such rights are portrayed as negative rights because they signalled constraints on the power of the state. 2) The second-generation view took shape during the Russian Revolution and was closely aligned with the concept of welfare in Western nations. They are known as positive rights because they are fundamentally economic, social and cultural in nature, and they call upon governments to respect, promote and fulfil these rights. 3) The third generation of human rights, as Vasak held, is a response to global interdependence. States can no longer singlehandedly fulfil their international obligations on human rights; Instead, they must work together to address a spectrum of common issues, including

136   *International human rights regimes*

peacekeeping, environmental protection and development. Swiss jurist Harro von Senger (1993), on the other hand, focuses on the "human" component of human rights and states that the theory of "three generations of human rights" advanced by Vasak is an example of the Western approach in which the development of the "right" component is overstressed. He believes that in the history of human rights, there are "two periods of rights", with the Universal Declaration of Human Rights adopted on December 10, 1948, serving as the turning point of the two. The first period (before 1948) is known as the period of non-universal human rights, or a period marked by the bestialization of non-European people. During this time, human rights and freedoms were conferred with distinction to race and colour. For example, women, indigenous peoples, coloured individuals and slaves were excluded from the scope of the adjective "human". The second period (since 1948) is the period of universal human rights, during which the word "human" evolved from the abstract and general to the concrete and eventually the universal (p. 253). Meanwhile, the division of human rights proposed by Norberto Bobbio, an Italian political philosopher, also has bearing on this discussion. Bobbio (1996) traced the evolution of human rights through three significant stages. The first stage can be traced to the earliest reflections in philosophical theories and writings. The second stage witnessed the transition from theory to practice, from the recognition of human rights to their implementation. As a result, the generality of human rights gave way to the concreteness of human rights. The Universal Declaration of Human Rights in 1948 heralded the beginning of the third stage, during which time human rights became both universal and concrete (pp. 15–16). Although these scholars have tried in different ways to signpost the evolution of human rights, they have failed to explain the formation of international human rights regimes. In light of their universality, the founding of the United Nations in 1945 may be viewed as a starting point for international human rights regimes to take shape. To date, we observe the following three phases.

The first phase witnessed the creation and initial development of international human rights regimes, marked by the adoption of the UN Charter and the Universal Declaration of Human Rights. Although the UN Charter is not an international instrument dedicated to human rights, it starts with a clear statement in the preamble of its goal to safeguard human rights. This sets the tone for the fundamental purposes and goals for international human rights regimes. Article 1(3) of the Charter clearly states that "promoting and encouraging respect for human rights and for fundamental freedoms for all" is one of the purposes of the United Nations. The Universal Declaration of Human Rights, adopted at the UN General Assembly in October 1948, further promoted the development of modern international human rights regimes. It is not a legally binding agreement between countries around the world, but according to Cassese (2001):

> The *Declaration* remains a lodestar, which has guided the community of States as they gradually emerged from the Dark Age when the possession of armies, guns, and warships was the sole factor for judging the conduct

of States, and there were no generally accepted principles for distinguishing good from evil in the world community.

(pp. 358–359)

Article 28 of the Declaration states that "everyone is entitled to a social and international order in which the rights and freedoms set forth in this Declaration can be fully realized". Article 30 states that:

> Nothing in this *Declaration* may be interpreted as implying for any State, group or person any right to engage in any activity or to perform any act aimed at the destruction of any of the rights and freedoms set forth herein.[3]

As the first international instrument on human rights, the Universal Declaration of Human Rights laid the foundation for the practice of human rights protection in the international community. Its principles have also been reiterated on various international occasions, such as the 1968 World Conference on Human Rights held in Tehran and the 1993 conference held in Vienna, and in both occasions universal respect for the Declaration was advocated.

The second phase saw the formalisation of international human rights regimes, marked by the adoption of the International Covenant on Civil and Political Rights (ICCPR) and the International Covenant on Economic, Social and Cultural Rights (ICESCR). After a long period of development, the idea of institutionalising human rights with joint efforts of the international community gained popularity. No longer dominated by Western pre-conceptions, international standards for human rights protection have borne greater universality and are increasingly recognised and accepted by the vast majority of countries. On the one hand, the Universal Declaration of Human Rights embodies the spirit and values for the ICCPR and the ICESCR; on the other hand, the latter two covenants further substantiate, universalise and legalise the "human rights" listed in the Universal Declaration of Human Rights. During the second phase, several human rights issues were addressed from the perspective of international regimes, and "international human rights, thus, have become constitutive elements of a modern and 'civilized' statehood" (Risse & Ropp, 1999, p. 234). The ICCPR is the embodiment of the human rights of the first generation. The Western liberal concept of human rights is reflected in the constitutions of almost all the contemporary countries as well as most of the international declarations and covenants adopted after World War II. The ICESCR covers the human rights stated in Articles 22–27 of the Universal Declaration of Human Rights, all of which are human rights of the second generation.[4] Denoting rights to, rather than freedom from, the second generation of human rights include the right to social security, the right to work, the right to education, the right to health, etc. They are interpreted as the benefits governments are responsible for; in other words, society has an obligation to provide public goods, such as social services, health care and education. In short, during this phase, international human rights regimes were established, with the ICCPR and the ICESCR at their core.

138   *International human rights regimes*

The third phase witnessed the deepening of international human rights regimes, marked by the UN Declaration on the Right to Development and the founding of the UN Human Rights Council. Western countries emphasise civil and political rights over the economic, social and cultural rights. The protection of the latter depends on overall development level. In other words, only when developing countries have fully realised their potential for development can they better implement the ICESCR. However, the international economic order before the 1980s severely restricted the growth of developing countries. In 1977, to support the struggle for the establishment of a new international economic order, at the 33rd session of the UN Commission on Human Rights, developing countries proposed for the first time that the right to development should be established as a human right. In March 1981, the 37th session adopted a resolution to set up the Working Group of Governmental Experts on the Right to Development, the task of which was to study the scope and contents of the right to development as well as the most effective means to ensure its realisation. From 1981, the Working Group started to work on a draft of the Declaration on the Right to Development. After a long period of research and debate, the final Declaration was adopted by the General Assembly by Resolution 41/128 on December 4, 1986. The Declaration on the Right to Development declares the right to development as "an inalienable human right" and that "every human person and all peoples are entitled to participate in, contribute to and enjoy economic, social, cultural and political development". This Declaration also states that the right to development implies "the full realization of the right of peoples to self-determination" as well as "the exercise of their inalienable right to full sovereignty over all their natural wealth and resources". It emphasises that "effective international co-operation" is essential in promoting the faster development of developing countries. The recognition from the Declaration that development is a human right contributes to yet another major conceptual breakthrough that, together with self-determination, complements Western emphasis on individual rights. This recognition is also a follow-up action taken by developing countries to implement the ICESCR. The Declaration reflects developing countries' new understanding of human rights and these nations' appeal for the protection of human rights within each country. All these inject new ideas into the international human rights protection and constitute the core of "the third generation of human rights"—collective human rights.

The establishment of the UN Human Rights Council in 2006 is of epoch-making significance in international human rights regimes. In March 2005, in his report on reforms, *In Larger Freedom: Towards Development, Security and Human Rights for All*, the late UN Secretary-General Kofi Annan proposed that a human rights council be established. After a year of painstaking consultations, the General Assembly finally adopted Resolution 60/251 by voting, which set the basic framework for the UN Human Rights Council. The establishment of the Council shows that the international community had been closely following and attached greater importance to human rights issues than they did previously. Resolution 60/251 made it clear that "peace and security and human rights are interlinked and mutually reinforcing". It signalled that human rights, together with development and security would be henceforth listed as the "three pillars" of the UN system. It reaffirmed that "all human rights are universal, indivisible, interrelated, interdependent and mutually reinforcing, and that all human rights must be treated in a fair and equal manner, on the same footing and with the same emphasis". Given the importance of human rights, the Human Rights Council was no longer a subsidiary of the Economic and Social Council but rather was elevated to the status of a subsidiary organ of the General Assembly. In addition, the Human Rights Council set up a Universal Periodic Review mechanism that, based on equal treatment for all, would periodically review each member state's fulfilment of its human rights obligations and commitments. In short, the establishment of the Human Rights Council promoted the development of international human rights regimes, both in terms of the status of human rights and the measures taken to review the implementation of human rights in member states.

The aforementioned development phases of international human rights regimes are based simply on a rough division. It should be noted that the analysis of human rights based on "generations" need not imply a hierarchy therein. An earlier generation may not be more important, and a later generation need not be superior. According to the United Nations (2005), "persistent false distinctions between civil and political rights, and economic, social and cultural rights, and lack of understanding of the legal nature and content of economic, social and cultural rights have undermined effective action on economic, social and cultural rights" (p. viii). The three phases are progressive, indivisible, interdependent and mutually complementary. The two groups of rights, namely "civil and political rights and economic, social and cultural rights, should be put together rather than separated" (Scott, 1989, p. 851). These rights "form an interdependent and synergistically interactive system of guarantees, rather than a menu from which one may freely pick and choose" (Donnelly, 1986, p. 607). The indivisible relationship among human rights was clearly articulated and reaffirmed at the UN World Conference on Human Rights, held in Vienna[5] in 1993. In addition, in the development of international human rights regimes, the international community has also issued several declarations and covenants on human rights (see Table 5.1). Together they constitute the current institutional framework for the protection and promotion of international human rights.

5.1.3 The relationship between human rights and public health

Human rights and public health were once two distinct domains, the former belonging to the political and the latter to the medical. However, with the progress in the modern human rights movement and an expanded list of the determinants of public health, the two seemingly unrelated areas have become increasingly intertwined and mutually influencing (see Figure 5.1).

The structural links between health and human rights are emerging in ever wider areas. Changes in the discourse of "health and human rights" have revealed the unequivocal relationship between the two. Therefore, through conceptual, analytical, strategic and programmatic work, the two distinct areas can be linked

140 *International human rights regimes*

Table 5.1 Current Major International Declarations and Covenants on Human Rights (in chronological order)

No.	Title	Year
1	Convention Concerning Forced or Compulsory Labour	1930
2	UN Charter	1945
3	Convention on the Prevention and Punishment of the Crime of Genocide	1948
4	Universal Declaration of Human Rights	1949
5	Convention for the Suppression of the Traffic in Persons and of the Exploitation of the Prostitution of Others	1949
6	Geneva Convention (I) for the Amelioration of the Condition of the Wounded and Sick in Armed Forces in the Field	1949
7	Geneva Convention (II) on Wounded, Sick and Shipwrecked of Armed Forces at Sea, 1949 and its commentary	1949
8	Geneva Convention (III) on Prisoners of War	1949
9	Geneva Convention (IV) on Civilians	1949
10	Convention Relating to the Status of Refugees	1950
11	International Convention on the Elimination of All Forms of Racial Discrimination	1963
12	International Covenant on Civil and Political Rights	1966
13	International Covenant on Economic, Social and Cultural Rights	1966
14	Protocol Relating to the Status of Refugees	1967
15	Declaration on the Use of Scientific and Technological Progress in the Interests of Peace and for the Benefit of Mankind	1975
16	Declaration on the Rights of Disabled Persons	1975
17	Convention on the Elimination of All Forms of Discrimination Against Women	1979
18	Declaration on the Protection of All Persons from Being Subjected to Torture and Other Cruel, Inhuman or Degrading Treatment or Punishment	1984
19	Declaration on the Right to Development	1986
20	Convention on the Rights of the Child	1989
21	Indigenous and Tribal Peoples Convention	1989
22	International Convention on the Protection of the Rights of All Migrant Workers and Members of Their Families	1990
23	Principles for the Protection of Persons with Mental Illness and the Improvement of Mental Health Care	1991
24	United Nations Principles for Older Persons	1991
25	Declaration on the Rights of Persons Belonging to National or Ethnic, Religious and Linguistic Minorities	1992
26	Standard Rules on the Equalization of Opportunities for Persons with Disabilities	1993
27	Declaration on the Elimination of Violence against Women	1993
28	The Universal Declaration on the Human Genome and Human Rights	1997
29	Declaration on the Right and Responsibility of Individuals, Groups and Organs of Society to Promote and Protect Universally Recognized Human Rights and Fundamental Freedoms	1998
30	Guiding Principles on Internal Displacement	1998
31	Maternity Protection Convention	2000

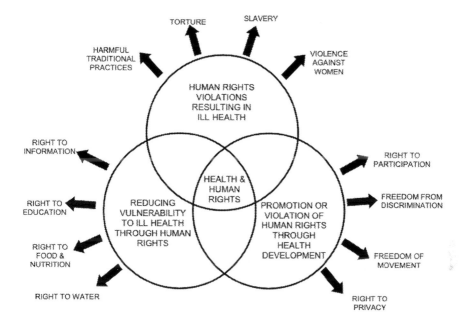

Figure 5.1 Linkages Between Human Rights and Public Health

and move forward together. In recent years, human rights have gradually become one of the focal points in studies regarding health and development issues. In fact, the level of explicit and institutional political commitment to health and human rights has never been stronger. This commitment manifests not only in the United Nations but also more importantly in governmental and non-governmental levels both domestically and internationally. Promoting and protecting health and respecting, protecting and fulfilling human rights are inextricably linked. The links between human rights and public health are best illustrated in the preamble to the Constitution of the World Health Organization, which states that "the enjoyment of the highest attainable standard of health is one of the fundamental rights of every human being without distinction of race, religion, political belief, economic or social condition" (WHO, 2020, p. 1). By implication, to violate civil rights on the bases of race, religion, political relief, gender and so forth is to render illusory the right to enjoy the highest attainable standard of health. Promotion and protection of human rights is "a prerequisite to health and wellbeing" (Gruskin et al., 2007, p. 452). Public health governance efforts which take human rights into account are more effective than those which ignore or violate such rights (Menon-Johansson, 2005).

The impact of human rights on public health can be construed positively and negatively. First, respecting and protecting human rights contribute to public health promotion. The protection of human rights is "the way to protect the public's health. The protection of a full range of human rights is the key to protecting

142 *International human rights regimes*

public health" (Jürgens & Cohen, 2007, p. 7). Governments have the responsibility to protect two groups of human rights: The first group comprises civil and political rights, including the right to life, freedom of information, freedom of movement, freedom of association, equality, freedom of speech and the right to participate. The second group consists of economic, social and cultural rights, including the right to education, development, the right to enjoy the benefits of scientific progress and its applications, the right to just and favourable conditions of work and the right to be free from hunger. Almost all these rights are closely related to public health. For example, rather than attempting to cover up the truth, a public health crisis can only be effectively managed if a government informs the public in a timely manner to ensure people's right to information. Further, if people's right to education is ensured and their general level of education is improved, they will be better equipped with public health knowledge and thus collectively improve public health conditions. The close link between human rights and public health is also reflected in the fight against HIV/AIDS. At the UN High Level Meeting on HIV/AIDS in 2006, world leaders reaffirmed that "the full realization of all human rights and fundamental freedoms for all is an essential element in the global response to the HIV/AIDS pandemic" (Jürgens & Cohen, 2007, p. 1). In short, human rights protection and public health governance share common goals. Human rights protection results in effective public health governance, and public health governance involves the protection of all types of human rights. Human rights "transcend almost every other right" (Gruskin et al., 2007, p. 450).

Second, human rights violations are not conducive to public health governance. Human rights violations "always have a negative impact on health" (Brundland G. H., 1998). Discrimination based on race, colour, gender, language, religion and so forth has exacerbated the situation in global health governance. Taking the global AIDS epidemic as an example, discrimination and human rights violations are not only the consequence of AIDS but also the cause of AIDS (Mann & Gruskin, 1999, p. 445). Violations of human rights have "exacerbated the AIDS epidemic" (Csete, 2004, p. 83). In the early 1990s, a UN special rapporteur on the prevention of discrimination against people with HIV/AIDS revealed that "discrimination against persons with HIV infection or AIDS remains widespread and occurs at all levels of society, including government, public and private institutions, and among individuals and communities" (Gostin & Lazzarini, 1997, p. 75). Despite other social roots of the human rights violations against people with HIV/AIDS, racial discrimination is the very reason behind the international community's inaction on the scourge of AIDS in Africa. As Peter Piot, then executive director of UNAIDS, put it when he was asked to comment on the international community's inaction on the AIDS epidemic in Africa, "if this would have happened in the Balkans, or in Eastern Europe, or in Mexico, with white people, the reaction would have been different" (Gellman, 2000, p. 5). Believing that health problems in Africa in the early 1990s were caused by overpopulation, the US government at the time insisted that AIDS-related deaths in Africa could lead to a decline in population, which in the end would be conducive to Africa's economic development

(Gellman, 2000). That this view is no longer popular is too little, too late. AIDS runs rampant in Africa and has triggered a global health crisis. Take the right to enjoy the benefits of scientific progress and its applications as another example: Since 2001, one of the key contributors to public health problems in developing countries, including AIDS, tuberculosis and malaria, are the high prices of medications brought by the TRIPS Agreement, preventing those who need treatment from obtaining affordable and effective medications. In the end, people's right to enjoy the benefits of scientific progress and its applications becomes a pipe dream, thereby further exacerbating global health crises.

If democracy is suppressed and human rights are ignored, it is impossible for citizens in any country to enjoy development and health. Respecting and protecting human rights will have a positive impact on public health promotion. The manner in which international human rights norms are implemented is bound to have a significant impact on global health governance (see Table 5.2). The integration of strategies on human rights in global health governance shows that establishing international human rights regimes has become the only viable approach for global health governance. Also described as a human rights–based approach, it has been increasingly used in global health governance. It has also been adopted by institutional actors in other international regimes. For example, the World Bank has incorporated health and human rights considerations in its regulations and rules pertaining to public health (World Bank, 1998). In 2006, the issue of health-related human rights was mentioned in the 11th Global Program of Work of the World Health Organization, demonstrating the importance WHO attaches to the relationship between health and human rights (WHO, 2006). The IHR (2005), which entered into force in 2007, also incorporates principles of human rights into the norms and standards used in health governance. For example, Article 32 of the IHR stipulates that "in implementing health measures under these Regulations, States Parties shall treat travellers with respect for their dignity, human rights and fundamental freedoms and minimize any discomfort or distress associated with such measures". Simplicity of language aside, the human rights provisions in the IHR bring into light the importance of human rights considerations in global health governance and further strengthen the link between health and human rights. The clarification and implementation of the human rights–based approach enable the concept of international human rights regimes to be applied to the area of global health governance and play in it an important role (see Table 5.2). The lack of attention to human rights in global health governance "is an omission that, if ignored, may be too high a price to pay" (Gruskin et al., 2007, p. S18).

5.2 ICCPR and ICESCR and their links with global health governance

The international community adopted The Universal Declaration of Human Rights after World War II in 1948. The Cold War loomed as the world set about making the Articles in this Declaration legally binding instruments, polarising

144   *International human rights regimes*

Table 5.2 Potential Impact of Major International Human Rights Regimes on Public Health

Major international human rights regimes	Time of its entry into force	A partial list of its potential impact on public health
Universal Declaration of Human Rights	1948	Everyone has the right to security in the event of sickness, disability or other lack of livelihood in circumstances beyond his control; patients with infectious diseases have the right to education.
International Covenant on Economic, Social and Cultural Rights	1976	Patients with infectious diseases and pathogen carriers have the right to work, the right to health, the right to an adequate standard of living, the right to education and the right to enjoy the benefits of scientific progress.
International Covenant on Civil and Political Rights	1976	Patients with infectious diseases and pathogen carriers have the right to liberty and security of person, the right to freedom of movement, the right to privacy, the right to freedom of association with others, the right to marry and the right to found a family.
International Convention on the Elimination of All Forms of Racial Discrimination	1969	Everyone, without distinction as to race, colour or national or ethnic origin, has the right to public health, medical care, social security and social services.
Convention on the Elimination of All Forms of Discrimination Against Women	1981	Discrimination against women increases the risk of getting infectious diseases, such as HIV/AIDS, and women's equal access to health care should be promoted.
Convention on the Rights of the Child	1990	AIDS orphans' rights.
Convention Against Torture and Other Cruel, Inhuman or Degrading Treatment or Punishment	1987	Patients with infectious diseases shall not be subjected to torture or to cruel, inhuman or degrading treatment or punishment. Inhuman treatment is not conducive to the control of infectious diseases.
Declaration on the Right to Development	1986	The vast majority of developing countries bear most of the burden of infectious diseases but lack the economic and technological resources needed to treat infectious diseases. The accessibility of essential medicines needs to be taken care of.
Declaration of Alma-Ata	1978	The people have the right and duty to participate individually and collectively in the planning and implementation of their health care. Health is a fundamental human right.

notions of human rights into two camps. The Western bloc argued that civil and political rights should take precedence, whereas economic and social rights were mere aspirations while the Eastern bloc, led by the Soviet Union, contended that rights to food, health and education should be of paramount importance, with civil and political rights of secondary consideration. However, as a matter of fact, "all human rights are universal, indivisible and interdependent and interrelated. The international community must treat human rights globally in a fair and equal manner, on the same footing and with the same emphasis".[6] It is true that there are huge divergences among different national and regional identities, as well as among different historical, cultural and religious backgrounds, but every country, regardless of its political, economic and cultural system, is obliged to promote and protect all human rights and freedoms. Therefore, in 1966, the international community created two different international covenants—the International Covenant on Civil and Political Rights (ICCPR) and the International Covenant on Economic, Social and Cultural Rights (ICESCR). Together, they have not only given substance to the 1948 Universal Declaration of Human Rights but have also laid the foundation for other international human rights instruments. As two mutually reinforcing drivers in international human rights regimes, they have exerted significant impact on global health governance.

5.2.1 The ICCPR and global health governance

Many of the rights governed in the ICCPR are connected to public health, including the right to freedom of information, the right to liberty and the right to privacy. The interaction between these human rights and public health governance has far-reaching implications for countries with respect to strategies for implementing human rights with a goal to better promote global health governance.

5.2.1.1 The right to freedom of information

The right to freedom of information, or the right to know, is the right of citizens to receive, seek and obtain the information held by the government. During the legislative campaign for information disclosure in the press in the 1940s, American scholar Kent Cooper coined the term "the right to know" and used it for the first time in a speech in 1945. In 1946, the UN General Assembly adopted the expression "freedom of information" in its Resolution 59, which declared it as a fundamental human right and emphasised that it is the key to all freedoms that the UN is committed to safeguarding. Article 19 of the Universal Declaration of Human Rights further reaffirms that "everyone has the freedom to seek, receive and impart information and ideas through any media".[7] Article 19(2) of the ICCPR stipulates that everyone shall have "the freedom to seek, receive and impart information and ideas of all kinds".[8] In a country based on the rule of law, the right to freedom of information is a self-explanatory right because citizens have a right to know what their representatives are doing and what they have done. This right can be secured

146　*International human rights regimes*

only when citizens have access to accurate and timely government information. The democratic deficit in governance will decrease only when informed citizenry takes part in any governance efforts. When the late US President Lyndon Johnson signed the Freedom of Information Act on July 4, 1966, he stressed in the accompanying statement that "a democracy works best when the people have all the information that the security of the Nation permits". Amartya Sen (1999), the winner of the 1998 Nobel Prize in Economics, also pointed out that accurate public information can not only provide officials with impetus to resolve crises, but also reveal whether the measures they have taken are sufficient enough. Therefore, in public health governance, governments should protect and not interfere with an individual's right to obtain information on public health crises. Moreover, they have an obligation to inform their citizens of the truth about public health issues. They must keep the public informed about outbreaks of infectious diseases or other public health crises. UNDP (2000) believes that "information and statistics are a powerful tool for creating a culture of accountability and for realizing human rights" (p. 10). A government hesitant to disclose or which even deliberately holds back information pertaining to public health problems from its citizens is an irresponsible government. Such irresponsible behaviour will only spawn rumours unconducive to finding effective solutions to public health problems. What happened in the SARS outbreak shows that the violation of the right to freedom of information will inevitably lead to the violation of a series of other fundamental rights. To guarantee people's access to adequate information is an indispensable part of global health governance. Information on health policies and resources are essential to the monitoring of public health policies and citizens' participation in the process of policymaking.

5.2.1.2　*The right to freedom of association with others*

In *Democracy in America*, Tocqueville (1996) wrote:

> Among the laws that govern human societies, there is one that seems more definitive and clearer than all the others. For men to remain civilized or to become so, the art of associating must become developed among them and be perfected in the same proportion as equality of conditions grows.
>
> (p. 640)

Association is a natural human tendency. People usually follow a certain sequence of steps to solve a problem, from working on the problem on their own to seeking help from their families then to forming or participating in groups and to setting up formal organisations. Civil societies organised on the freedom of association with others have a more solid moral foundation than formal public organisations. Article 20(1) of the Universal Declaration of Human Rights stipulates that "everyone has the right to freedom of peaceful assembly and association".[9] Article 22(1) of the ICCPR stipulates that "everyone shall have the right to freedom of association with others, including the right to form and join trade unions for the protection of

International human rights regimes 147

his interests; No restrictions may be placed on the exercise of this right".[10] Regarding the right to freedom of association with others, a government's obligation to its citizens comprise two types: On the one hand, this government has a negative obligation that is, the government is obliged to allow its citizens' association-based activities and to recognise their ability to act on their own as well as their way of arranging their lives by associating. On the other hand, this government also has a positive obligation; that is, this government shall protect its citizens' freedom of association and regulate association-based activities through a series of institutional arrangements. Positive obligations can further take several forms. The government may make laws to safeguard citizens' freedom of association, it may formulate related fiscal and tax policies to support the development of non-profit organisations or it may provide a participation channel for associations and other types of NGOs to contribute to politics and social governance. Setting up a non-governmental public health organisation is a typical example of the right to freedom of association with others. NGOs can play an irreplaceable role in the current global health governance, especially in areas such as notification of outbreaks, testing, medical technical assistance, response planning and public health agenda setting. Governments shall not interfere with or limit such rights of their citizens. Likewise, by restricting people's personal freedom, mandatory quarantines or compulsory supervision on patients with infectious diseases and pathogen carriers often stop them from enjoying the right to freedom of association with others. In addition, some governments often use various excuses to ban or suppress organisations founded by people who share a similar history of infectious diseases, and by their supporters and sympathisers, as a way to express their views and safeguard their interests, such as AIDS organisations. At the 2007 World Economic Forum in Dalian, China, Peter Piot, former executive director of UNAIDS, stressed the importance of NGOs in public health governance and argued that no country in the world could successfully stop AIDS without allowing civil society to play its role.

5.2.1.3 The right to freedom of movement

Article 13(1) of the Universal Declaration of Human Rights stipulates that "everyone has the right to freedom of movement and residence within the borders of each state".[11] Article 12(1, 2, 4) of the ICCPR also stipulates that:

> Everyone lawfully within the territory of a State shall, within that territory, have the right to liberty of movement and freedom to choose his residence; Everyone shall be free to leave any country, including his own; No one shall be arbitrarily deprived of the right to enter his own country.[12]

In other words, a government shall not restrict citizens' freedom of movement on the grounds of their health conditions. But restrictions on personal freedom of patients with infectious diseases are extremely common. For example, in Germany, a federal judge once claimed that it was necessary to place patients living with HIV in isolation (Garrett, 1997). In the decade after HIV/AIDS was first

148 *International human rights regimes*

identified, 104 countries adopted various types of restrictive laws in relation to the disease. When HIV testing made it possible to identify carriers of the disease, the number of such laws soared (Mann et al., 1992). As a result, many patients who are most in need of AIDS-related services and information are afraid to disclose their health conditions for fear of being isolated or having their personal freedom restricted, which in the end increases the possibility of further spread of the epidemic. More controversially, many countries around the world have restricted foreign patients with infectious diseases from entering their countries. If we continue to use HIV/AIDS as an example, many countries, including the United States, have adopted similar bans prohibiting people with HIV infections from entering their countries, hoping to keep AIDS outside their borders. However, these restrictions have proved to be both futile and counterproductive. Just like what Gostin and Lazzarini (1997) once pointed out, such restrictions treat people differently based solely on their health status, "offend the non-discrimination principles", may "interfere with international cooperation" on infectious disease control, often "lead other countries to retaliate with their own limitations" and "substantially affect a broad scope of human endeavours" such as "family unity" (e.g. husband and wife are not living in the same country) and "access to specialized health care" (e.g. patients travel abroad for treatment) (p. 87).

Nevertheless, not all restrictions on the free movement of individuals due to public health concerns are on equal grounding of legitimacy. Quarantines and isolations intended to cope with serious infectious diseases (e.g. Ebola, SARS) may have interfered with peoples' right to freedom of movement, but these measures are viewed as lawful based on international human rights instruments because they are taken essentially to protect the public good. By contrast, if a country restricts the right to freedom of movement of people with HIV/AIDS on the grounds of protecting national security or maintaining public order, the legitimacy of such restriction is debatable.

5.2.1.4 *The right to liberty*

Article 3 of the Universal Declaration of Human Rights stipulates that "everyone has the right to life, liberty and security of person".[13] Article 9(1) of the ICCPR stipulates that "everyone has the right to liberty and security of person; No one shall be subjected to arbitrary arrest or detention".[14] But in these two articles, the right to liberty are not stated as an absolute right, which means that when personal liberty clashes with emergency measures taken in a public health crisis, personal liberty can be somewhat restricted according to related provisions of laws. For example, in *Jacobson v. Massachusetts* in the United States in 1905, Jacobson argued that mandatory government sanitation measures, specifically mandatory smallpox vaccinations, had violated his constitutional right to liberty and security. The US Supreme Court held that mandatory vaccinations did not violate Jacobson's right to liberty, because the liberty enshrined in the US Constitution was not stated as an absolute right for each person at all times and in all circumstances. "There are manifold restraints to which every person is necessarily subject for the common good. The public interest in preventing smallpox out- weighed Jacobson's

International human rights regimes   149

individual rights" (Fidler, 1999, p. 172). For infectious diseases that can spread quickly and easily from person to person, countries around the world have more or less taken similar measures to quarantine patients and restrict their personal liberty. For example, patients with suspected SARS infections were subjected to mandatory quarantines for medical observation. However, concerns do arise over whether other kinds of public health measures imposed on citizens violate their right to liberty, such as compulsory medical treatment, physical examinations and premarital check-ups. Take containment of AIDS as an example: When a government uses public health security as an excuse to impose isolations on people with HIV/AIDS and to restrict their personal liberty, such restrictions are not justified. It is recommended in *HIV/AIDS and Human Rights: International Guidelines* released by the Office of the High Commissioner for Human Rights and UNAIDS (2006) that HIV testing of individuals should be performed with the specific informed consent of that individual, and "exceptions to voluntary testing would need specific judicial authorization, granted only after due evaluation of the important considerations involved in terms of privacy and liberty". In short, in public health governance, a public health measure should not only be based on the scientific principles of public health governance but also take people's right to liberty into consideration.

5.2.1.5 The right to equality

Equality and non-discrimination are essential to citizens' access to healthy life. Although citizens' access to healthy life is affected by the quality of health care and levels of economic development, national public health policies must reflect the "equality of opportunity"; that is, a country must build a society in which the value of life is recognised and respected, and all patients have access to treatment as a manifestation of social justice. This is the reason why the principle of non-discrimination in health protection is explicitly affirmed in almost all international covenants. The right to equality is the central theme characterising the ICCPR, of which Article 26 stipulates that:

> All persons are equal before the law and are entitled without any discrimination to the equal protection of the law. In this respect, the law shall prohibit any discrimination and guarantee to all persons equal and effective protection against discrimination on any ground such as race, colour, sex, language, religion, political or other opinion, national or social origin, property, birth or other status.[15]

Equality is the key to the protection and realisation of human rights. Although the ICCPR does not explicitly state that citizens should not be denied the right to equality based on their health status, the term "or other status" in Article 26 indicates that citizens' health status must not be used to justify discrimination. It was pointed out by the UN Commission on Human Rights (1995) that:

> Discrimination on the basis of AIDS or HIV status, actual or presumed, is prohibited by existing international human rights standards and that the

150 *International human rights regimes*

term "or other status" in non-discrimination provisions in international human rights texts can be interpreted to cover health status, including HIV/AIDS.

5.2.2 The ICESCR and global health governance

In view of the significant correlation between public health governance and a country's society, culture, politics, laws and economy, it is necessary to examine the impact of the International Covenant on Economic, Social and Cultural Rights (ICESCR), a major international human rights regime, on public health governance. It encompasses the right to social security, the right to be free from hunger, the right to health, the right to education and the right to enjoy the benefits of scientific progress and its applications.

5.2.2.1 The right to social security

The right to social security refers to the right of citizens to obtain social resources and services from the state and society when they face social risks that threaten their survival. This right enables them to survive and achieve a reasonable standard of living. Article 9 of the ICESCR stipulates that "the States Parties to the present Covenant recognize the right of everyone to social security, including social insurance".[16] Quality social security services in the field of public health in all countries around the world is the foundation of effective global health governance. Governments have the obligation to provide their citizens with sound social security systems in the field of public health. However, in many countries, especially Third World countries, the commercialisation of basic public health services such as childhood immunisation and the prevention and treatment of infectious diseases, coupled with the lack of sound public health statutes, have resulted in an acute shortage of public goods in public health governance at the national level. Among the world's poor, "2.4 billion are still using unimproved sanitation facilities"[17] and "more than 880 million people lack access to health services" (UNDP, 1999, p. 22). In the field of infectious disease control, the lack of social security would cause the rampant spread of tuberculosis, cholera, malaria and other infectious diseases, which in turn give rise to frequent public health crises. Reasons for the lack of social security can be attributed to government's pure indifference to the right to social security and to the physical constraints brought by the economic backwardness of some countries, particularly developing countries.

5.2.2.2 The right to be free from hunger

Article 11(2) of the ICESCR stipulates that:

The States Parties to the present Covenant, recognizing the fundamental right of everyone to be free from hunger, shall take, individually and through international co-operation, the measures, including specific programs, which are needed: (a) To improve methods of production, conservation and distribution

International human rights regimes 151

of food by making full use of technical and scientific knowledge, by disseminating knowledge of the principles of nutrition and by developing or reforming agrarian systems in such a way as to achieve the most efficient development and utilization of natural resources; (b) Taking into account the problems of both food-importing and food-exporting countries, to ensure an equitable distribution of world food supplies in relation to need.[18]

This means that the right to food and the right to be free from hunger require the states parties to undertake the obligation to provide the necessary food supplies for those in need. However, due to natural disasters, wars or sanctions imposed by other countries, many citizens in developing countries are living in hunger. Severe acute malnutrition could trigger a series of public health crises. According to Oxfam, an international charity, as many as one billion people worldwide are now living below the starvation line. According to the UN, one-sixth of the world's population has no access to adequate food; one-fifth has no access to clean drinking water; 29 countries are facing severe hunger, with 800 million people being chronically hungry, and 200 million children under the age of five are suffering from severe acute malnutrition.[19] Such appalling food shortages make the right to be free from hunger pure wishful thinking and undermine the efficiency of global health governance. The solution to the problem lies not only in poor countries' self-saving efforts but also in rich countries' fulfilment of moral obligations to famine-stricken countries to secure their citizens' right to be free from hunger.

5.2.2.3 The right of everyone to education

The right to education is a fundamental human right. Humans at the very beginning of their life possess no better survival skills than animals. But humans are endowed with certain attributes that distinguish them from animals, the most important of which is the capacity for education. The education level of citizens is closely related to the overall health status in a country. Article 13(1) of the ICESCR stipulates that "the States Parties to the present Covenant recognize the right of everyone to education".[20] In other words, each state party has the obligation to take all necessary measures to ensure that citizens have access to a certain level of education. In some countries, however, people with infectious diseases, including hepatitis B carriers and AIDS patients, are denied the right to education. This not only constitutes discrimination against people with infectious diseases but also deprives them of the precious opportunity to learn health care knowledge.

5.2.2.4 The right to enjoy the benefits of scientific progress
and its applications

All scientific and technological progress should be placed at the service of all mankind, the benefits of which should also be shared by all. Article 15(1.b) of the ICESCR stipulates that "the States Parties to the present Covenant recognize the right of everyone to enjoy the benefits of scientific progress and its applications".[21] However, in public health governance, one of the biggest obstacles for people to

152　*International human rights regimes*

exercise this right is the TRIPS Agreement of the World Trade Organization. It specified that medicine patents in developed countries would be valid for as long as 20 years, a decision that has made medicines prohibitively expensive and pharmaceutical companies in developed countries wallow in profits. However, people in many poor countries face threats from diseases simply because they cannot afford expensive medicines or vaccines. The TRIPS Agreement, led by developed countries, prevents people in poor countries from enjoying the benefits of scientific progress and its applications. As a result, the inaccessibility of essential medicines and vaccines has caused public health crises in many developing countries. This is also the result of Western countries' intellectual hegemony through abuse of the "rules of the game" of WTO. The United States has always sought to implement the TRIPS Agreement through various bilateral negotiations so that it can price medicines and vaccines at a level that is virtually out of the reach of people in poor countries. This is a deprivation and violation of human rights.

In 2000, the United Nations Economic and Social Council (2000) added a 20-page document on "the right to the highest attainable standard of health" to the ICESCR. It is a general comment on its Article 12. In paragraph 43, it is stated that states parties have a core obligation to ensure the satisfaction of, at the very least, minimum essential levels of health care. For example, the provision of essential drugs, as defined under the WHO Action Program on Essential Drugs, is part of the core obligation. Paragraph 47 stipulates that:

> If resource constraints render it impossible for a State to comply fully with its Covenant obligations, it has the burden of justifying that every effort has nevertheless been made to use all available resources at its disposal in order to satisfy, as a matter of priority, the obligations outlined above. It should be stressed, however, that a State party cannot, under any circumstances whatsoever, justify its non-compliance with the core obligations set out in paragraph 43 above, which are non-derogable.

In addition, state parties have an obligation to help other countries to fully realise their citizens' right to health. In paragraph 39, it is stated that:

> States Parties should ensure that the right to health is given due attention in international agreements and, to that end, should consider the development of further legal instruments. In relation to the conclusion of other international agreements, States parties should take steps to ensure that these instruments do not adversely impact upon the right to health. Similarly, States Parties have an obligation to ensure that their actions as members of international organisations take due account of the right to health.

5.2.3　*Justified restraints on human rights in public health governance*

Rousseau, one of the Enlightenment philosophers, famously claimed "man is born free, but he is everywhere in chains" (Rousseau, 1980, p. 8). Although people around the world are entitled to the freedoms and rights stipulated in the two international covenants on human rights, enjoyment of such rights are invariably "chained". A key factor in deciding whether these "chains" are justified in global health governance is whether they meet the Siracusa Principles on the Limitation and Derogation of Provisions in the International Covenant on Civil and Political Rights and the guidelines of WHO. The Siracusa Principles refers to the informal interpretation of the "derogation measures" stipulated in Article 4 and other restrictive provisions in the ICCPR provided by the UN Human Rights Committee at the Expert Meeting held in Siracusa, Italy, in 1984.[22] According to the Siracusa Principles, only if governments of states parties to the two covenants were to impose limits on the rights of their citizens, with such an arrangement being the last resort, will a government's action be considered legal but still subject to the following conditions: The relevant limits on civil rights have been stipulated in accordance with the law and are implemented in accordance with the law; they serve the judicial purpose of protecting the public interest; it is necessary for such limits to be imposed in a democratic society to achieve certain objectives; there is no less invasive or restrictive approach to achieving the same goal; the limits are not imposed without reason or in an unreasonable or discriminatory manner. In addition, as is clearly stated in Principles 25 and 26, governments may limit certain rights on the ground of public health. Thus, states parties are allowed to "take measures dealing with a serious threat to the health of the population or individual members of the population. These measures must be specifically aimed at preventing disease or injury or providing care for the sick and injured". At the same time, governments shall have "due regard to the international health regulations of the World Health Organization".[23]

Therefore, public health may be invoked by the governments of states parties in international human rights regimes as a ground for interfering with the rights and freedoms of their citizens only when certain prerequisites are met. To avoid violating human rights in the name of protecting public health, member states must take measures that limit human rights as a last resort and must follow the due procedures stipulated in international human rights regimes. Quarantines or isolations imposed in response to serious infectious diseases (e.g. Ebola, SARS) may have interfered with peoples' right to freedom of movement, but these interferences are lawful and are in accordance with international human rights instruments because such interferences are sometimes necessary to protect the public good. If a country restricts the right to freedom of movement of people with HIV/AIDS or puts them in prison, and if a country refuses to allow doctors to treat dissidents or does not provide anti-epidemic measures to certain groups, then these measures run counter to the norms of international human rights regimes. In addition, public health measures adopted by governments should be based on scientific evidence and argumentation and in accordance with the guidelines of the WHO. For example, mandatory isolation precautions are necessary for SARS patients, but when the same measures are applied to AIDS patients or patients with a hepatitis B infection, they may go against scientific research results and against the guidelines of WHO. In sum, if effective global health governance is to be achieved, any public health policy or measure must be formulated and implemented with human

154 *International human rights regimes*

rights considerations because the promotion and protection of human rights are inseparably linked with the promotion and protection of health.

5.3 The right to health and global health governance

The right to health is an externalised illustration of the intricate relationship between health and human rights. People's right to health, as the term suggests, is the metric to gauge the efficiency of global health governance. In 1946, WHO included the right to health for the first time in the preamble of its Constitution. In 1948, the Universal Declaration of Human Rights adopted by the United Nations formally established the right to health as a fundamental human right. The international community's claims for the right to health are also reflected in other international human rights regimes. In a sense, the extent to which the right to health is realised has become an important criterion for measuring the effectiveness of global health governance.

5.3.1 Definition of the right to health

The right to health has been "one of the poor relations in the UN human rights system" for many years (Hunt, 2002, p. 1878). Although the right to health has now become an important discourse in global health governance, as a notion it is rather vague and contentious in academia, leading not to consensus but rather to a system of viewpoints as complicated and grand as the Tower of Babel.[24] A few reasons account for this phenomenon. On one hand, people usually confuse the concept of public health with other concepts, such as health care, primary health care, medical services and medical care. On the other hand, WHO provides a broad definition of health: "health is a state of complete physical, mental and social well-being and not merely the absence of disease or infirmity". Although many international public health documents and declarations feature the right to health as an area of concern, none of them gives a specific and clear definition.

The *Report of the Special Rapporteur on the right of everyone to the enjoyment of the highest attainable standard of health* defines the right to health as "an inclusive right, extending not only to timely and appropriate health care, but also to the underlying determinants of health, such as access to safe and potable water and adequate sanitation, healthy occupational and environmental conditions, and access to health-related education and information, including on sexual and reproductive health."[25] According to WHO, it is a legal obligation of states to ensure access to timely, acceptable and affordable health care of appropriate quality as well as to providing for the underlying determinants of health, such as safe and potable water, sanitation, food, housing, health-related information and education and gender equality.[26] Although the two definitions are slightly different, they both illustrate the substance of the right to health. The right to health is not the right to be healthy, for no government can make every citizen free from ailments regardless of the state of policies for public health protection. Nor can it keep everyone away from all possible causes of human diseases because an individual's health may be affected by his or her genetic factors, susceptibility to disease, pursuit of unhealthy or dangerous lifestyles and so forth. Besides, a government is under no obligation to protect people from health problems arising from personal habits, such as fasting to lose weight. The right to health does not require governments of poor countries to offer expensive health services not financially feasible. Instead, the right to health is the right of citizens to the enjoyment of the highest attainable standard of health. To this end, citizens have the right to necessary facilities, goods, services and conditions, including health care and basic determinants of health, such as clean water, adequate and safe food, adequate hygiene and housing, a healthy work environment and natural environment, information on diseases, disease-related education and so forth (see Figure 5.2). We see from the historical development of public health that emphasis on the provision of sanitation facilities is not enough to promote human health. "Adequate attention needs to be paid to the improvement of sanitation and other environmental conditions" (Toebes, 1999, p. 8). There is also a need for governments and public authorities to develop relevant policies and action plans to make health care available to all in the shortest possible time.

5.3.2 The development of the right to health

In traditional society, health issues were believed to fall within the private rather than the public domain. Health was understood to be the absence of ailments. It was not until the beginning of industrialisation in the West that health conditions were mentioned in laws. For example, the Moral Apprentices Act of 1802 and the Public Health Act of 1848 in the United Kingdom were both adopted to ease the social pressures caused by poor working conditions.

When public health became a social issue, people's understandings of the concept of health also changed. The Universal Declaration of Human Rights adopted by the United Nations General Assembly in 1948 reflects people's aspirations to make the right to health a universal human right (Gruskin et al., 2007). The right to health was recognised for the first time after WHO was established in 1948. Later, the right to health was mentioned and reaffirmed in various international and regional covenants on human rights, such as Article 25 of the Universal

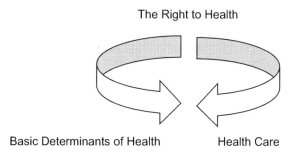

Figure 5.2 Components of the Right to Health

156 *International human rights regimes*

Declaration of Human Rights, Article 33 of the American Declaration of the Rights and Duties of Man, Article 11 of the European Social Charter, Article 12 of the International Covenant on Economic, Social and Cultural Rights and Article 16 of the African Charter on Human and Peoples' Rights.

In 1978, the Declaration of Alma-Ata on Primary Health Care reaffirmed that the right to health is a universal right. Signatory countries pledged to develop a complete health care system to ensure an effective and equitable distribution of health resources. They also emphasised that they had a responsibility for the health of their citizens, "which can be fulfilled only by the provision of adequate health and social measures".[27] This Declaration further developed the basis for the provision of primary health care and implicitly pointed to the significance of the protection of the right to health. Although it is just a declaration, it has not only shown the commitment of member countries to respect the right to health but has also provided an overall policy framework for the realisation of the right to health. In accordance with the spirit of this Declaration, signatory countries launched the "Health for All by the year 2000" initiative.

Article 6 of the Maastricht Guidelines on Violations of Economic, Social and Cultural Rights, adopted by the international community in January 1997, states that "the failure of States to provide essential primary health care to those in need may amount to a violation".[28] It is clearly stated in the Maastricht Guidelines that states have the obligation to realise their citizens' right to health. This is in line with the provision stipulated in the International Covenant on Economic, Social and Cultural Rights General Comment No. 3 that every state party must ensure the satisfaction of minimum essential levels of primary health care. It is also enshrined in the Constitution of WHO that "there is a baseline below which no individuals in any country should find themselves".[29] The Declaration of Alma-Ata on Primary Health Care pointed out that primary health care is the key to the implementation of international obligations. With primary health care, the goal that all peoples of the world should attain "a level of health that will permit them to lead a socially and economically productive life" can be achieved. Primary health care not only "constitutes the first element of a continuing health care process", but also "forms an integral part both of the country's health system, of which it is the central function and main focus, and of the overall social and economic development of the community".[30] This Declaration also calls on governments to examine domestic policies, strategies and plans of action to ensure primary health care for all. The concept of the right to health has been developed in a series of subsequent international documents and declarations on public health, such as the Ottawa Charter for Health Promotion (1986),[31] the World Health Assembly Resolution: Health Promotion (1998)[32] and the Bangkok Charter for Health Promotion in a Globalized World (2005).[33] In short, the development of the right to health is a process in which the notion is constantly being updated. The right to health is no longer just an individual private right but is also a social right, which means that in addition to citizens being responsible for their own health, governments shall have a positive obligation to safeguard their citizens' right to health. In other words, governments have the responsibility to ensure the realisation of the right to health and play an important role in public health services.

5.3.3 The goal of the right to health at the international level

The right to health is a fundamental human right, which is not only linked to but also depends on many other human rights. Many international human rights regimes have not only expounded on the definition and concept of the right to health but also further stipulated the specific goals and steps to realise it. The goals of the right to health at the international level are illustrated in the following aspects.

First, the Universal Declaration of Human Rights points out the relationship between health and other human rights, such as the right to food, housing, medical care and social services. The Declaration takes a broad view on the right to health, suggesting that the realisation of the right to health is closely related to the efficiency of governments in fulfilling their public service functions. For example, Article 25(1) stipulates that:

> Everyone has the right to a standard of living adequate for the health and well-being of himself and of his family, including food, clothing, housing and medical care and necessary social services, and the right to security in the event of unemployment, sickness, disability, widowhood, old age or other lack of livelihood in circumstances beyond his control.[34]

Second, the International Covenant on Economic, Social and Cultural Rights explicitly recognises the right to health as a right to be enjoyed by people and proposes specific steps in different aspects that a government can take to realise it. For example, Article 12 stipulates:

1 The States Parties to the present Covenant recognize the right of everyone to the enjoyment of the highest attainable standard of physical and mental health.
2 The steps to be taken by the States Parties to the present Covenant to achieve the full realization of this right shall include those necessary for:

   (a) The provision for the reduction of the stillbirth-rate and of infant mortality and for the healthy development of children;
   (b) The improvement of all aspects of environmental and industrial hygiene;
   (c) The prevention, treatment and control of epidemic, endemic, occupational and other diseases;
   (d) The creation of conditions which would assure to all medical service and medical attention in the event of sickness.

Third, the International Convention on the Elimination of All Forms of Discrimination Against Women requires states parties to guarantee the right to health on a basis of equality of men and women. It includes, in particular, provisions on proper prenatal care and breastfeeding care. For example, Article 12 stipulates:

1 States Parties shall take all appropriate measures to eliminate discrimination against women in the field of health care in order to ensure, on a basis of

158   *International human rights regimes*

equality of men and women, access to health care services, including those related to family planning.

2   Notwithstanding the provisions of paragraph I of this article, States Parties shall ensure to women appropriate services in connection with pregnancy, confinement and the post-natal period, granting free services where necessary, as well as adequate nutrition during pregnancy and lactation.

Fourth, the Convention on the Rights of the Child recognises the right to health that all children should enjoy. For example, Article 23 stipulates:

1   States Parties recognize that a mentally or physically disabled child should enjoy a full and decent life, in conditions which ensure dignity, promote self-reliance and facilitate the child's active participation in the community.

2   States Parties recognize the right of the disabled child to special care and shall encourage and ensure the extension, subject to available resources, to the eligible child and those responsible for his or her care, of assistance for which application is made and which is appropriate to the child's condition and to the circumstances of the parents or others caring for the child.

3   Recognizing the special needs of a disabled child, assistance extended in accordance with paragraph 2 of the present article shall be provided free of charge whenever possible, taking into account the financial resources of the parents or others caring for the child, and shall be designed to ensure that the disabled child has effective access to and receives education, training, health care services, rehabilitation services, preparation for employment and recreation opportunities in a manner conducive to the child's achieving the fullest possible social integration and individual development, including his or her cultural and spiritual development.

4   States Parties shall promote, in the spirit of international cooperation, the exchange of appropriate information in the field of preventive health care and of medical, psychological and functional treatment of disabled children, including dissemination of and access to information concerning methods of rehabilitation, education and vocational services, with the aim of enabling States Parties to improve their capabilities and skills and to widen their experience in these areas. In this regard, particular account shall be taken of the needs of developing countries.

In addition, the Convention on the Rights of the Child also proposes steps to implement the protection of children's right to health. For example, Article 24 stipulates:

1   States Parties recognize the right of the child to the enjoyment of the highest attainable standard of health and to facilities for the treatment of illness and rehabilitation of health. States Parties shall strive to ensure that no child is deprived of his or her right of access to such health care services.

2 States Parties shall pursue full implementation of this right and, in particular, shall take appropriate measures:

(a) To diminish infant and child mortality;
(b) To ensure the provision of necessary medical assistance and health care to all children with emphasis on the development of primary health care;
(c) To combat disease and malnutrition, including within the framework of primary health care, through, inter alia, the application of readily available technology and through the provision of adequate nutritious foods and clean drinking-water, taking into consideration the dangers and risks of environmental pollution;
(d) To ensure appropriate pre-natal and post-natal health care for mothers;
(e) To ensure that all segments of society, in particular parents and children, are informed, have access to education and are supported in the use of basic knowledge of child health and nutrition, the advantages of breastfeeding, hygiene and environmental sanitation and the prevention of accidents;
(f) To develop preventive health care, guidance for parents and family planning education and services.

3 States Parties shall take all effective and appropriate measures with a view to abolishing traditional practices prejudicial to the health of children.
4 States Parties undertake to promote and encourage international co-operation with a view to achieving progressively the full realization of the right recognized in the present article. In this regard, particular account shall be taken of the needs of developing countries.

The right to health is also reflected in other international human rights covenants, including the Convention on the Elimination of All Forms of Racial Discrimination, the Convention Relating to the Status of Refugees and the International Convention on the Protection of the Rights of All Migrant Workers and Members of Their Families, Geneva Conventions, the Declaration on the Protection of Women and Children in Emergency and Armed Conflict, Standard Minimum Rules for the Treatment of Prisoners, the Declaration on the Rights of Mentally Retarded Persons, the Convention on the Rights of Persons with Disabilities and the Declaration of Commitment on HIV/AIDS. Each includes provisions which have directly and indirectly addressed different aspects of the right to health. In addition, there also exists a large number of instruments on human rights at the regional and national levels, such as the European Social Charter, the African Charter on Human and Peoples' Rights and the Additional Protocol to the American Convention on Human Rights in the Area of Economic, Social and Cultural Rights. For example, Article 11 of the European Social Charter touches on the right to protection of health, which stipulates that states parties shall take appropriate measures to "provide advisory and educational facilities for the promotion of health", prevent diseases and so forth. Article 13 also requires governments

160 *International human rights regimes*

to provide adequate social or medical assistance to any citizen who is without adequate resources, which to some extent underlines the relationship between the right to health and the right to equality. Nevertheless, the right to health in international human rights regimes still needs to be implemented at the national level. The right to health, as one of the fundamental human rights, has been incorporated into the constitutions or laws of most member countries (see Figure 5.3).

5.4 International human rights regimes in global health governance: some limitations

By incorporating public health into human rights norms, international human rights regimes provide a new framework and a guideline for actions to promote public health for countries across the world. The human rights–based approach signals the return of a human-centred approach in global health governance. At the same time, "integrating a human-rights approach into public health is both an essential requirement for the realization of health for all—or, for example, the MDG goals—and a *sine qua non* for a world operating on social justice" (London, 2008, p. 66). Combining the two lends public health governance more moral support.

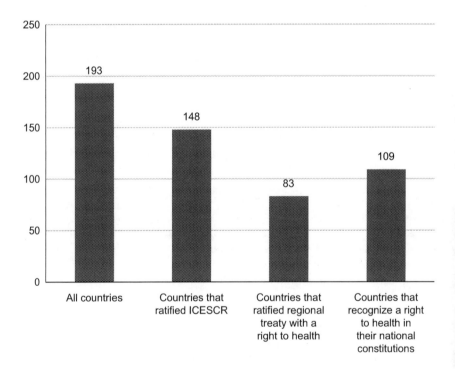

Figure 5.3 National Recognition of a Right to Health

Source: Kinney, E. D. (2001). The International Human Right to Health: What Does This Mean for Our Nation and World? *Indiana Law Review*, 34, p. 1465.

International human rights regimes 161

However, given the inherent weaknesses of the international human rights mechanisms and the economic gap between the Global North and the Global South, the role of human rights regimes in global health governance has been severely restrained. In many developing countries, especially in southern Africa, human rights provisions that are critical for public health governance remain on paper only. Putting them in action has proven to be exceedingly difficult. Violations of human rights triggered by public health crises are commonplace, in turn leading to more public health crises. The prevalence of HIV/AIDS infections is a typical example of this vicious cycle. As an overview, there are several factors limiting the role of the international human rights regimes in global health governance.

5.4.1 Lack of mandatory enforcement mechanisms

Any effective implementation of international norms requires a certain enforcement body; international human rights mechanisms are no exception to this rule. To monitor or implement human rights norms universally, the international community has set up several instruments and institutions. They are commonly divided into two categories. One is UN charter-based bodies, which are given the widest mandate to raise awareness, foster respect for human rights protection and respond to violations of human rights. The UN Commission on Human Rights is the most important body in this category. However, "as a general rule, states are reluctant to couple a strong instrument with a powerful and effective enforcement body" (Mutua, 1998. p. 216). Since the birth of the Universal Declaration of Human Rights in 1948, the mandate and purpose of the UN charter-based bodies are restricted to functions such as "to research", "to promote", "to incentivize" and "to urge and to recommend" (Liu, 2000, p. 75). As a result, bodies of this type do not have the legal-binding authority to enforce implementation of human rights related to public health.

The other type encompasses treaty-based bodies, such as the Human Rights Council founded on the International Covenant on Civil and Political Rights. Theoretically speaking, since bodies of the second type have jurisdiction over specific treaties, they are empowered to monitor and enforce international human rights norms. However, "in reality, such bodies have few powers, a fact which generally renders them weak" (Mutua, 1998, p. 216). Two reasons lead to the lack of mandatory enforcement of treaty-based bodies. First, these bodies require member states to report whether human rights are protected, respected and upheld, but they cannot visit each member state to verify the credibility of such reports. In other words, information on how member states have complied with relevant norms are furnished by members themselves. This makes their supervisory functions illusory. Second, enforcement capacity from these bodies are further under the interference of political influence. Human rights issues are highly sensitive. It is difficult to avoid political interference from big powers when implementing relevant norms. For example, the Human Rights Commission can trace its weak enforcement power to an overall politicised atmosphere during its inception. Similarly, when the International Covenant on Civil and Political Power was

162   *International human rights regimes*

formulated in the 1950s and 1960s, due to the deep ideological divide at that time, the International Human Rights Commission lacked "teeth" since the very beginning. As a human rights scholar observes, during the Cold War "language related to the purpose and power of human rights institutions remains to be discussed, and the compromises reached on these irreconcilable views are inevitably expressed in simplistic and ambiguous terms" (Steiner, 2000, p. 17). Therefore, the Commission on Human Rights is vague on the purpose and scope of power of these institutions, not least on the enforcement power of the international human rights regimes. In short, "many official international human rights bodies such as the Human Rights Committee (HRC) are basically weak and ineffectual" (Mutua, 1998, p. 211). It is therefore not difficult to imagine the role these regimes can play in monitoring member states' implementation of human rights related to public health governance, including the right of health, equality and the right to knowledge.

5.4.2 *Vagueness on the right to health*

Of all the human rights enshrined by the international human rights regimes, right to health is the most closely related to public health governance. The degree to which the right to health is ensured determines the efficiency of public health governance. However, lack of clarity in the scope and meaning of this right has made relevant norms and standards fuzzy. Therefore, member implementations vary in quality. In general, such vagueness is reflected in two ways.

First, it is vague as a concept. The Constitution of WHO has provided a description of the right to health. Article 12 of the International Covenant on Economic, Social and Cultural Rights also states: "The States Parties to the present Covenant recognize the right of everyone to the enjoyment of the highest attainable standard of physical and mental health". The right to health is thus seen as a right to reach the highest and attainable standard of health. In reality, however, both definitions are too general in scope. Ruth Roemers (1989), a well-known American public health expert, even believes the phrase "right to health" is absurd because it connotes the guarantee of perfect health (p. 17). In fact, the definition provided in Article 12 of the International Covenant on Economic, Social and Cultural Rights is similarly vague, in part because it has always been a controversial issue to ensure access to health care services. There is no consensus on specific obligations member states must undertake in providing their citizens with health care, let alone obligations to provide the right to health. Some believe the right to health merely describes a strong yearning for a mysterious and ideal society rather than a right per se. Others believe that right to health only exists as a piece of "soft law" whose content is so broad and vague that its actual meaning and content is difficult to articulate. No wonder some scholars have lamented this lack of clarity by saying, "the right to health is a concept that is frequently used but the meaning is quite unclear" (Yue, 2007, p. 1).

Second, the accountability mechanism to achieve the right to health is unclear. WHO believes that as with other human rights, member states are obligated to respect, protect and enforce the right to health. But without a member state's voluntary assistance and proactive intervention, it is virtually impossible to truly achieve the right to health. To some extent, realisation of people's right to health depends on the scope and extent of a member state's obligations. Since the right to health "creates rights and obligations, it needs effective accountability mechanisms" (Hunt, 2006, p. 604). Such accountability obviously lies with the government of a member state. Theoretically speaking, if a government fails to fulfil its obligation to provide the right to health, it should be held accountable. Nevertheless, it is difficult to hold a government responsible for its actions. As one of the two main international human rights conventions, Article 2(1) of the International Covenant on Economic, Social and Cultural Rights stipulates that member states are obliged to "take steps, to the maximum of [their] available resources, with a view to achieving progressively the full realization of the rights recognized in the present Covenant".[35] This provision is vague, imprecise and too broad. In the phrase "to the maximum of [their] available resources", two conflicting adjectives ("maximum" and "available") are used to describe a vague noun, "resources". "Maximum" denotes idealism, whereas "available" stands for realism. While "Maximum" is the most common phrase used in human rights protection, "available" provides leeway for a member state to opt out of their obligations to ensure the right to health. The standard phrase "available resources" is often used by member states as a readily made excuse to confer or deprive their citizens of their economic, social and cultural rights. This ambiguous wording provides an "escape hatch" for states when it comes to their obligations regarding implementing and ensuring the realisation of relevant rights. In other words, a state always has an excuse to evade accountability. No wonder people are led to believe in an unfortunate truth: The right to health is just an illusion.

5.4.3 North–South divide

If the vagueness of the right to health leads to the failure in its implementation and consequently to failure in global health governance, will things improve if the aim and paradigm of the right to health shift from the International Covenant on Economic, Social and Cultural Rights to other international norms or "soft laws"? The Declaration of Alma-Ata, which was adopted in 1978 at the initiative of WHO, made it clear that it wanted to achieve the goal of "Health for All by 2000". This is by far the most systematic and clear definition on global health challenges (including the definition on the right to health). The Pan-American Health Organization believes that the goal of "'Health for All by 2000' is the most specific and useful definition on the programmatic right to health. It expresses the consensus that a state shall be held responsible for the health for its citizens" (Hernán & Connor, 1989, p. 603). However, in most developing countries, this ambitious goal has fallen through. Given the Declaration of Alma-Ata's clarity on the goal to improve the health of the population of developing countries, how did it end in failure? One of the most important reasons has to do with the current North–South Divide. Chinese scholar Huiping Xiong holds that right to health is

164 *International human rights regimes*

not guaranteed because there exists a poverty of such right. The right to health is distributed asymmetrically between the rich and the poor. The power of the rich may trample over, clash or result in the lack of the right of the poor. What's happening under the hood is that "the gap between the rich and the poor is getting wider" (Xiong, 2007, p. 73). The wealth gulf that exists between developing and developed countries is an important trigger for the global health crisis. Most of the world's poor population is in developing countries. For them, provisions for basic sanitation and health conditions, such as adequate nutrition, safe drinking water and rudimentary sanitation facilities, are not guaranteed, let alone the right to health. The most obvious gap between the North and South in public health is the "10/90 gap". Out of the total worldwide resources devoted to health research, as little as 10% is dedicated to solving public health issues that are faced by as many as 90% of the world's population. For instance, the total expenditure on health research in the world was US$160 billion in 2005, of which 97% was invested in developed countries as opposed to 3% spent in and low- and middle-income countries.[36] Southeast Asian countries, with 12% of the global total health workers, carry 29% of the global disease burden. African countries, with 3% of health workers, carry 24% of the global disease burden. In contrast, the United States only has 10% of the global burden of disease, but its health and medical personnel account for 37% of the global total (WHO, 2007). These shocking disparities have only shown signs of widening. The North–South Divide is also reflected in the Declaration of Alma-Ata: "The existing gross inequality in the health status of the people particularly between developed and developing countries as well as within countries is politically, socially and economically unacceptable and is, therefore, of common concern to all countries".[37] The failure of the international regimes to close the North–South Divide has not only defeated the ultimate goal of the Declaration of Alma-Ata but also spelt doom for all efforts seeking to enunciate the right to health in a practical and feasible manner.

5.4.4 *Biases and discriminations in international human right regimes*

Yasuaki (2003) pointed out that "for a long time, the manner in which human rights are questioned, discussed and assessed has been dominated by Europe and the United States" (p. 162). The Europe-and-America-centric view of international human rights regimes has also affected global health governance, especially in terms of which of the two international human rights conventions should be given more weight. The International Covenant on Civil and Political Rights and the International Covenant on Economic, Social and Cultural Rights are both closely related to public health governance, especially to the realisation of the right to health. To protect human rights, developing countries focus more on fighting the economic, social and cultural constraints, whereas Western countries, which dominate human rights discourses, pay more attention to citizens' civil and political rights. As Fidler (2000) argued, "although the inseparable and interdependent nature of these two rights is now generally accepted in the United Nations, the reality in practice is that economic, social and cultural rights are

International human rights regimes 165

still largely ignored" (p. 300). This negligence cannot meaningfully help achieve global health governance. For example, for AIDS patients to be given personal freedom and political rights but not access to necessary medication they need is a half-hearted response to public health problems.

More importantly, Western developed countries tend to "emphasize the universality, but not the collectivity, of human rights" (Jiang, 2002, p. 73). In their view, the right to development is the right to implement "all individual rights" rather than "all national rights". In contrast, the developing countries emphasise shared responsibility, especially the responsibility of developed countries to assist developing countries. If such assistance mechanisms are not established, and if the development rights and opportunities for development are not guaranteed for the developing world, developing countries cannot solve public health and safety issues on their own. Rather regrettably, developed countries are quick to criticise human rights violations and political repressions of the developing world, but when their opportunities come to help the developing world protect their human rights, by, for instance, providing economic assistance (including vaccines, medication and advanced treatments), they would be rather content to resort to lip service. A person who is disease-ridden, poverty-stricken and lacking in means to even afford his aspirin can make but little use of his right to vote and freedom of speech. The current international mechanisms "have profoundly affected the realization of human rights, especially in countries that are poor and weak" (Pogge, 2005, p. 197). Similarly, the current international development regimes dominated by developed countries have greatly affected the realisation of the right to health in developing countries. According to UNDP (1994):

Despite all out technological breakthroughs, we still live in a world where a fifth of the developing world's population goes hungry every night, a quarter lacks access to even a basic necessity like safe drinking water, and a third lives in a state of abject poverty—at such a margin of human existence that words simply fail to describe it.

(p. 2)

This condition explains why we need to review and recommit ourselves to the realisation of their economic, social and cultural rights, rather than emphasising their civil and political rights. Fidler (1996) pointed out that:

Today, the attention being generated on emerging or recurrent infectious diseases comes mainly from the developed world, which fears the spread of infectious diseases from the developing world. Developing states need massive financial and technical assistance to deal with endemic diseases more than rules to prevent their diseases from travelling to the developed world.

(p. 500)

Developed countries should aid developing countries in all possible ways, acknowledge developing world's rights to development and thereby gradually

166 *International human rights regimes*

close the North–South Divide. They ought to pay equal attention to the International Covenant on Civil and Political Rights and the International Covenant on Economic, Social and Cultural Rights to helping developing countries achieve economic and social development. Only in this way can there be good external conditions for effective global health governance.

Summary

Human rights protection and public health governance cannot be achieved without each other's support. The human rights–based approach and the requirement used in global health governance not only illustrate the importance of human rights regimes for public health governance but also show that global health governance is itself an effort to protect human rights and by nature a human-centred endeavour. The right to health, in particular, is an instantiation of how human rights protection has been incorporated into public health governance. However, due to the huge public health gap between the North and South and the double standards used in human rights protection in developed countries, efforts to achieve the right to health consist of more rhetoric than action. The non-mandatory enforcement of international human rights regimes means it is challenging to get public health–related human rights protection enforced at the national level. This calls for the creation of good internal and external incentives to better implement the human rights–based approach in global health governance. On one hand, developed countries need to aid developing countries and work hard to close the public health gap between the North and South, thereby enhancing the capability of developing countries to achieve the right of health and other international human rights norms. On the other hand, there is a need to strengthen the effectiveness of relevant international human rights regimes, thereby increasing their compliance pull. The efficiency of global health governance can only be raised, and the human rights concerns solved, if countries around the world are empowered and driven to implement international human rights norms.

Notes

1 See *Health and Human Rights*. Retrieved from www.emro.who.int/pdf/afg/programmes/hhr.pdf?ua=1.
2 UN Commission on Human Rights, once a subsidiary organ of the United Nations Economic and Social Council (ECOSOC), was reorganised into the Human Rights Council. The Council was no longer a subsidiary of the ECOSOC but rather elevated to the status of a subsidiary organ of the General Assembly, showing that the international community had attached greater importance to human rights issues than they did previously.
3 See *The Universal Declaration of Human Rights*. Retrieved from www.un.org/en/universal-declaration-human-rights/.
4 See *the International Covenant on Economic, Social and Cultural Rights*. Retrieved from www.ohchr.org/en/professionalinterest/pages/cescr.aspx.
5 In 1993, the Vienna Declaration and Programme of Action was adopted by the UN at the World Conference on Human Rights in Vienna. Article I(5) reaffirms that "all

International human rights regimes   167

human rights are universal, indivisible and interdependent and interrelated". See: United Nations. (1993, July 12). *Vienna Declaration and Programme of Action*. Retrieved from www.ohchr.org/en/professionalinterest/pages/vienna.aspx.

6   See *Vienna Declaration and Programme of Action*.
7   See Article 19 of the Universal Declaration of Human Rights. Retrieved from www.un.org/en/universal-declaration-human-rights/.
8   See Article 19(2) of the International Covenant on Civil and Political Rights. Retrieved from www.ohchr.org/en/professionalinterest/pages/ccpr.aspx.
9   See Article 20(1) of the Universal Declaration of Human Rights.
10 See Article 22(1) of the International Covenant on Civil and Political Rights.
11 See Article 13(1) of the Universal Declaration of Human Rights.
12 See Article 12(1, 2, 4) of the International Covenant on Civil and Political Rights.
13 See Article 3 of the Universal Declaration of Human Rights.
14 See Article 9(1) of the International Covenant on Civil and Political Rights.
15 See Article 26 of the International Covenant on Civil and Political Rights.
16 See Article 9 of the International Covenant on Economic, Social and Cultural Rights. Retrieved from www.ohchr.org/EN/ProfessionalInterest/Pages/CESCR.aspx.
17 See Global Action for United Nations Millennium Development Goals. Retrieved from www.un.org/chinese/millenniumgoals/unsystem/target10.htm.
18 See Article 11(2) of the International Covenant on Economic, Social and Cultural Rights.
19 See *Report on G8 Finance Ministers Meeting: Debt relief for poor countries*. Retrieved from www.g8.utoronto.ca/evaluations/2005compliance_interim/2005-06_g8-i-comp_debt.pdf.
20 See Article 13(1) of the International Covenant on Economic, Social and Cultural Rights.
21 See Article 15(1.b) of the International Covenant on Economic, Social and Cultural Rights.
22 See Article 4 of the International Covenant on Civil and Political Rights for "derogation measures".
23 See Principle 25 and 26 of Siracusa Principles on the Limitation and Derogation of Provisions in the International Covenant on Civil and Political Rights.
24 See the story of the Tower of Babel in Genesis 11:1–9. The story of its construction explains the existence of diverse human languages. According to the story, people around the world used to have one language and a common speech. They agreed to build a tower tall enough to reach heaven, and the tower was built quickly. But the Lord came and said, "if as one people speaking the same language they have begun to do this, then nothing they plan to do will be impossible for them". So, the Lord disrupted their work by confusing their language so that they could no longer understand one another. The tower was never completed.
25 See "Report of the Special Rapporteur on the Right of Everyone to the Enjoyment of the Highest Attainable Standard of Physical and Mental Health". Retrieved from www.ohchr.org/en/issues/health/pages/srrighthealthindex.aspx.
26 See the Right to Health. Retrieved from www.who.int/news-room/fact-sheets/detail/human-rights-and-health.
27 See the Declaration of Alma-Ata. Retrieved from www.who.int/publications/almaata_declaration_en.pdf.
28 See The Maastricht Guidelines on Violations of Economic, Social and Cultural Rights. Retrieved from www.ohchr.org/Documents/Publications/training12en.pdf.
29 See Global Strategy for Health for All by the Year 2000. Retrieved from www.who.int/publications/i/item/9241800038.
30 See the Declaration of Alma-Ata.
31 See the Ottawa Charter for Health Promotion. Retrieved from www.who.int/healthpromotion/conferences/previous/ottawa/en/.

168 *International human rights regimes*

32 See the World Health Assembly Resolution: Health Promotion. Retrieved from www. who.int/healthpromotion/wha51-12/en/.
33 See the Bangkok Charter for Health Promotion in a Globalized World. Retrieved from www.who.int/healthpromotion/conferences/6gchp/bangkok_charter/en/.
34 See the Universal Declaration of Human Rights.
35 See Article 2 of the International Covenant on Economic, Social and Cultural Rights.
36 See "Health Research Spending Tops US$160 Billion, Yet Investment Fails to Meet the Needs of Developing Countries". Retrieved from www.globalforumhealth.org/filesupld/press%20releases/PressReleaseMFF08.pdf.
37 See the Declaration of Alma-Ata.

References

Bobbio, N. (1996). *The Age of Rights*. Cambridge: Polity Press.

Cassese, A. (2001). *International Law*. New York: Oxford University Press.

Csete, J. (2004). Missed Opportunities: Human Rights and the Politics of HIV/AIDS. *Development*, 47(2), 83–90.

Davidson, S. (1993). *Human Rights*. Buckingham: Open University Press.

Donnelly, J. (1986). International Human Rights: A Regime Analysis. *International Organization*, 40(3), 599–642.

Donnelly, J. (1997). *International Human Rights*. Boulder, CO: Westview Press.

Fidler, D. P. (1996). Mission Impossible? International Law and Infectious Diseases. *Temple International & Comparative Law Journal*, 10(2), 493–502.

Fidler, D. P. (1999). *International Law and Infectious Diseases*. New York: University Press.

Fidler, D. P. (2000). *International Law and Public Health: Materials on and Analysis of Global Health Jurisprudence*. New York: Transnational Publishers Inc.

Garrett, L. (1997). *Microbes versus Mankind: The Coming Plague*. New York: Foreign Policy Association.

Gellman, B. (2000, July 5). Death Watch: The Global Response to AIDS in Africa. *Washington Post*.

Gostin, L. O., & Lazzarini, Z. (1997). *Human Rights and Public Health in the AIDS Pandemic*. Oxford: Oxford University Press.

Gruskin, S., Ferguson, L., & Bogecho, D. O. (2007). Beyond the Members: Using Rights-Based Perspectives to Enhance Antiretroviral Treatment Scale-Up. *AIDS*, 21(Supplement 5), S13–S19.

Gruskin, S., Mills, E. J., & Tarantola, D. (2007). History, Principles, and Practice of Health and Human Rights. *The Lancet*, 370(9585), 449–455.

Henkin, L. (1990). *The Age of Rights*. New York: Columbia University Press.

Hernán, L. F.-P., & Connor, S. S. (1989). *The Right to Health in the Americas: A Comparative Constitutional Study*. Washington, DC: Pan American Health Organization.

Hunt, P. (2002). The Right to Health: From the Margins to the Mainstream. *The Lancet*, 360(9348), 1878.

Hunt, P. (2006). The Human Right to the Highest Attainable Standard of Health: New Opportunities and Challenges. *Transactions of the Royal Society of Tropical Medicine and Hygiene*, 100(7), 603–607.

Jiang, G. (2002). *International Law in Evolution*. Beijing: Law Press·China.

Jürgens, R. E., & Cohen, J. (2007). *Human Rights and HIV/AIDS: Now More Than Ever: 10 Reasons Why Human Rights Should Occupy the Center of the Global AIDS Struggle*. Law and Health Initiative, Public Health Program, Open Society Institute. Retrieved from www.aidslaw.ca/site/wp-content/uploads/2013/04/MoreThanEver-ENG.pdf?lang=en

Kinney, E. D. (2001). The International Human Right to Health: What Does This Means for Our Nation and World? *Indiana Law Review*, 34, 1457–1475.

Li, L., & Wan, E. (1992). *Human Rights Theory and International Human Rights*. Wuhan: Wuhan University Press.

Liu, J. (2000). From Human Rights Declaration to ICCPR and ICESCR: A Historical Look. In J. Wang, H. Liu, & L. Li (Eds.), *Human Rights in 21st Century*. Beijing: Law Press China.

London, L. (2008). What Is a Human Rights-Based Approach to Health and Does It Matter? *Health and Human Rights*, 10(1), 65–80.

Mann, J. M. (1997). Health and Human Rights: If Not Now, When? *Health and Human Rights*, 2(3), 113–120.

Mann, J. M., & Gruskin, S. (1999). *Health and Human Rights: A Reader*. New York: Routledge.

Mann, J. M., Tarantola, D. J. M., & Netter, T. W. (1992). *AIDS in the World*. Cambridge, MA: Harvard University Press.

Menon-Johansson, A. S. (2005). Good Governance and Good Health: The Role of Societal Structures in the Human Immunodeficiency Virus Pandemic. *BioMed Central International Health and Human Rights*, 5(1), 4.

Mutua, M. W. (1998). Looking Past the Human Rights Committee: An Argument for De-Marginalizing Enforcement. *Buffalo Human Rights Law Review*, 4, 211–260.

Office of the High Commissioner for Human Rights and UNAIDS. (2006). *HIV/AIDS and Human Rights: International Guidelines*. Retrieved from www.ohchr.org/Documents/Publications/HIVAIDSGuidelinesen.pdf

Pogge, T. W. (2005). Human Rights and Global Health: A Research Program. *Metaphilosophy*, 36, 182–209.

Risse, T., & Ropp, S. C. (1999). International Human Rights Norms and Domestic Change: Conclusions. In T. Risse, S. C. Ropp, & K. Sikkink (Eds.), *The Power of Human Rights* (pp. 234–278). Cambridge: Cambridge University Press.

Roemers, R. (1989). The Right to Health Care. In L. F.-P. Hernán & S. S. Connor (Eds.), *The Right to Health in the Americas: A Comparative Constitutional Study*. Washington, DC: Pan American Health Organization.

Rousseau, J.-J. (1980). *The Social Contract* (Z. He, Trans.). Beijing: The Commercial Press.

Scott, C. (1989). Interdependence and Permeability of Human Rights Norms: Towards a Partial Fusion of the International Covenants on Human Rights. *Osgoode Hall Law Journal*, 27(4), 769–851.

Sen, A. (1999). *Development as Freedom*. New York: Alfred A. Knopf.

Senger, V. H. (1993). *From the Limited to the Universal Concept of Human Rights: Two Periods of Human Rights*. Goldbach: Keip.

Steiner, H. J. (2000). Individual Claims in a World of Massive Violations: What Role for the Human Rights Committee? In P. Alston & J. Crawford (Eds.), *The Future of UN Human Rights Treaty Monitoring*. Cambridge: Cambridge University Press.

Tocqueville, A. D. (1996). *Democracy in America* (G. Dong, Trans.). Beijing: The Commercial Press.

Toebes, B. C. A. (1999). *The Right to Health as a Human Right in International Law*. Intersenti-Hart, Groningen: School of Human Rights Research.

United Nations. (2005). *Economic, Social and Cultural Rights: Handbook for National Human Rights Institutions*. New York: United Nations.

170 *International human rights regimes*

United Nations Commission on Human Rights. (1995, March 3). *Discrimination in the Context of Human Immune Deficiency Virus (HIV) or Acquired Immune Deficiency Syndrome (AIDS)*. Geneva: United Nations.

United Nations Development Programme. (1994). *Human Development Report 1994*. New York: Oxford University Press.

United Nations Development Programme. (1999). *Human Development Report 1999*. New York: Oxford University Press.

United Nations Development Programme. (2000). *Human Development Report 2000*. New York: Oxford University Press.

United Nations Economic and Social Council. (2000, August 11). *CESCR General Comment No. 14: The Right to the Highest Attainable Standard of Health (Art. 12)*. New York: United Nations.

WHO. (2006). *Engaging for Health: The 11th Global Programme of Work, 2006–2015: A Global Health Agenda*. Geneva: WHO.

WHO. (2007). *World Health Statistics*. Geneva: WHO.

WHO. (2020). *Constitution of the World Health Organization*. Geneva: WHO. Retrieved from http:// www.who.int/gb/bd/PDF/bd46/c-bd46_2.pdf

World Bank. (1998). *Development and Human Rights: The Role of the World Bank*. Washington, DC: World Bank.

Xiong, H. (2007). On Right to Health from Poor Economics Perspective: Poverty of the Right to Health and Its Governance. *Social Science Research*, 6, 36–39.

Yasuaki, O. (2003). *Human Rights, Nations and Civilization* (Z. Wang, Trans.). Beijing: SDX Joint Publishing Company.

Yue, Y. (2007). On National Obligation to Provide Right to Health to Citizens. *Chinese Medical Ethics*, 3, 99–102.

6 Biological Weapons Convention (BWC) and global health governance

The development of modern biotechnology is a double-edged sword. Its benefits are as bountiful as its concomitant perils. The most noteworthy risk of biotechnology is the development and application of bioweapons. It is believed that "a lethal pathogen might ultimately threaten the entire world population" (Steinbruner, 1997, p. 89). Given the ever-growing threat of terrorism, there is also "a growing opportunity for terrorists to acquire and use bioweapons" (Blix, 2006, p. 112). Using biotechnology for biological weapons puts global health security in serious jeopardy. International cooperation on biotechnology under the BWC also exerts significant influence on the capacity of developing countries to respond to public health crises. Therefore, as the most important international regime in bioweapons control, the BWC has been influential in global health governance. Strengthening the effectiveness of the BWC will greatly promote global health governance while "the international community can ill afford to perpetuate its careless custody of the norm against biological weapons" (Smithson, 2004a, p. 175).

6.1 Background and stages of the development of the BWC

The BWC is the first international norm in the history of mankind to ban an entire category of weapons of mass destruction. It is also an important part of the international disarmament system and the UN-centred international collective security framework. However, since it entered into force in 1975, the BWC has revealed some inherent flaws. Its development, therefore, has been largely a process to amend these deficiencies.

6.1.1 Historical background to the development of the BWC

Biological weapons, also known as germ weapons, use biological toxins or infectious agents to kill humans, animals or plants. Biological weapons can be classified in three ways. According to the type of biological agents used, they are divided into bacterial weapons, viral weapons and toxin weapons. Effect-wise, they can be divided into infectious biological weapons which can be transmitted between humans or infected targets, and non-infectious biological weapons which only directly affect the targets. Operationally, they are categorised as either lethal

172 *BWC and global health governance*

weapons or incapacitating weapons. The use of biological weapons in warfare has been around for hundreds of years. In the Roman Empire, for example, soldiers would contaminate wells and springs with human and animal bodies to infect their enemies. According to historical records, the earliest "biological ballistic missiles" were used in 1346, when the Tartars hurled plague-infected cadavers over the walls of Caffa (now Feodosia, Ukraine) to end the siege.[1] In particular, during World War I, the wide use of poison gas inflicted so much harm to human society that it prompted the international community to prohibit the use of biological and chemical weapons in war. In 1925, the Protocol for the Prohibition of the Use in War of Asphyxiating, Poisonous or Other Gases and of Bacteriological Methods of Warfare, also known as the Geneva Protocol, was signed and subsequently entered into force in 1928, thereby becoming the first international regime for the arms control of biological weapons in history.

As the first international regime to ban biological weapons, the Geneva Protocol placed restrictions on the use of biological weapons in three ways. First, it banned their use only in armed conflicts between ratifying members states of the Protocol. In other words, the use of biological weapons was not expressly prohibited when one or both countries at war were non-ratifying member states. Second, the Geneva Protocol did not prohibit the research, development, production and stockpiling of biological and chemical weapons. Therefore, it did not limit member states' ability to produce biological weapons through their own scientific and technological advances. Third, several signatories raised their reservations about the Geneva Protocol because it allowed parties to use biological weapons in retaliation to the first use of their enemies.[2] In this sense, this not only makes the Geneva Protocol a "no-first-use" agreement but also allows governments to freely develop and stockpile biological weapons. Deterrence works only when a country has credible ability to retaliate against the hostile country that uses biological and chemical weapons. The Geneva Conventions have thus turned into a trigger for the arms race in biological weapons. As an international norm prohibiting the use of biological weapons, the Geneva Protocol plays a limited role in this regard. In the early 1940s, for example, Japan conducted extensive bacteriological weapons tests in China and released viruses such as anthrax and plague.[3] The United States, the United Kingdom and the Soviet Union also developed biological weapons. The United States and the Soviet Union had the most ambitious programs; the biological agents they studied included viruses for anthrax, smallpox and plague, among others.

6.1.2 Stages of development of the BWC

The Geneva Protocol failed to effectively prevent Japan, the Soviet Union and the United States from developing biological weapons. With the change in the international situation and the development of biotechnology, control of biological weapons was put back on the UN's agenda. In 1969, US President Richard Nixon unilaterally announced the suspension of all offensive biological weapons programmes, which created necessary international political conditions to establish a new biological weapons control regime. In the same year, the United Kingdom proposed a draft convention on the prohibition of the use of biological weapons in war. On September 28, 1971, 12 countries, including the United States, the United Kingdom and the Soviet Union, submitted a drafted text of the BWC to the United Nations General Assembly. The United States, the United Kingdom and the Soviet Union, the three parties in possession of biological weapons, signed the convention into law in 1972. On March 26, 1975, the BWC entered into force. It consisted of a preamble and 15 articles. Its preamble reaffirmed the principles and objectives of the 1925 Geneva Protocol on the prohibition of the use of biological weapons in war by parties and provided that a Review Conference would be held every five years. Signatories have subsequently held eight Review Conferences on the BWC, in 1980, 1986, 1991, 1996, 2001, 2006, 2011 and 2017. As of January 2020, the BWC membership comprised 183 states parties and four signatory states, with ten non-signatory states.

The BWC is a milestone in international arms control because it is the first treaty to outlaw an entire class of weapons and the first to require actual disarmament through the elimination of stockpiles.[4] Compared to the Geneva Protocol, the BWC added a clause prohibiting "the development, production, stockpiling, acquisition, or retention" of biological weapons. However, although the BWC is an improvement over the Geneva Protocol, it is still the result of compromise among member states, especially between the United States and the Soviet Union at the time. These compromises, coupled with the blurred line between the peaceful use of biological agents and their use for military purposes, have given rise to many inherent flaws of the BWC. For example, the BWC does not have a mechanism to verify the status of research and development of biological weapons in various countries; it does not involve provisions for the verification of breach of contract. There is no prohibition on the research of biological weapons, and it allows member states to use biological agents peacefully. It does not contain lists of biological agents and threshold quantities; it only prohibits the development, production and stockpiling of biological weapons and fails to mention the prohibition of the use of biological weapons.[5] In addition, the effectiveness of this international regime was further constrained by the national enforcement of the BWC and the universality of its membership. The subsequent development of the BWC revolves around efforts to address these inherent defects. The formulation of the Protocol on the effective enforcement of the BWC marks the most important watershed moment in the history of this international regime. Accordingly, the development of the BWC can be divided into three stages: the pre-Protocol period, the Protocol period and the post-Protocol period.

6.1.2.1 Pre-Protocol period (1981–1991)

The prevention of biological weapons calls for further international cooperation, mainly for the following reasons: The rapid development of life sciences may lead to unpredictable and dangerous consequences; the BWC, which was signed in 1972, lacked a mechanism to monitor, verify and ensure its implementation

174 *BWC and global health governance*

and enforcement; many countries either did not have domestic legislation or found it difficult to strictly enforce national legislation and other related laws to ensure compliance with the BWC's obligations; the abuse of biological defence programs may have a negative impact. For example, the illegal development and retention of technologies related to biological weapons may be used in the name of biological defence programs; the modern economy was more susceptible to bioterrorism. In short, at that time, the BWC failed to effectively prohibit member states from developing biological weapons. The 1979 Sverdlovsk incident in the Soviet Union is a case in point.[6] All of the previously mentioned reasons have forced member states to be more attentive to the apparent absence of compliance clauses in the Convention. There are two major developments at this stage to enhancing the BWC's effectiveness.

First, member states added provisions to Article 5 regarding consultation and cooperation within the framework of the United Nations. Article 5 of the BWC stipulates that "the States Parties to this Convention undertake to consult one another and to co-operate in solving any problems which may arise in relation to the objective of, or in the application of the provisions of, the *Convention*". It suggests that the United Nations should be used as a negotiation and cooperation framework, but it did not specify procedures or the specific circumstances in which the Article should or might be invoked. Thus, at the 1980 Review Conference of the BWC, member states agreed on more specific procedures under Article 5: Any state party shall have the right to request that a consultative meeting be convened, which would help to solve problems and deal with the concern about the implementation expressed by parties.[7] The subsequent Review Conferences held in 1986 and 1991 added more details to the procedures, including the scope, organisation and cost of consultative meetings. Furthermore, both conferences emphasised the possibility of states parties to initiate appropriate international procedures within the framework of the United Nations and in accordance with its Charter.[8] Such possibility was again reaffirmed at the 1996 Review Conference.

Second, member states discussed the possibility to set up confidence-building measures (CBMs) for the BWC. Confidence-building measures were intended to "prevent or reduce the occurrence of ambiguities, doubts and suspicions".[9] As part of the BWC, the proposal for CBMs, which aimed to enhance the relevant exchange of information and transparency among member states, was adopted at the second Review Conference in 1986. These measures mainly included the exchange of data on research centres and laboratories that meet very high national or international safety standards (Biosafety Level 4), the exchange of information on all outbreaks of infectious diseases, encouragement of the publication of results of biological research directly related to the Convention and the active promotion of contacts between scientists engaged in biological research. The third Review Conference, which took place in 1991, expanded the CBMs and established their main forms and required the states parties to submit annual reports on seven specific activities by April 15 of each year.[10]

6.1.2.2 The Protocol period (1991–2001)

In the early 1990s, with the exposure of the biological weapons programmes of Iraq and the Soviet Union, concerns arose about verification measures in the BWC. Although the BWC prohibits the development, production and stockpiling of bacteriological, biological and toxin weapons, it lacked effective measures to verify the compliance of each member state. Although Article 5 of the BWC stipulated that states parties could seek consultations within the UN framework or lodge complaints with the UN Security Council, the veto power of the permanent members of the Security Council made it almost impossible to investigate such a breach. In short, the absence of verification measures made it a "lame convention". In view of these reasons, at the third Review Conference in 1991, member states decided to establish an ad hoc group of governmental experts to identify and examine potential verification measures from a scientific and technical standpoint. In 1993, the Group of Governmental Experts (GGE) issued a final report, which recommended that compliance with the Protocol require a combination of notification from states parties and on-site inspections. In 1994, the UN convened a Special Conference of the States Parties to the BWC in Geneva and decided to establish an ad hoc group to replace the GGE. The Ad Hoc Group (AHG) was tasked with reviewing possible measures to strengthen the BWC, including possible verification measures, and with drafting protocols that could be made into legally binding instruments.

In accordance with its mandate, the AHG convened a total of 24 meetings from 1995 to July 2001 to discuss the main issues in the draft Protocol, such as the verification mechanism, verification measures, the framework of the protocol, export control, international cooperation and the list of biological warfare agents. In July 2001, the AHG proposed a compromise solution on all major outstanding issues. However, the US delegation rejected the draft Protocol on the grounds that it would not effectively address the threat of biological weapons and could harm US national security and commercial interests. Donald Mahley (2001), head of the US delegation, claimed that:

> The draft Protocol will not improve our ability to verify BWC compliance. It will not enhance our confidence in compliance and will do little to deter those countries seeking to develop biological weapons. In our assessment, the draft *Protocol* would put national security and confidential business information at risk.

The move by the United States scuttled the international community's efforts to establish a formal verification mechanism for the BWC. As Michael Nguyen (2006), a US biological weapons expert, put it: "Ten years of work devoted to preparing for and then negotiating a draft protocol to establish a standing verification organisation for the treaty collapsed" (p. 16). Graham Pearson, professor of international security at the University of Bradford in the United Kingdom, also

176 *BWC and global health governance*

believed that the draft Protocol would have strengthened member states' ability to counter the proliferation of biological weapons, but the US rejection had literally killed the Convention.[11]

6.1.2.3 Post-Protocol period (2001–present)

On December 7, 2001, John Bolton, the US Under Secretary for Arms Control and International Security Affairs, announced that the United States had agreed to hold annual meetings, starting in November 2002, to consider and assess progress made by the member states in their implementation of the new measures or mechanisms to effectively strengthen the BWC (Rissanen, 2002). In exchange, however, the United States demanded that the Review Conference should agree to terminate the AHG's mandate. The US rejection sent a clear message: Further work on a compliance instrument was unacceptable to the United States and must stop; the United States was against any motion that implied "creeping institutionalization". This proposal sent shock waves through the meeting room. To prevent outright failure, Tibor Tóth, the Chair of the AHG, declared the adjournment of the Review Conference until the following year. In September 2002, the United States proposed that the scheduled two-week resumption of the conference be reduced to one half-day at which the decision would be made simply to convene another Review Conference in 2006. At the Review Conference reconvened on October 15 of the same year, member states discussed various proposals for improvement, but in view of the strong resistance from the United States, the Review Conference evaded to have any discussions on verification and compliance issues altogether and instead reached a modest consensus in some other areas, including from 2003 until 2005, holding annual one-week meetings in Geneva, and holding additional two-week-long expert meetings to discuss a number of specific aspects of the BWC's enforcement, such as biological security, national penal legislation, international surveillance of disease, responses to suspicious outbreaks of disease or alleged use of biological weapons and codes of conduct for scientists.[12] At the sixth Review Conference on December 8, 2006, because the United States refused to discuss any proposals or mechanisms that might hamper the expansion of biological defence, the Review Conference found it hard to achieve a major breakthrough. One of the main outcomes of this conference was the establishment of a standing Implementation Support Unit (ISU), which replaced the Conference Secretariat to provide administrative support for the BWC and its CBMs.

6.2 Links between the BWC and public health

On the face of it, the BWC and public health belong to different domains. At the international level, biological weapons security and public health security are governed by different regimes. Given that biological defence and the arms control policy of biological weapons are traditional security topics, they are governed by the BWC, while as public health issues, disease prevention and control is under the mandate of WHO. However, due to the development of biological science and

BWC and global health governance 177

technology and the emergence of bioterrorism, "this strict separation has become increasingly blurred" (Kelle, 2007, p. 217). As the late UN Secretary-General Kofi Annan (2006b) said: "These developments have transformed the environment in which the *Convention* operates, and altered ideas about its role and potential". In other words, the BWC should no longer seek only to control biological weapons among member states but rather play an important role in the governance of global health security in a broad sense. Therefore, "the convention is most usefully seen not as part of a WMD non-proliferation regime, but rather as part of an expanded response to disease-based security threats in general" (Enemark, 2005, p. 111). In general, the BWC and public health are connected to each other in the following three ways.

6.2.1 The emergence of bioterrorism

Although the use of biological weapons appeared in human history a long time ago and terrorist activities are nothing new, the connection between the two has never been so close and intimidating. "The increased risk of terrorist organisations and non-state actors seeking weapons of mass destruction" is the "most serious challenge" facing the international community (Zhang, 2003). The same is true of the threat posed by terrorist organisations seeking biological weapons. Annan (2006a) once described bioterrorism as "the most important under-addressed threat relating to terrorism" and called on the international community to pay attention to "'designer' disease[s] and pathogen[s]". Member states' compliance with the BWC is of critical importance to prevent bio-terrorism because the most likely sources for biological weapons acquisition by terrorists are states. Fortunately, there is no evidence that terrorists have or will soon be able to independently develop such weapons. No country would risk its own security to furnish biological weapons to terrorists. Terrorists would sooner buy, steal or invade a national biological project than replicate the costly and time-consuming development process of biological weapons (Rosenberg, 2007). There is evidence that shows the anthrax spores used in the 2001 bioterrorist attacks in the United States may have come from samples provided to certain laboratories in the United States by the US Army Medical Research Institute for Infectious Diseases (USAMRID) (Broad & Miller, 2001). Therefore, the effectiveness of the BWC is determined to a great extent by whether it can successfully prevent bioterrorism.

If bioterrorism strikes, public health authorities will be on the front line to respond to such a crisis. The report by the UN secretary-general's High-Level Panel on Threats, Challenges and Change (2004) stated that a well-equipped public health defence system holds the key to address the potential threat of bioterrorist attacks. Public health systems are essential to the effective defence of biological weapons. The primary responsibility for the public health community is to quickly identify the presence of a biological attack and deal with it afterwards (Katz, 2002). One study found that identification up to 24 hours of an anthrax attack targeting 100,000 people and prompt distribution of medical resources to targets may still result in a death toll of 5,000 people and US$128 million worth

178 BWC and global health governance

of economic damage. If the anthrax attack is not identified within six days and only preventive antibiotics are provided to the population exposed to the attack, as many as 33,000 people could lose their lives, and economic costs would be as high as US$26.3 billion (Kaufmann et al., 1997). This shows how important the public health sector is in responding to bioterrorism. For example, after the anthrax terrorist attack in the United States in 2001, it was not the United States Department of Defence, but the United States Centres for Disease Control and Prevention, that took the first response. In the spring of 2002, in preparation for the 55th World Health Assembly, the Secretariat of WHO published a report titled "Deliberate Use of Biological and Chemical Agents to Cause Harm". It pointed out that, to respond to the previously mentioned incidents, the WHO should "strengthen the disease alert and response systems at all levels, as such a system will detect and respond to diseases that may be deliberately caused (WHO, 2002). In response to potential biological attacks, WHO published "Public Health Response to Biological and Chemical Weapons" in 2004. The Department of Communicable Disease Surveillance and Response of the Secretariat of WHO also launched the Programme for Preparedness for Deliberate Epidemics (PDE). In short, if the BWC is not effectively implemented, it will simply fuel the emergence of bioterrorism, making corresponding public health response measures extremely critical. The rise of bioterrorism has forged and strengthened the link between the BWC and public health (see Figure 6.1).

6.2.2 The impact of the BWC on public health responses

Biotechnology is different from nuclear fission technology. While the latter has few other uses than to develop nuclear weapons, the development of biotechnology not only can be used to develop biological weapons, but it also holds the key to public health security. Therefore, restricting the development and progress of biotechnology will hinder the development of new treatments and vaccines that are needed in tackling public health issues, such as infectious diseases. The control of biological agents required by the BWC will inevitably affect the progress of biotechnology. Some scientists argue that when attempting to prevent the intentional or malicious use of biological research, "increased government oversight of basic life sciences research would 'kill' the research" (Kahn, 2007, p. 12).

In addition, Article 10 of the BWC stipulates that:

> The States Parties to this Convention undertake to facilitate, and have the right to participate in, the fullest possible exchange of equipment, materials and scientific and technological information for the use of bacteriological

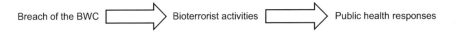

Figure 6.1 Linkages Between the BWC and Public Health

(biological) agents and toxins for peaceful purposes. Parties to the BWC in a position to do so shall also co-operate in contributing individually or together with other States or international organisations to the further development and application of scientific discoveries in the field of bacteriology (biology) for the prevention of disease, or for other peaceful purposes.

This *Convention* shall be implemented in a manner designed to avoid hampering the economic or technological development of States Parties to the *Convention* or international co-operation in the field of peaceful bacteriological (biological) activities, including the international exchange of bacteriological (biological) agents and toxins and equipment for the processing, use or production of bacteriological (biological) agents and toxins for peaceful purposes in accordance with the provisions of the *Convention*.

Although these provisions stipulate that all countries have the obligation to promote international cooperation in the peaceful use of biotechnology, developed countries have strived to weaken the effectiveness of the provisions on international cooperation and have also restricted the transfer of biotechnology to developing countries on grounds of biosafety. Developing countries, on the other hand, maintain that to promote international cooperation in the field of biology, all discriminatory export control measures should be eliminated, and a fair and reasonable export control mechanism should be established within the BWC's framework. They emphasise the importance of scientific and technological cooperation in the field of biotechnology and the importance of full and equal technology transfer. To counter developing countries' calls to scrap existing export control arrangements, at the fifth Review Conference, US representative John Mahley claimed the BWC was "a disarmament, not a trade treaty" (Rissanen, 2001, p. 6). In fact, one of the reasons given by the United States for having rejected the draft protocol to the BWC is that it is detrimental to American commercial interests. No wonder Cuba argued that "the rest of the world was being held hostage to the 'hegemonic' interests of the United States" (Rissanen, 2001, p. 32). To improve global disease surveillance and control, member states should take measures and do all they can to promote the exchange of equipment, data and scientific and technological information, and to promote technology transfer to developing countries in particular. Only in this way can the BWC play an active role in global health governance rather than becoming a tool for developed countries to control biotechnology exports to developing countries.

6.2.3 BWC and public health: different means towards the same end

The establishment of the BWC is "to exclude completely the possibility of bacteriological (biological) agents and toxins being used as weapons for the sake of all mankind".[13] The global health policy is also designed to protect humans from bacterial diseases. The two share the same goal, which is to achieve biosecurity. Therefore, it is important to promote the coordination and integration of biological weapons policies and public health policies. According to Fidler

180 BWC and global health governance

(2008), "effective biosecurity policy and governance requires, nationally and globally, the integration of security and public health" (p. 8). Such integration is necessary for global health governance, both in practice and in rulemaking. On the prevention, detection and response to disease outbreaks, there is considerable overlap between the areas of concern covered in the BWC and the practice of global health policy. As C. F. Chyba (2001), an American biological weapons expert, says: "Biological security must address both the challenge of biological weapons and that of infectious disease" (p. 2349). Understanding the potentially catastrophic biological threats posed by natural infectious diseases and biological weapons is "critical to formulating an effective biosecurity strategy" (Grotto & Tucker, 2006, p. 1). In particular, in the context of the increasing threat posed by bioterrorism and emerging infectious diseases, the international community should pay more attention to and strengthen global health capacity building "in order to provide the basis for an effective global defence against bioterrorism and natural outbreaks of deadly infectious disease" (United Nations, 2004, p. viii). In short, biological weapons and the global health threat posed by natural outbreaks intertwine and constitute an unprecedented policy challenge, posing threats that require countries in the world to no longer confine the issue of biological weapons to traditional security as they work to improve the BWC. In terms of global public health, the WHO should not confine itself to a traditional "technical approach". Only by combining biological weapons policies with public health policies can the world jointly promote global health governance.

Mark Wheelis, a microbiologist at the University of California, once warned that "biology is in the midst of what can only be described as a revolution. This technology will have great power both for peaceful and hostile uses" (2004, p. 6). This change highlights the necessity and urgency for the international community to improve on the BWC. Countries around the world, especially countries strong in biotechnology, should incorporate the increasingly significant international norm to better comply with the BWC and actively carry out international cooperation on the peaceful use of biotechnology so that they may help countries with less-advanced biotechnological resource become more capable of responding to public health crises. This is the only approach to achieving public health security in this interdependent world.

6.3 BWC: deficiencies and dilemmas

To strengthen the effectiveness and function of the Biological Weapons Convention, the international community has to date convened a total of six review conferences in Geneva. However, due to the BWC's inherent deficiencies, the different priorities of developed and developing countries, and the "biosecurity dilemma" between member states, little progress has been made from these conferences. Some scholar even believed that "the more complete truth is that little will be done in Geneva to ensure security from intentionally inflicted disease"(Kellman, 2006, p. 235). In view of the BWC's significant impact on global health issues such as bioterrorism and recurrent infectious diseases, it is necessary to systematically examine factors that have restricted the BWC's role. It is also an urgent challenge for the international community to deal with the BWC's inherent flaws.

6.3.1 Deficiencies of the BWC

Since it entered into force in 1975, the BWC has never succeeded in "bringing an end" to biological weapons programmes in some of its member states. The exposure of the biological weapons programmes by the Soviet Union and by Iraq in the early 1990s put the BWC in crisis. In recent years, the United States has also carried out its own biological defence activities, including building highly classified facilities to develop bioweapons. The international community is thus all the more concerned about potential violations of the BWC by the United States (Warrick, 2006). All these examples illustrate the deficiencies in the enforcement and regulatory design of the BWC.

6.3.1.1 Absence of legally binding verification mechanisms

Zanders (1996) pointed out that "ever since governments began considering a formal ban on BW development and possession, verification was seen as an almost insurmountable obstacle" (p. 35). On August 6, 1968, in its working paper on biological warfare, the United Kingdom suggested that:

> Consideration might be given to the possibility that a competent body of experts, established under the auspices of the United Nations, might investigate allegations made by a party to the Convention which appeared to establish a prima facie case that another party had acted in breach of the obligations established in the *Convention*. The *Convention* would contain a provision by which parties would undertake to co-operate fully in any investigation and any failure to comply with this would be reported to the Security Council.
> (Stockholm International Peace Research Institute, 1971, p. 255)

Unfortunately, this proposal was not accepted by member states. When the United States and the Soviet Union reached a consensus on a draft protocol of the BWC in 1971, it did not contain any provisions on verification measures. The absence of a legally binding and well-established procedure in the BWC meant that biological weapons policies made by member states might be unpredictable and that member states may easily become victims of arbitrary acts or face accusations by other member states. The BWC has failed to play its due role in addressing the threats brought by state and non-state actors and in coping with scientific and technological developments. Therefore, the absence of verification measures has become a focal concern of member states since the BWC entered into force.

The anthrax virus leak in the Soviet Union in 1979 demonstrates that without verification measures, the BWC would simply become toothless for some member states. Its lack of enforcement power is made more apparent by the exposure of the biological weapons programmes conducted by the Soviet Union and by

182 BWC and global health governance

Iraq in the early 1990s. After the collapse of the Soviet Union, concerned about Russia's biological weapons, the United States, the United Kingdom and Russia, sat down to establish a trilateral verification mechanism among these three major powers of bioweapons. However, due to the mutual distrust between the United States and Russia, this mechanism did not last long. At the same time, the United Nations Special Commission (UNSCOM) also tried to verify Iraq's biological weapons programmes, but to little avail.

Tucker (2004b) suggested that "the only way to put real 'teeth' in the *Convention* is through the negotiation of legally binding agreements that create enforceable obligations and deter violations" (p. 13). Recognising the need to strengthen the BWC, the 1991 Review Conference agreed to set up a group of government verification experts to conduct a systematic study of biological monitoring techniques. From March 1992 to September 1993, this group convened four meetings. In 1994, the United Nations established a new multilateral negotiating forum called the Ad Hoc Group (AHG) to work on a legally binding instrument to augment the power of the BWC and to design relevant verification measures.[14] However, as major powers of bioweapons, the United States and Russia remained ambivalent towards the verification measures for the BWC. US officials maintained that there was no way to effectively verify member compliance of the BWC, so they strongly opposed to using "verification" to describe any legally binding instrument (Lacey, 1994, p. 55). The US rejection of the draft Protocol in 2001 showed its reluctance to implement a legally binding international instrument for the verification of biological weapons. In view of this rejection, the 2006 Review Conference did not address the protocol on verification measures at all. Seen from this perspective, under the current international political environment, it is almost impossible for the international community to reach consensus on a protocol on verification measures. It is as J. Littlewood, a US expert on biological weapons, concluded: "When one considers the negotiations on the BWC Protocol together with the developments in international policies from 1991 through the present day, the fundamental lesson for the Convention is a simple one: There will be no BWC Protocol" (Littlewood, 2005, p. 232).

6.3.1.2 Lack of confidence-building measures

The purpose of confidence-building measures (CBMs) is to "reinforce or support an established treaty obligation or provide mechanisms to prevent default or verify compliance" (Holst, 1983, p. 5). Based on the stringency of confidence-building measures, they can be classified as voluntary measures, legally binding measures and politically binding measures. Among the three, legally binding CBMs are the most effective, followed by politically binding ones, then voluntary ones.

CBMs are a tool for arms control. For the BWC to play a better role in the prohibition of biological weapons, member states have also established a series of CBMs. Nicolas Isla, a researcher at the Hamburg Centre for Biological Arms Control at Hamburg University, believes that "a good starting point for building confidence in compliance is to increase transparency" (Isla & Hunger, 2006, p. 19).

At the second Review Conference in 1986, member states reached an agreement, which required members to report annually on CBMs related to biological weapons. The third Review Conference in 1991 revised and expanded this agreement. However, only a small number of countries implemented CBMs. These politically binding measures required member states to report to the United Nations Department of Disarmament Affairs (UNODA) on specific activities each year, including data on research centres and laboratories; information on national biological defence research and development programmes; information on outbreaks of infectious diseases and similar occurrences caused by toxins; publication of results and promotion of use of knowledge; information on legislation, regulations and other measures; declaration of past activities in offensive and/or defensive biological research and development programmes and information on vaccine-production facilities.[15] Annual declarations are collated by the UNODA and distributed back to the member states (in their respective languages, thus no translation is required).

To increase the effectiveness of CBMs, the BWC's AHG has been trying to develop a legally binding protocol since 1995. However, since the United States rejected the Protocol in 2001, there has not been any legally binding CBM among member states. The political mistrust between developed and developing countries, especially between the United States and Iran and between the United States and Russia, has made these politically binding CBMs highly unpredictable. The take-up of voluntary CBMs fared even worse. From 1987 to 1995, only 70 out of 139 member states had submitted declarations, and only 11 had participated in all exchanges of information (Kelle, 1997, p. 141).

New biotechnological developments and opaque biodefense activities will create or aggregate traditional security risks. With bioterrorism and infectious diseases becoming a global threat, member states of the BWC should adopt more effective CBMs to increase transparency in their biological programs. This will help reduce mutual suspicion and mistrust. Nevertheless, since "the level of transparency of biodefense programs has become one of the hottest controversies in contemporary biosecurity policy" (Fidler, 2008, p. 90), the prospects for effective CBMs in this area are not encouraging.

6.3.1.3 Absence of organisational support for the BWC

International treaties and organisations can provide post-conference support, function as a communication channel and a clearing house for information exchange and provide a platform for members to interact with each other. Of the three international instruments on weapons of mass destruction, the BWC has the weakest enforcement record. While the NPT is subject to monitoring and verification by the International Atomic Energy Agency (IAEA), and the CWC is subject to inspections by the Organisation for the Prohibition of Chemical Weapons (OPCW), there is no such legally binding instrument to ensure the BWC's enforcement, not even a standing secretariat. As a result, the BWC has become a toothless regime. It has become extremely difficult for member states to verify and monitor the BWC's enforcement.

184 *BWC and global health governance*

To make up for this deficiency, the Weapons of Mass Destruction Commission, led by Hans Blix (2006), recommended that member states to the BWC should establish a standing secretariat to handle organisational and administrative matters related to the treaty, such as Review Conferences and expert meetings. At the sixth Convention Review Conference held in December 2006, member states agreed to establish an Implementation Support Unit (ISU) consisting of three full-time staff members to provide administrative support and CBMs within the Geneva Branch of the United Nations Office for Disarmament Affairs. In terms of administrative support, the ISU needs to perform the following tasks: provide administrative support to and prepare documentation for meetings agreed by the review conference; facilitate communications among contracted parties and, upon request, with international organisations; facilitate contact between member states and intergovernmental, international and non-governmental organisations, including relevant sectors of industry and the scientific and academic communities; maintain liaisons with the designated national focal points of contact in the governments of states parties and support, as appropriate, member states' efforts to implement the decisions and recommendations of the Review Conference. ISU's CBM-related tasks include receiving and distributing CBMs to/from member states, sending information notices to member states regarding their annual submissions, compiling and distributing data on CBMs and reporting on participation at each meeting of the member states, developing and maintaining a secure website on CBMs accessible only to member states and serving as an information exchange point for assistance related to the preparation of CBMs.

It can be seen from these functions that setting up such a mechanism will not contribute significantly to the BWC's enforcement. As the unit's mandate will be limited to the previously mentioned tasks, the ISU is dwarfed by the CWC and the Treaty on the Non-Proliferation of Nuclear Weapons. In some respects, the ISU could even backfire. Consider CBMs instituted to enhance the transparency. The ISU should create an electronic spreadsheet for member states to fill and, after obtaining the consent of member states who have submitted the information, post the completed form on a secure website and make it accessible for all member states. Without express consent from member states, the information supplied shall not be circulated to any other individuals and organisations. This means that NGOs and other international organisations are denied access to the CBMs established by the member states, which is not conducive to promoting the transparency of the CBMs. As a result, the "support" the ISU is meant to provide is trivial in practice. It can only serve as an ad hoc secretariat at best, let alone monitor or verify the BWC's enforcement.

6.3.2 *Three dilemmas that lead to the defects of the BWC*

Reasons for the defects in the BWC are manifold. They mainly include problems from collective action due to the anarchy in international politics, the dual-use dilemma of biotechnology and the biosecurity dilemma in the security perception of countries.

6.3.2.1 Problems of collective action

International regimes are born because countries need to interact with each other in the international system. The anarchic state of the international community is ripe for problems of collective action. In the preface Olson wrote for Todd Sandler's book *Collective Action: Theory and Applications*, he noted that all social science research is based on two laws. The first law is that "when each individual considers only his or her interests, a collectively rational outcome emerges automatically"; The second law is that "sometimes, the first law doesn't hold: no matter how intelligently each individual pursues his or her interest, no socially rational outcome can emerge spontaneously" (Sandler, 1992, p. vii). Obviously, the outcomes of the BWC and its Protocol belong to the second scenario. For the entire international community, the ideal outcome of the BWC is that all member states would abide by all its provisions and eventually achieve global biosecurity. However, as countries have different interests and priorities regarding the specific implementation of the BWC, it is difficult for them to reach consensus on those differences, thereby trapping the BWC's enforcement into problems of collective action. Western countries, led by the United States, tend to emphasise Article 3 of the BWC, which concerns the prevention of the proliferation of biological weapons, including export controls and restrictions on technology transfer. In contrast, non-aligned countries, led by India and Iran, are demanding strict enforcement of Article 10, which advocates international cooperation and technological exchanges in the peaceful use of biotechnology. Article 10 therefore runs into potential conflict with Article 3. Non-aligned countries have been protesting that the export controls imposed by developed countries have hindered the exchange and development of biotechnology, while Western countries have always maintained that export controls are part of Article 3 and use it to set up "Australian Group (AG)", an informal forum of their own.

According to Chevrier (1995, p. 216), "it is logical to conclude that in any trade-off among issues, each group of countries is unlikely to concede where its interests are strongest" (p. 216). Given the conflict of interests between developed countries and non-aligned countries, it is difficult to take collective action to improve the BWC's enforcement, especially "when there is no leader nation that plays a major role in the contingency" (Sandler, 2004, p. 7). For example, the United States, a major power of bioweapons, refuses to accept the Protocol, while Russia, another major power, is also ambivalent about the Protocol, thus exacerbating the global collective action problems in the BWC's enforcement.

6.3.2.2 Biosecurity dilemma

The security dilemma is "the most fundamental concept of all in security studies, and it is at the centre of international politics" (Wheeler & Booth, 1992, p. 29). The heart of the security dilemma argument is that an increase in one state's security results in a decrease in perceived security of others because the defensive measures taken by one state may be considered a threat by another.[16] The same

186 *BWC and global health governance*

can be applied to the biosecurity dilemma. When a country's defensive biological plan is considered offensive by another, it has no other choice but to implement a hedging strategy that may lead to an arms race between the two, resulting in a common insecurity. In general, there are two main reasons for the biosecurity dilemma.

First, the difference between defensive and offensive biological research and developmentlies primarily in their intentions. However, intentions are difficult to define, so a safer choice is for countries to make appropriate responses based on the capabilities of their potential opponents rather than intentions they express. As a result, these countries also develop defensive biological programmes, which in turn are considered offensive by their opponents, thus resulting in a vicious circle. According to Leitenberg (2002), "if many states feel more pressure to engage in research and development, the world would have slipped from an envelope into an arms race" (p. 23). In other words, the failure to identify intentions causes the biosecurity dilemma.[17] For example, before the conclusion of the BWC, the Nixon administration unilaterally announced its abandonment of the biological weapons programmes, while the Soviet Union, being a member state of the BWC, still went on to develop ambitious biological programmes after the BWC entered into force. An important reason, according to the Soviet Union, was that it did not believe the United States would give up its offensive biological weapons programmes. Just as Ken Alibek, a former Soviet biological warfare expert, claimed: "We didn't believe a word of Nixon's announcement. Even though the massive US biological munitions stockpile was ordered to be destroyed, we thought the Americans were only wrapping a thicker cloak around their activities" (1999, p. 234).

Second, potential opponents may worry that other countries will make new breakthroughs in their research in response to new biological weapons, which will in turn put them at a disadvantage. This will result in biological arms race or even prolonged biotechnology competition with undefined military implications. In an arms race of bioweapons, countries will compete to gain an advantage in the field of biological sciences and "ramp up their own R&D activities as a hedge against technological surprise and the unpredictability of future adversaries—a 'keeping up with the Joneses' effect" (Grotto & Tucker, 2006, p. 43). Under such circumstances, it is only natural for the BWC to be thrown out the window by member states.

Ever since the anthrax attack in 2001, the US federal government's annual budget for biodefense surged from US$414 million in 2001 to US$7.6 billion in 2005 (Schuler, 2004). Its spending on biodefense research and development increased even further in recent years. In September 2001, the *New York Times* revealed that the United States was conducting some type of test for bioweapons. Soon other member states and arms control experts claimed the move was a violation of the BWC and could lead to a new round of bioweapons arms race (Miller et al., 2001). On July 30, 2006, the *Washington Post* reported that the US Department of Homeland Security implemented a highly confidential "Biological Threat Characterization Program" (Warrick, 2006). The programme aimed to "understand new scientific trends that may be exploited by our adversaries to develop biological weapons" (The White House, 2004, p. 4). In the program, researchers mimicked the major steps a state or terrorist would take to create a biological arsenal to better understand the threat, which included anthrax bacteria spore attacks and highly deadly super viruses that evolved from ordinary viruses. Jonathan B. Tucker, a senior researcher at the Monterey Institute of International Studies, believes that "the laboratory characterization of putative biological threats run the risk of becoming a self-fulfilling prophecy that undermines US national security" (2006, p. 197). Research of this kind will raise suspicions in other countries, weaken the effectiveness of the BWC and increase the risk of genetically altered viruses and related technologies being leaked to proliferators and terrorists. Third, the United States' own actions raise suspicions about its own compliance with the BWC and "fosters a 'biological security dilemma' that could lead to a new biological arms race" (Tucker, 2004a, p. 14). The United States cannot make people not suspect its violation of the BWC. Susan Wright (2004) of the University of Michigan also believes America's overreaction to biological defence risks could produce a race for novel biological weapons that might be wildly out of control. It is not too difficult to understand why the United States rejected the draft Protocol to the BWC. Trade secret protection was a convenient shield over plans to develop bioweapons. It would be difficult for other countries to take the BWC seriously when they believe the United States violated the BWC by developing offensive bioweapons programmes.

6.3.2.3 Dual-use dilemma of biotechnology

The dual-use dilemma arises in the context of research in the biological and other sciences as a consequence of the fact that one and the same piece of scientific research sometimes has the potential to be used for harm as well as for good (Miller & Selgelid, 2007). Another important reason why the BWC is difficult to implement is that due to the dual-use nature of biotechnology some provisions are rendered ambiguous. Article I of the BWC, for example, provides that:

> Each State Party to this *Convention* undertakes never in any circumstances to develop, produce, stockpile or otherwise acquire or retain microbial or other biological agents, or toxins whatever their origin or method of production, of types and in quantities that have no justification for prophylactic, protective or other peaceful purposes. Weapons, equipment or means of delivery designed to use such agents or toxins for hostile purposes or in armed conflict.

However, it does not provide the definition of "peaceful purposes". Take the smallpox virus as an example. It is at the same time a lethal bioweapon and a necessary ingredient for vaccines. At the moment, the United States and Russia are the only two countries that have stockpiles of smallpox samples. Since smallpox was eradicated in 1980, WHO urged both countries to destroy their samples, but they have not yet done so, citing scientific research as the reason. Therefore, there are still many grey areas regarding the peaceful use of biotechnology. In this

188 *BWC and global health governance*

sense, some people think the BWC is unverifiable by nature. As Amy Smithson (2004b), a researcher at the Stimson Centre in Washington and the Centre for Strategic and International Studies, puts it:

> Policymakers, industry officials and the general public are commonly told that the BWC is "unverifiable" due to the complex, dual-use nature of biological materials, equipment, and technologies and the claim that inspections would automatically reveal sensitive defence or business information. These assertions hang in the air unchallenged.
>
> (p. vii)

The dual-use nature of biological weapons technology makes it extremely difficult to prevent the proliferation of biological weapons. Therefore, the non-verifiability of the BWC, which results from the dual use of biotechnology, has become the technical bottleneck restricting the establishment of a verification mechanism for the BWC and a major reason for the United States to reject the Protocol to the BWC.

Summary

The defects caused by the dilemmas mentioned earlier have seriously restricted the functioning of the BWC, "to the extent that it, as an arms control regime, is less and less valued" (Becker, 2007). However, with the development of biotechnology, the outbreaks of various emerging infectious diseases and the increasingly serious threat of bioterrorism, the importance of the BWC in global health governance is also being felt. "Upholding the BWC is an essential part in achieving global biosecurity" (Atlas & Reppy, 2005, p. 52). Therefore, how to strengthen the effectiveness of the BWC has become an urgent task for the international community. For now, although it remains almost impossible to establish a legally binding verification mechanism and a formalised international organisation for the BWC, it would be a stretch to think the BWC has been completely "sidelined". Instead, this situation only underscores the need for member states to take other proactive measures to enhance its effectiveness. The international community has been making considerable efforts in this regard. The UN Security Council adopted Resolution 1540 in 2004, and the IHR (2005) went into effect in 2007. Resolution 1540 affirms:

> Its resolve to take appropriate and effective actions against any threat to international peace and security caused by the proliferation of nuclear, chemical and biological weapons and their means of delivery, in conformity with its primary responsibilities, as provided for in the United Nations Charter.[18]

It states that the Security Council has the authority to act on the implementation of the BWC. Article 7 of the IHR (2005) also stipulates that:

If a State Party has evidence of an unexpected or unusual public health event within its territory, irrespective of origin or source, which may constitute a public health emergency of international concern, it shall provide to WHO all relevant public health information.

By implication, public health incidents caused by biological weapons should also be reported to WHO. At the same time, Article 14 of the IHR (2005) provides that:

In cases in which notification or verification of, or response to, an event is primarily within the competence of other intergovernmental organisations or international bodies, WHO shall coordinate its activities with such organisations or bodies in order to ensure the application of adequate measures for the protection of public health.

In other words, in a bioterrorist attack, WHO should coordinate its activities with the newly established Implementation Support Unit of the BWC. The IHR "have also become a part of the international regimes that deal with bioweapons threats" (Fidler & Gostin, 2008).

Resolution 1540 affirms that "prevention of proliferation of nuclear, chemical and biological weapons should not hamper international cooperation in materials, equipment and technology for peaceful purposes while goals of peaceful utilization should not be used as a cover for proliferation".[19] In other words, preventing the proliferation of biological weapons should not be used as an excuse by developed countries to curb biotechnology development in developing countries. International co-operation on biotechnology based on Article 10 of the BWC can improve the capacity of developing countries to respond to global health security crises, which in turn will encourage more countries to join the regime. In addition, better functioning of the BWC depends on the internalisation of its norms by member states. In other words, it is essential for member states to enact relevant legislation on biosecurity at the national level. More importantly, all countries in the world, especially the major powers of biological weapons, should not treat the BWC as merely a non-proliferation treaty because all member states are prohibited from acquiring biological weapons. Only in this way can the international community exclude completely the possibility of bacteriological (biological) agents and toxins being used as weapons for the sake of all mankind.

Notes

1 For the history of biological warfare before World War I, see Wheelis (1999).
2 For example, the United Kingdom, France and the Soviet Union, among others, made the reservations that the Protocol would no longer be binding on any enemy or its allies if they failed to comply with the provisions. See Geneva Protocol 1925. Retrieved from https://fas.org/nuke/control/geneva/intro.htm.
3 For more details on Japan's bacteriological weapons plan, see Harris (1995).
4 See Article 3 of the BWC. Retrieved from http://disarmament.un.org/treaties/t/bwc/text.

5 The BWC did not explicitly prohibit the use of biological weapons. Member states only reaffirmed at the fourth Review Conference that "the use by the States Parties, in any way and under any circumstances, of microbial or other biological agents or toxins, that is not consistent with prophylactic, protective or other peaceful purposes, is effectively a violation of Article I of the convention". However, this did not become part of the BWC, but merely an extension of Article 1. Retrieved from www.un.org/press/en/1996/19961206.dc2572.html.

6 The incident occurred on April 2–3, 1979, when an explosion at an underground test site of a microbial centre in Sverdlovsk during weapons testing resulted in the release of weapons-grade anthrax, killing hundreds of residents of the area in a single week.

7 See BWC/CONF.I/10. Retrieved from www.brad.ac.uk/acad/sbtwc/btwc/rev_cons/1rc/docs/conf/BWC_Co nf.I_10_E.pdf.

8 See BWC/CONF.III/23. Retrieved from www.unog.ch/bwcdocuments/1991-09-3RC/BWC_CONF.III_23.pdf.

9 See "Second Review Conference of the Parties to the Convention on the Prohibition of the Development, Production and Stockpiling of Bacteriological (Biological) and Toxin Weapons and on Their Destruction: Final Document". (1986). Retrieved from www.un.org/disarmament/wmd/bio/.

10 The report should include: data on research centres and laboratories; information on vaccine-production facilities; information on national biological defence research and development programmes; declaration of past activities in offensive and/or defensive biological research and development programmes; information on outbreaks of infectious diseases and similar occurrences caused by toxins; publication of results and promotion of use of knowledge and contacts; information on legislation, regulations and other measures.

11 See "The US Rejection of the Protocol at the Eleventh Hour Damages International Security Against Biological Weapons". Retrieved from www.sussex.ac.uk/Units/spru/hsp/documents/cbwcb53-Pearson.pdf.

12 See BWC/CONF.V17 (2002). Retrieved fromwww.sussex.ac.uk/Units/spru/hsp/documents/cbwcb53-Pearson.pdf www.unog.ch/bwcdocuments/2001-11-5RC/BWC_CONF.V_17.pdf.

13 See the preamble of the BWC.

14 These verification measures mainly include: 1) Notification: Member states regularly notify and disclose relevant information related to the BWC and evaluate member states' activities related to biological weapons; 2) Conversation with staff: If done properly, the peaceful motives of the inspected equipment items can be verified and clues about secret activities related to biological weapons can be found; 3) On-site inspection: Inspectors shall inspect equipment, safety measures, animal equipment, containers and waste disposal. Since all bioweapon equipment is dual-use and routine on-site inspections are announced in advance, it is difficult to find non-convertible evidence of breaches, but the inspection team shall be able to identify whether the characteristics of the equipment are consistent with the R&D or production plan notified by the country; 4) On-site verification of critical equipment necessary for the development, testing and production of biological weapons. Although all of these devices are dual-use, they can be used as a marker when something suspicious happens; 5) Sampling and marking (on-site): The scope of sampling includes the equipment used for R&D, production and stockpiling, dust inside buildings, soil outside buildings, wastewater from factories and plants and animals used for R&D and production of reagents. On-site sampling is one of the most controversial issues in the formulation of the protocol because it may disclose information concerning commercial confidence and national security.

15 See BWC/CONF.III/23. Retrieved from www.unog.ch/bwcdocuments/1991-09-3RC/BWC_CONF.III_23.pdf.

16 For more details on the security dilemma, see Jervis (1976).

BWC and global health governance   191

17 For more information on the biosecurity dilemma, see Koblentz (2004).
18 See UN Security Council Resolution 1540, S/RES/1540. (2004). Retrieved from https://undocs.org/S/RES/1540 (2004).
19 See UN Security Council Resolution 1540, S/RES/1540. (2004).

References

Alibek, K. (1999). *Biohazard*. New York: Random House.
Annan, K. (2006a, April 27). *Report of the UN Secretary-General: Uniting Against Terrorism: Recommendations for a Global Counter-Terrorism Strategy*. Retrieved from www.un.org/unitingagainstterrorism/sg-terrorism-2may06.pdf
Annan, K. (2006b, November 20). *Remarks to the Sixth Review Conference of the Biological Weapons Convention*. Retrieved from www.un.org/apps/sg/sgstats.asp?nid=2311
Atlas, R. M., & Reppy, J. (2005). Globalizing Biosecurity. *Biosecurity and Bioterrorism: Biodefense Strategy, Practice, and Science*, 3(1), 51–60.
Becker, U. (2007). *Light at the End of the Tunnel? The Sixth Review Conference of the Biological Weapons Convention*. Frankfurt: Peace Research Institute.
Blix, H. (2006). *Weapons of Terror: Freeing the World of Nuclear, Biological and Chemical Arms*. Stockholm: The Weapons of Mass Destruction Commission.
Broad, W. J., & Miller, J. (2001, December 2). Inquiry Includes Possibility of Killer from a US Lab: An Insider Would Fit the FBI's Official Profile of an Anthrax Suspect. *New York Times*.
Chevrier, M. I. (1995). From Verification to Strengthening Compliance: Prospects and Challenges of the Biological Weapons Convention. *Politics and the Life Sciences*, 209–219.
Chyba, C. F. (2001). Biological Security in a Changed World. *Science*, 293(5539), 2349–2349.
Enemark, C. (2005). Infectious Diseases and International Security: The Biological Weapons Convention and beyond. *The Nonproliferation Review*, 12(1), 107–125.
Fidler, D. P., & Gostin, L. O. (2008). *Biosecurity in the Global Age: Biological Weapons, Public Health, and the Rule of Law*. Redwood City, CA: Stanford University Press.
Grotto, A. J., & Tucker, J. B. (2006). *Biosecurity: A Comprehensive Action Plan*. Washington, DC: Centre for American Progress.
Harris, S. H. (1995). *Factories of Death: Japanese Biological Warfare, 1932–1945 and the American Cover-Up*. London and New York: Routledge.
Holst, J. J. R. (1983). Confidence-Building Measures a Conceptual Framework. *Survival*, 25(1), 2–15.
Isla, N., & Hunger, I. (2006). BWC 2006: Building Transparency through Confidence Building Measures. *Arms Control Today*, 36(6), 19–22.
Jervis, R. (1976). *Perception and Misperception in International Politics*. Princeton: Princeton University Press.
Kahn, L. H. (2007). Government Oversight and the Life Sciences. *Bulletin of the Atomic Scientists*, 12.
Katz, R. (2002). Public Health Preparedness: The Best Defence against Biological Weapons. *Washington Quarterly*, 25(3), 69–82.
Kaufmann, A. F., Meltzer, M. I., & Schmid, G. P. (1997). The Economic Impact of a Bioterrorist Attack: Are Prevention and Postattack Intervention Programs Justifiable? *Emerging Infectious Diseases*, 3(2), 83.

192 BWC and global health governance

Kelle, A. (1997). Developing Control Regimes for Chemical and Biological Weapons. *The International Spectator*, 32(3–4), 137–157.

Kelle, A. (2007). Securitization of International Public Health: Implications for Global Health Governance and the Biological Weapons Prohibition Regime. *Global Governance*, 13(2), 217–235.

Kellman, B. (2006). Notes from a BWC Gadfly. *Biosecurity and Bioterrorism: Biodefense Strategy, Practice, and Science*, 4(3), 231–236.

Koblentz, G. (2004). Pathogens as Weapons: The International Security Implications of Biological Warfare. *International Security*, 28(3), 84–122.

Lacey, E. J. (1994). Tackling the Biological Weapons Threat: The Next Proliferation Challenge. *Washington Quarterly*, 17(4), 53–64.

Leitenberg, M. (2002). Biological Weapons and Bioterrorism in the First Years of the Twenty-First Century. *Politics and the Life Sciences*, 21(2), 3–27.

Littlewood, J. (2005). *The Biological Weapons Convention: A Failed Revolution*. Aldershot, Hampshire: Ashgate Publishing Ltd.

Mahley, D. (2001, July 25). *Statement by the United States to the Ad Hoc Group of Biological Weapons Convention States Parties*. Retrieved from https://2001-2009.state.gov/t/isn/bw/rmks//index.htm

Miller, J., Engelberg, S., & Broad, W. J. (2001). US Germ Warfare Research Pushes Treaty Limits. *New York Times*, 4, A1.

Miller, S., & Selgelid, M. J. (2007). Ethical and Philosophical Consideration of the Dual-Use Dilemma in the Biological Sciences. *Science and Engineering Ethics*, 13(4), 523–580.Nguyen, M. (2006). BWC Verification: A Decade-Long Detour? *Arms Control Today*, 36(4).

Rissanen, J. (2001). A Turning Point to Nowhere? BWC in Trouble as US Turns Its Back on Verification Protocol. *Disarmament Diplomacy*, 59, 11–17.

Rissanen, J. (2002). Left in Limbo: Review Conference Suspended on Edge of Collapse. *Disarmament Diplomacy*, 62, 18–45.

Rosenberg, B. H. (2007). A Counter-Bioterrorism Strategy for the New UN Secretary-General. *Disarmament Diplomacy*, 84, 29–35.

Sandler, T. (1992). *Collective Action: Theory and Applications*. Ann Arbor, MI: University of Michigan Press.

Sandler, T. (2004). *Global Collective Action*. Cambridge: Cambridge University Press.

Schuler, A. (2004). Billions for Biodefense: Federal Agency Biodefense Funding, FY2001–FY2005. *Biosecurity and Bioterrorism: Biodefense Strategy, Practice, and Science*, 2(2), 86–96.

Secretary-General's High-Level Panel on Threats, Challenges and Change. (2004). *A More Secure World: Our Shared Responsibility*. New York: United Nations.

Smithson, A. (2004a). Biological Weapons: Can Fear Overwhelm Inaction? *The Washington Quarterly*, 28(1), 165–178.

Smithson, A. (2004b). Resuscitating the Bioweapons Ban: US Industry Experts' Plans for Treaty Monitoring. *Center for Strategic and International Studies*, 11.

Steinbruner, J. D. (1997). Biological Weapons: A Plague Upon All Houses. *Foreign Policy*, 109, 85–96.

Stockholm International Peace Research Institute. (1971). *The Problem of Chemical and Biological Warfare, Volume IV: CB Disarmament Negotiations 1920–1970*. Stockholm: Almqvist & Wiksell.

Tucker, J. B. (2004a). Biological Threat Assessment: Is the Cure Worse Than the Disease? *Arms Control Today*, 34(8), 14.

Tucker, J. B. (2004b). Strengthening the BWC: A Way Forward. *Disarmament Diplomacy*, 78, 24–30.

Tucker, J. B. (2006). Avoiding the Biological Security Dilemma: A Response to Petro and Carus. *Biosecurity and Bioterrorism: Biodefense Strategy, Practice, and Science*, 4(2), 195–199.

United Nations. (2004). *United Nations Secretary-Genernal's High-Level Panel on Threats, Challenges and Change, A More Secure World: Our Shared Responsibility*. New York: United Nations.

Warrick, J. (2006). The Secretive Fight against Bioterror. *Washington Post*, 30, p. A1.

Wheeler, N., & Booth, K. (1992). The Security Dilemma. In J. Baylis & N. S. Rengger (Eds.), *Dilemmas of World Politics: International Issues in a Changing World* (pp. 29–60). Oxford: Oxford University Press.

Wheelis, M. (1999). Biological Warfare before 1914. In E. Geissler & J. E. v. C. Moon (Eds.), *Biological and Toxin Weapons: Research, Development and Use from the Middle Ages to 1945*. Oxford: Oxford University Press.

Wheelis, M. (2004). Will the "New Biology" Lead to New Weapons? *Arms Control Today*, 34(6), 6.

The White House. (2004). *Biodefense for the 21st Century*. Washington, DC: The White House.

WHO. (2002). *Deliberate Use of Biological and Chemical Agents to Cause Harm*. Geneva: WHO.

Wright, S. (2004). Taking Biodefense Too Far. *Bulletin of the Atomic Scientists*, 60(6), 58–66.

Zanders, J. P. (1996). Verification of the BTWC: Seeking the Impossible or Impossible to Seek? *Proceedings of the Conference*, 3(3), 38–45.

Zhang, Y. (2003, December 30). Turn Challenges Into Opportunities and Seek Security through Cooperation. *PLA Daily*.

7 China's role in global health governance

Efficient global governance depends on an adequate supply of global public goods, but most global public goods follow a summation process. Put differently, all countries must contribute for the good to emerge. According to Kaul (2003), "global public goods thus can be seen as comprising national public goods plus international cooperation" (p. 284). National public goods, or national building blocks, are an essential part of global public goods. In the same vein, global public goods for health comprise national public health products plus international public health cooperation. A country's responsibility therefore is reflected through its contribution to global health governance in the form of more global public goods. China's active participation and consequent provision of global public goods for health are instantiations of its ideal to make the world a harmonious place. It has carried out different levels of health governance efforts. This chapter first describes the diplomatic process through which China participated in global health governance; it then examines problems regarding this participation.

7.1 China's engagement in global health governance

Global health governance is achieved mainly through global health cooperation. Through coordinated efforts from countries around the world, global health governance can solve transnational public health security issues and produce global public goods for health. Specifically, global health governance uses public health diplomacy to overcome problems of collective action. The relevant norms and practices used by WHO and WTO, for example, are all results of diplomatic and collaborative efforts.

Although public health and diplomacy seem like quite different domains, this difference belies the deep connection between the two fields. In fact, with the emergence of public health crises, such as SARS, HIV/AIDS and the anthrax attacks, the two domains are becoming more intertwined than ever. Foreign policy and global health are "working together towards common goals" and are "protecting and promoting public health as part of the foreign policy agenda has taken special significance" (Chan et al., 2008). The securitisation of global health issues means global health issues have become more prominent in foreign policies. Public health diplomatic strategies are now increasingly popular concerns for policymakers. This is illustrated in the mission of the Foreign Policy and Global Health (FPGH), an initiative launched by the foreign ministers of Brazil, France, Indonesia, Norway, Senegal, South Africa and Thailand, seeks to promote the use of a health lens in formulating foreign policy to work together towards common goals. Global health diplomacy is a concept both old and young. It is old because public health diplomacy has been around since the mid-19th century; it is young because it was not long ago that it came to be analysed as a concept. Public health diplomacy involves political movement that can not only improve domestic and international health conditions but also maintain and improve international relations. Richard Horton, editor-in-chief of the well-known British medical journal *The Lancet*, believes public health is now the most important foreign policy issue of our time. He identifies four advantages in using health as an instrument of foreign policy: First, health is strategically correct; second, focusing on health will produce unequivocally positive benefits—social cohesion, equity and a strengthened national infrastructure; third, focusing on health is a valuable diplomatic tool in its own right to promote good bilateral relations and to signal good leadership; finally, focusing on health will encourage trust between nations and across global multilateral organisations (Horton, 2006). In short, global health diplomacy refers to international cooperation conducted by a nation to safeguard the health of its own citizens and the health of other countries' citizens. Global health diplomacy can encompass a broad range of actors, including governmental actors (e.g. ministries of foreign affairs, ministries of health), inter-governmental organisations and nongovernmental organisations. Global health diplomacy is also a collective joint governance initiative taken by countries worldwide to achieve global health security. China sees itself as a stakeholder in global health security and holds international public health cooperation in high regard. Public health security threats affect not only human safety, but also economic, political, environmental and social safety. All countries must figure out how to deal with these non-traditional security challenges. Public health diplomacy is a necessary path to achieve global health security. In the shared endeavours to achieve global health governance, China has emerged as an important contributor and leader. Dr Sue Desmond-Hellmann, CEO of the Bill & Melinda Gates Foundation, believes "China has shown extraordinary leadership in promoting global health security and the health and well-being of the poor".[1] Overall, China has used public health diplomacy to promote global health governance on three levels.

7.1.1 China's global health diplomacy

China has a long history of participation in global health diplomacy. At the conference to set up the United Nations held in San Francisco from April 25 to June 26, 1945, China's representatives, together with Brazil's, jointly submitted a proposal to set up an international health organisation. This proposal laid the foundation for the World Health Organization. China later became one of the organisation's founding members. China's global health diplomacy is shown in its full participation in the building and shaping of global health security mechanisms. Before the

196 *China's role in global health governance*

Cold War, China's diplomacy centred around traditional national security concerns. After the Cold War, with the emergence of transnational infectious diseases such as avian flu and HIV/AIDS, public health issues entered into China's diplomatic work. But somehow, they were still not a priority in foreign policy. This lack of attention was reflected at the UN General Assembly Special Session on Drugs (UNGASS) convened in New York in May 2001, when China, contrary to many other countries, sent a delegation to attend the meeting headed by its Minister of Health as opposed to higher-level government representatives. It was not until the outbreak of SARS that public health became a focal point in China's foreign policy. Through WHO, China began to work with more countries to bring SARS under control. In November 2006, China's candidate, Margaret Chan, was elected as the new WHO director-general. It was the first time that a Chinese candidate was nominated and elected as the chief of a specialised UN agency. It was a great moment of victory for China's local public health diplomacies. Generally speaking, China's public health diplomacy at the global level focuses on the following areas.

7.1.1.1 Engagement in the construction of global health security regimes

Global health regimes are the most important actors in global health governance. A participant and contributor to international public health norms, China has played an important role in making global health policies and in the implementation of public health initiatives.

As "the directing and coordinating authority on international health work", WHO is at the heart of global health governance. As one of the founding members of WHO, China has been involved in developing WHO's standards, norms and practices all along. WHO became a familiar name to every Chinese person during the SARS outbreak. China worked closely with WHO to finally overcome the SARS crisis. In the post-SARS era, China set more store by its partnership with WHO. On May 20, 2003, China Vice-Premier Wu Yi led a high-level delegation to attend the World Health Assembly, signalling to the international community that China had recognised the country was growing more interdependent with the world in the context of globalisation. Previously, during the lengthy process of negotiations that led to China's admission to WTO, China had outdated views of sovereignty that regarded national economy as a country's top priority. Its close collaboration with WHO and other countries once again reflects China's flexible view towards national sovereignty issues. In view of the limitations and inadequacy of the old IHR in addressing emerging public health crises, China has actively participated in the discussion of their revision and was able to achieve consensus with all member states of WHO. In August 2003, China endorsed the Declaration on the Implementation of the TRIPS Agreement and Public Health within WTO's framework, under which newly approved measures such as compulsory licensing of pharmaceutical patent rights and parallel imports have greatly expanded drug accessibility to developing countries. On January 17, 2017, Chinese President Xi Jinping visited the WHO headquarters in Geneva and met with its director-general, Dr Margaret Chan. That was the first time a Chinese head of state visited WHO, further demonstrating the importance China attaches to global health governance today. President Xi pointed out that health issues are global challenges; advancing global health is an important part of implementing the 2030 Agenda for Sustainable Development. China would like to use its cooperation with WHO as a model and actively participate in WHO's efforts in tackling various challenges. China welcomes WHO's engagement in the Belt and Road initiative to jointly build a Health Silk Road. China is willing to strengthen its cooperation with WHO and work towards building a community of shared future for mankind.[2] During the visit, President Xi and Director-General Chan witnessed the signing of a series of agreements, including the Memorandum of Understanding between the Government of the People's Republic of China and WHO on Cooperation in the Health Field of the "Belt and Road". In addition, China has carried out all-round cooperation with WTO. For instance, China has helped to resolve misalignment between the intellectual property agreements adopted by WTO and the availability of drugs to many developing countries. China has also ratified the two UN human rights conventions, thus providing a legal basis for China to adopt a human rights approach in public health governance.

Furthermore, China has proposed a series of public health security initiatives within the UN framework. On October 27, 2003, the 58th Session of the General Assembly adopted by consensus the draft resolution on Strengthening Global Health Capacity Building. The resolution, which was submitted by China and signed by 156 countries, reflects the common interests and aspirations of the international community. It urges all countries to further integrate public health under their national economic and social development strategies in line with the United Nations Millennium Development Goals, to continuously improve the public health system and to strengthen international cooperation. It also calls on member states to pay attention to the "bird flu" epidemic and be more active in related international cooperation. It encourages UN member states and specialised agencies to provide developing countries with technical and other assistance to help strengthen their public health capacity building. The adoption of this resolution would promote international public health cooperation and address new non-traditional security threats. Since public health issues have become more globalised and public health exerts more impact on international security, China, on January 31, 2006, proposed to build an International Association of National Public Health Institutes. The Association was designed to promote exchanges and mutual development of public health agencies in various countries through technical cooperation, expert resource sharing and policy advocacy. Its goal is to improve people's health by strengthening the function and collaboration of national public health institutions. In short, China's participation in constructing these global health international regimes not only serves its own public health security but also contributes to global health governance.

7.1.1.2 China's contribution to global health governance programs

In November 2006, Dr Margaret Chan was elected the seventh director-general of WHO. It was the first time an ethnically Chinese candidate was elected to the top

198 *China's role in global health governance*

office of an important international organisation since China resumed its legal status at the United Nations in 1971. The election marks a milestone for China's public health diplomacy. It also reflects China's contribution to the cause of global public health. In addition, since 1990, China has been dispatching military medical professionals to the United Nations peacekeeping operations. These peacekeepers have made great efforts to promote local public health in host countries.

As the largest developing country in the world, China is not affluent. However, it spared no efforts to fund global health programs. At the 60th World Health Assembly, the Chinese government announced it would donate US$8 million to WHO. The money would be used to help developing countries in Africa and other regions to build and improve disease surveillance networks, enhance disease prevention and treatment capabilities and facilitate responses to public health emergencies.[3] As proof of China's determination and willingness in joining the global fight against HIV/AIDS, tuberculosis and malaria, China pledged to donate a total of US$10 million to the Global Fund to Fight AIDS, Tuberculosis and Malaria. The donations would come in five equal instalments each year starting from 2003. At the opening ceremony of the Ministerial Meeting of the International Fundraising Conference on Avian Influenza Prevention and Control held in Beijing in 2006, the Chinese government announced it would contribute US$10 million to global avian influenza prevention and control. In the same year, China also provided avian influenza virus samples to related international organisations for research purposes. In short, China's provision of human, material and financial assistance to WHO has demonstrated its determination to work with WHO and the wider international community to achieve global health governance.

7.1.2 *China's regional public health diplomacy*

Regional public health cooperation carries no less weight in China's diplomacy. As people and goods flow more frequently between neighbouring countries and regions, peer pressure in public health governance between neighbours will prompt everyone in the region to strengthen public health cooperation. There are huge opportunities for all-round security, economic and cultural exchanges. Cooperation in health will also promote cooperation on other relevant fronts through "issue linkages". Being a stabiliser in regional economic development, China's active participation is essential. Working with other countries and regions in the area is also in line with China's national interest. China's regional cooperation efforts are centred around three regional organisations.

7.1.2.1 *Asia-Pacific economic cooperation*

The Asia-Pacific region has always been at high risk for new infectious diseases, such as avian influenza and SARS, pushing public health issues to the top of the agenda of the Asia-Pacific Economic Cooperation (APEC). As an important member in the Asia-Pacific region, China has contributed immensely in setting APEC's health agenda through the "consensus principle". The APEC Shanghai

Summit in 2001 published the APEC Strategy to Combat Epidemics. The Mexico Summit in 2002 unanimously agreed to establish a regional public health surveillance network and early warning system to allow quick response to epidemic outbreaks, in particular those arising from bioterrorism. Three APEC Ministerial Meetings on Avian and Influenza Pandemics were subsequently held in 2003, 2006 and 2007. In May 2003, in the spirit of seeking common ground, APEC signed the SARS Cooperation Action Plan, which specified short-, medium- and long-term goals to combat SARS, which signalled the start of APEC's comprehensive fight against SARS. At the 12th APEC Economic Leaders' Meeting in 2004, Chinese President Hu Jintao highlighted the threat of infectious diseases to human security and expressed his full support for APEC to strengthen cooperation in preventing and controlling infectious diseases. He stressed the need for information exchange and technical cooperation to help members improve their public health systems. At the 13th APEC Economic Leaders' Meeting on November 19, 2005, President Hu pointed out that avian flu is a challenge confronting the Asia-Pacific region and the rest of the world and that APEC members should work together to address the challenge. China strongly supported APEC's cooperation in bird flu prevention and control. In 2006, China participated in the drafting of the Ha Noi Declaration, which urged members to strengthen international cooperation on avian influenza and HIV/AIDS prevention and control. China's public health cooperation with other members within the APEC framework is conducive to promoting the disease defence capacity of the people in the region, improving health security in the region and forestalling outbreaks of infectious diseases.

7.1.2.2 Public health cooperation between China and East Asia

China has important stakes in East Asia. Public health cooperation in East Asia is guided by China's "good-neighbourly" diplomatic principle. To respond to non-traditional security threats in East Asia, in November 2002, China and ASEAN leaders signed the Joint Declaration on Cooperation in Non-Traditional Security Fields. The public health crises including SARS and bird flu in 2003 made China realise the importance of public health cooperation in East Asia. On April 29, 2003, during the fight against SARS, China and ASEAN countries jointly responded to the crisis by signing the China-ASEAN Joint Statement on Preventing SARS. All signatories agreed to establish a communication mechanism that acted as a timely and effective supplement to existing cooperation efforts in non-traditional security areas. China also invested RMB 10 million in a special fund to support various public health cooperation activities with ASEAN countries. On April 30, at the height of the SARS outbreak, Chinese Premier Wen Jiabao visited Thailand and attended a special high-level summit on SARS between China and the ASEAN countries. The visit demonstrated China's resolve to confront the epidemic. Chinese leadership's shuttle visits to ASEAN countries has amended the strained bilateral relationship and assured ASEAN countries, who were also afflicted with the disease, of China's commitment and responsibility in the region. By issuing the Joint Declaration of the People's Republic of China and ASEAN

200 *China's role in global health governance*

Leaders on October 10, 2003, China and the ASEAN countries reaffirmed the need to implement the agreement made between China and ASEAN leaders on SARS in April 2003 and strengthen public health cooperation. They jointly agreed to launch a 10+1 Public Health Cooperation Fund and the 10+1 Health Ministers' Meeting Mechanism. On March 2, 2004, the China–ASEAN Special Conference on the Prevention and Control of Avian Influenza was held in Beijing. A Joint Statement of the Special Session on Influenza was issued after the conference, which emphasised the need for strong leadership, political will, cross-sectoral collaboration and partnerships at both national and regional levels to deal with the epidemic.

In November 2004, ASEAN countries, together with China, Japan and South Korea, issued the Joint Ministerial Statement on Prevention and Control of Avian Flu in Bangkok, stressing the importance of cooperation between governments, international organisations and social groups to quickly curb the spread of the disease. On January 14, 2007, Wen Jiabao delivered a speech titled "Jointly Building a Peaceful, Prosperous and Harmonious East Asia" at the 10th ASEAN, China, Japan and South Korea Leadership Meeting. He pointed out in the speech that to further enhance 10+3 cooperation, East Asian countries should strengthen public health cooperation and establish a regional disease surveillance network, enabling countries in the region to better prevent and control infectious diseases and respond to public health emergencies. China's efforts for diplomatic cooperation in public health in East Asia would surely improve the overall development of the region. Such cooperation is also the precondition for APEC members to build a public health security cooperation mechanism in East Asia, which would further deepen the cooperation between China and East Asia. The cooperation and coordination between East Asian countries in the fight against SARS and avian influenza has not only created possibilities for future cooperation among countries in the area but also greatly promoted global health governance.

7.1.2.3 Shanghai Cooperation Organization

The Shanghai Cooperation Organization (SCO) is a Eurasian political, economic and security alliance. Created in the 21st century, this regional multilateral organisation has shifted its focus from solving traditional security issues (old territorial disputes) to responding to non-traditional security threats. The organisation is also a pioneer in China's cooperation with five other member states in the field of security. With the continuous spread of the public health security crisis in recent years, public health issues have also been put on the SCO's agenda. For example, on October 30, 2008, a regular meeting of the Council of Heads of Government (Prime Ministers) of the Shanghai Cooperation Organization was held in Astana. Prime Ministers attending the meeting reached consensus in six areas of social development cooperation, one of which was to require member states to carry out public health cooperation, especially in the areas of prevention, diagnosis and treatment.[4] China's international public health cooperation with other members within the framework of the SCO helps to further deepen connection among member states.

7.1.2.4 BRICS cooperation mechanism

"BRIC" was coined by Jim O'Neill, co-head of Global Economics Research at Goldman Sachs, in 2001. It is an acronym for the four fastest-growing emerging economies (Brazil, Russia, India and China). With their rising economic, political and developmental influence, the BRIC countries held their first formal annual summit in Russia in June 2009. At the end of 2010, South Africa was invited to join BRIC, marking the official birth of BRICS as a cooperation mechanism.

In recent decades, the BRICS countries have greatly increased their influence on the international stage. Together, they account for about 25% of the world's gross national income, more than 40% of the global population and about 40% of the global burden from disease (Huang, 2018). In July 2015, to better raise funds for infrastructure and sustainable development projects in emerging international economies, including in BRICS, the group set up the BRICS New Development Bank. This Bank is committed to the economic development of all developing countries, including the five countries within the group. Accounting for about 40% of the global disease burden, BRICS member states are at the same time subjects of and contributors to global health governance.

The BRICS countries play an increasingly important role in global health affairs. The BRICS Health Ministers Meeting was officially launched in July 2011. Through this cooperation mechanism, China has actively deepened its health cooperation with other BRICS countries. China has organised training courses on global health diplomacy in the BRICS countries, set up cooperation forums on pharmaceutical innovation and hosted events to share experience in the prevention and control of various infectious and chronic diseases. These efforts have raised the stature of BRICS countries in global health governance. The annual BRICS Ministers of Health Meeting has provided an institutionalised platform for member states to cooperate in the field of global health (See Table 7.1).

The theme of the seventh BRICS Health Ministers Meeting in 2017 is "Strengthening the construction of health systems and promoting the achievement of health-related sustainable development goals". The meeting adopted the Tianjin Communiqué that sought to strengthen BRICS countries' role in global health governance, to encourage members to share useful experiences in improving the health system and the quality of health services and to promote the achievement of health-related sustainable development goals. The participating countries promised to strengthen cooperation among BRICS countries, protect and promote people's health and achieve the 2030 Agenda for Sustainable Development. They expressed determination to continue cooperation in the field of health through technical working groups and the "BRICS Health Strategy Project Cooperation Framework". By tapping into each other's strengths and comparative advantages, cooperation among the BRICS countries will bring about global changes and make a positive contribution to the health of the people of BRICS and the rest of the world. In particular, Brazil, China and India have succeeded in producing low-cost medicines and vaccines. In just a few years, the BRICS countries have accumulated rich experience in achieving universal health

202 *China's role in global health governance*

Table 7.1 Annual Themes of the BRICS Health Ministers Meetings

Time	Host country	Communiqué issued	Theme
July 2011	China	Beijing Declaration	Health cooperation, technology exchange and drug accessibility
January 2013	India	Delhi Declaration	Disease surveillance, medical technology, chronic disease control and drug development
November 2013	South Africa	Cape Town Communiqué	Technical cooperation and experience sharing, health monitoring system, maternal and child health and medical technology progress
December 2014	Brazil	Communiqué of the IV BRICS Health Ministers	Ebola prevention and control, tuberculosis prevention and control, drug development and accessibility and cross-sectoral cooperation
October 2015	Russia	Russia Declaration	Disease surveillance, cooperation mechanism, tobacco control and mental illness
December 2016	India	Delhi Declaration	Health surveillance system, non-communicable disease control, drug research and development and cooperation of regulatory institutions
July 2017	China	Tianjin Communiqué	Traditional medicine, strengthening technical cooperation, global health governance, reducing child mortality and HIV/AIDS prevention and control

coverage and expanding access to low-cost drugs and vaccines. Their cooperation has set a model for low- and middle-income countries, thus contributing to global health governance.

7.1.3 *China's bilateral public health diplomacy*

Compared with global and regional public health diplomacy, bilateral public health diplomacy is marked by superior flexibility and diversity. Bilateral public health cooperation is not only an important part of global health governance but also consolidates comprehensive relations between the two states. China's bilateral public health diplomacy revolves around cooperation between China and the United States and between China and Africa.

7.1.3.1 Sino–US public health cooperation

Given the international status of the two countries, China and the United States are both stakeholders in each other's prosperity and are constructive partners. This is also true in the field of public health security. China and the United States have conducted extensive public health diplomatic cooperation. Wang (2007) characterises Sino–US public health cooperation as a functional issue between the two. Seen in this way, the degree and range of the exchanges the two have in solving functional issues often become an instrument in national policy and serve as indicators of bilateral relations. Public health cooperation between the two countries did not start until they resumed diplomatic relations in the 1970s. On June 2, 1979, China and the United States signed an unprecedented document, the Protocol on Sino–US Health Science and Technology Cooperation. In recent years, with the wide spread of infectious diseases, such as SARS, HIV/AIDS and avian influenza, public health problems brought by emerging and recurrent infectious diseases have gradually become prominent issues for various governments, often with grave implications for the economic and social development. After the SARS epidemic, China and the United States launched comprehensive cooperation in the field of public health with progress in a variety of domains and channels. In October 2005, Health Ministers from two countries signed a Memorandum of Understanding between the Ministry of Health of the People's Republic of China and the Department of Health and Human Services of the United States of America on Establishing a New and Renewed Infectious Diseases Cooperation Project in Washington, DC. The MOU sought to strengthen the two countries' ability to prepare for and respond to emerging infectious disease threats at all operational levels through more research on the epidemiology, prevention, control, diagnosis and treatment. Ultimately, the MOU aimed to raise the professional capabilities of medical and scientific researchers in China and the United States and their ability to detect, respond to and deal with emerging and recurrent infectious diseases in a timely manner. On December 5, 2008, the two countries jointly renewed the Protocol on Cooperation in the Field of Medicine and Public Health Science and Technology in the Ministry of Health of the People's Republic of China and the Ministry of Health and Human Services of the United States of America on the side lines of the fifth China–US Economic Strategic Dialogue Conference in Beijing. In addition to the public health diplomatic cooperation on the governmental level, public health cooperation through civil societies and the private sector is even more fruitful. The synergy achieved between multiple channels of public health cooperation not only promotes public health security but also provides a converging point in the comprehensive development of relations between the two countries. More importantly, they reflect the growing interdependence between the two countries.

7.1.3.2 China–Africa public health cooperation

The birth of new China in 1949 opened a new chapter in Sino–African relations. Since then, a great number of newly independent African countries have established diplomatic relations with China. There are frequent high-level exchanges of

204 *China's role in global health governance*

visits and personnel exchanges. Bilateral cooperation takes place in a wide range of areas; consultations and coordination of various international affairs are also on the rise. China–Africa public health cooperation is an important part of this relationship. The way it is carried out reflects the change in China's own concept of global health governance. In a way, China–Africa public health cooperation epitomises China's foreign health assistance model, driven not only by governmental but also in-depth civil participation. China not only has helped African countries achieve the Millennium Development Goals (MDGs) but will also help them achieve the 2030 Sustainable Development Goals in a wide-ranging manner. In 1964, China sent medical teams to Algeria, initiating China's public health diplomacy with Africa. During a visit to South Africa in April 2015, China's Foreign Minister Wang Yi said that helping African countries "establish and improve public health care system[s]" will be one of the three priority areas in China–Africa cooperation. On April 24, 2017, the Ministerial Forum on China–Africa Health Cooperation was held in Pretoria, the capital of South Africa. According to a statement issued after the conference, to better promote Sino–African public health cooperation, the two sides would focus on providing access to African health services and products, building capacity within African public health prevention and control systems, investing in adolescents and women and promoting health and cultural exchanges between China and Africa. On January 22, 2018, Chinese President Xi Jinping's special envoy Li Bin attended the inauguration of the Liberian President. Li is Minister of China's National Health and Family Planning Commission. This was the first time the head of China's Ministry of Health visited Africa as a special envoy, illustrating the importance China attaches to Africa's health development. Since the first medical teams arrived in Africa in 1963, a total of 20,000 Chinese medical professionals have come to work in Africa. They have given diagnosis and treatment to 210 million Africans from 50 countries. As a model of South–South cooperation, China–Africa health cooperation is an important part of China and Africa's partnership and epitomises the closeness of the countries' friendship. Many Chinese provinces also send their medical teams virtually every year (see Table 7.2)

The China–Africa Cooperation Forum, set up in 2000, provides an even more comprehensive framework for public health cooperation. Under this framework, China has strengthened the training of health personnel in African countries in the areas of traditional medicine, clinical medicine, disease control, rural health management and technology. In addition, both sides would send 5–6 groups of ministerial-level delegations to visit each other. The Chinese government has also taken measures to help African nations prevent and treat infectious diseases, including malaria, AIDS and bird flu, and has provided timely and necessary assistance. The two sides have also strengthened exchanges and cooperation in the prevention and treatment of infectious diseases, quarantines and public health emergencies. In particular, at the Beijing Summit of the Forum on China–Africa Cooperation in 2006, China made a number of pledges to aid Africa.

Episodes during the fight against the Ebola crisis, which struck western Africa in 2014, provide another demonstration of the significance of China and

Table 7.2 Medical Teams Sent by Chinese Provinces to African Countries

Chinese provinces	African countries
Fujian Province	Botswana
Gansu Province	Madagascar
Guangdong Province	Equatorial Guinea
Guangxi Autonomous Region	Niger, Cameroon
Henan Province	Zambia, Ethiopia, Eritrea
Hubei Province	Algeria, Lesotho
Hunan Province	Sierra Leone, Zimbabwe, Cape Verde
Inner Mongolia Autonomous Region	Rwanda
Jiangxi Province	Tunisia
Ningxia Autonomous Region	Benin
Qinghai Province	Burundi
Shanxi Province	Mauritania, Sudan, Guinea
Shandong Province	Tanzania, Seychelles
Shanghai	Morocco
Shaanxi Province	Cameroon, Togo, Djibouti
Sichuan Province	Mozambique, Guinea Bissau
Tianjin	Congo, Gabon
Yunnan Province	Uganda
Zhejiang Province	Mali, Namibia, Central Africa

Note: The Tibet Autonomous Region, the Xinjiang Autonomous Region, Guizhou Province and Hainan Province have not sent medical teams abroad. Other provinces not in the list have sent medical teams to countries other than Africa.

Africa's health cooperation and China's contribution to African regional health security. On December 26, 2013, the Ebola virus was first identified in a remote village in Guinea. In a short span of a few months, it had quickly spread to Liberia, Sierra Leone, Nigeria and Senegal. Outside Africa, Italy, Spain and the United States also reported some infections. On August 8, 2014, WHO declared the Ebola epidemic a "public health emergency of international concern". By June 10, 2016, there had been a total of 28,616 confirmed, suspected or suspicious cases found in West Africa, Guinea, Liberia and Sierra Leone. A total of 11,310 people had lost their lives, including more than 800 medical workers, further exacerbating the already fragile public health systems in the three countries. To help African countries fight Ebola, starting in April 2014, China provided three afflicted West African countries with RMB 750 million worth of humanitarian aid, the biggest-ever health aid in the history of China's foreign health assistance. Additionally, in human resources, China sent nearly 1,200 troops and medical personnel to the three most heavily stricken areas in Liberia, Sierra Leone and Guinea, as well as to seven neighbouring countries. Chinese medical aid teams which were already in Africa also actively participated in the control efforts. In total, Chinese medical workers tested 8,000 Ebola haemorrhagic fever samples and diagnosed and treated more than 900 patients. China also helped with the training of local medical personnel and boosted local public health capacity building.

206 *China's role in global health governance*

At the same time, China participated in and strongly supported the efforts made by the United Nations, WHO and the African Union to combat the disease. China has provided multiple rounds of funding to these multilateral institutions. China supported Resolution 2177 (2014) adopted at the 7268th meeting of the UN Security Council and proposed that the international community should establish the UN Mission for Ebola Emergency Response (UNMEER), the first emergency health mission in UN's history. China fully supported the UN secretary-general's proposal to hold an International Ebola Recovery Conference and to set up a High-level Panel on the Global Response to Health Crises. On September 26, 2014, at the UN High-Level Meeting on Response to Ebola Virus Disease Outbreak, China's Foreign Minister Wang Yi pointed out that epidemics know no borders and that Ebola is a common challenge for all countries around the world. All lives are equal. It is the mission of all mankind to defend the dignity of life. The international community should take further actions to rally and pursue the joint campaign against this outbreak. China supports WHO and the United Nations in continuing with their roles of mobilising global resources to combat the epidemic. At the same time, it is important that:

> We address both the symptoms and root causes of the outbreak. We need to both manage the crisis and remove the root causes of the epidemic. Efforts should be made to help Africa enhance its public health capacity and achieve even greater development.[5]

At the UN Security Council Emergency meeting on the Ebola virus outbreak, China's representative stressed that:

> We (China) will significantly increase input to and support for the medical and health efforts of the countries involved and help them establish a sound health care and epidemic prevention system as soon as possible. China will work hard to promote Africa's economic and social development, strengthen its infrastructure and public system capacity building, and strengthen Africa's ability to fight the epidemic.[6]

China's multilateral efforts in helping African countries fight the Ebola epidemic have received widespread recognition and appreciation from the international community.

Public health cooperation is an important part of China–Africa's overall cooperation in the field of non-traditional security. Through cooperation, China and Africa have jointly responded to today's public health threats. Moreover, they have also expanded the dimensions of the traditional China–Africa strategic partnership. China's public health assistance to Africa has significantly promoted local public health governance and expanded China's influence in Africa. Thompson (2005) believes that "China's public health diplomacy in Africa constitutes an important part of its soft power in Africa" (p. 3). Chen and Gao (2008) pointed out that "China demonstrates its responsibility by engaging in international exchanges and cooperation, developing its own health capability with the use of international resources and helping underdeveloped countries improve their people's health" (p. 38). Through different levels of China's public health diplomacy, China has acted by its duties as a regional power. It has become more capable and active in constructing today's global health security mechanisms. In an era when the world becomes ever more interdependent in public health security, China's public health diplomacy is a strategic choice that is mutually beneficial to China and to the rest of the world.

7.2 China's public health diplomacy and response to COVID-19

Public health crises, including emerging and recurrent infectious diseases and acts of bioterrorism, have presented grave challenges to human security, national security and international security. To effectively manage these crises, the international community has performed active public health diplomacy through multilateral public health mechanisms. The COVID-19 pandemic, which broke out in China at the end of 2019, has now affected more than 210 countries and regions around the world (Johns Hopkins Coronavirus Resource Centre, 2020), making it the most devastating public health crisis to the international community since World War II. It has posed unprecedented challenges to global political and economic development and put the global health governance regime under an unprecedented stress test. The Organization for Economic Cooperation and Development (OECD) estimates that COVID-19 will halve the rate of global economic growth in 2020 and plunge some countries into recession (Partington & Inman, 2020). According to WTO's annual trade forecast published on April 8, the COVID-19 pandemic represents an unprecedented disruption to the global economy and world trade (WTO, 2020). It predicts that world trade is expected to fall by between 13% and 32% in 2020, and the decline will likely exceed the slump brought on by the financial crisis of 2008. Some scholars even hold that COVID-19 will become the last straw to overwhelm economic globalisation (Niblett, 2020). China's public health diplomacy is an important building block of global health governance. As one of the most important national actors in global health governance, China has carried out global health diplomacy in a proactive manner and is committed to the prevention and treatment of COVID-19. It has become a champion of building a global community of health for all, a pillar of strength for countries with weaker public health systems and a provider of norms and technologies in the global fight against the pandemic.

7.2.1 China's role in the prevention and treatment of COVID-19

First, China serves as a champion in building a global community of health for all. In the history of human development, the lives and health of peoples of all countries have never been so interconnected and so mutually vulnerable as they are today. At the same time, peoples of all countries have never been so acutely aware that human beings living in the global village actually make up a community of shared future. COVID-19 has posed a common threat to the world, and no single country can escape unscathed on its own. The values underpinning a global community of health for all, which China has championed all along, have injected moral momentum into COVID-19 response. In the face of a severe global health crisis, our only hope to overcome this challenge lies in collective action and our belief in a community of shared future. At the Extraordinary G20 Leaders' Summit held on April 26, 2020, China's President Xi Jinping emphasised that China stands by its vision of building a community of shared future for mankind. China is more than willing to share its good practices, conduct joint research and development of drugs and vaccines and provide assistance where it can to countries hit by the growing outbreak (WHO, 2020). At the Virtual Event of the Opening of the 73rd World Health Assembly, President Xi delivered a speech titled "Fighting COVID-19 through Solidarity and Cooperation, Building a Global Community of Health for All". He pointed out that, since the outbreak, China has taken swift measures to control COVID-19 at its source. Although these measures entailed tremendous sacrifice, they bought time for the world to prepare and curbed the spread of the virus to other parts of the world. Beijing's declaration on these two occasions and its action fully illustrate how China has incorporated its vision of building a community of shared future for mankind in its public health diplomacy. Building a global community of health for all is not only an important initiative China has proposed to maintain the health and well-being of human beings, but it is also a philosophy upon which China is set forth to promote global health security.

Second, China serves as a pillar of strength for countries with weak public health systems. The achievement of global health security hinges on whether these countries can succeed in COVID-19 prevention and treatment. Developing countries with weaker public health systems in Asia, Latin America and, in particular, Africa will struggle to handle the daunting challenges posed by this pandemic. Helping these countries improve their capabilities is a top priority for global pandemic response. Therefore, it has become a focal point in China's public health diplomacy to, within its capacity, provide assistance to these countries. As of May 31, 2020, at the instruction of the Chinese government, Chinese foreign aid medical teams stationed in 56 countries have assisted their host countries in pandemic prevention and treatment. They have provided technical consultation and health education to local people as well as over 400 online and offline training sessions. China has sent a cumulative total of more than 56 billion masks, 250 million pieces of medical protective clothing, ventilators, testing equipment and reagents and other medical supplies to more than 150 countries and four international organisations. Most of these assistances were given for free. China has sent 29 teams of medical experts to 27 countries to help countries hit hardest by the pandemic. As WTO launched its Strategic Preparedness and Response Plan to mobilise funding for 13 African countries with frail prevention and control capabilities, China has responded to the call by donating more than US$50 million to WTO to help developing countries combat the disease. At the 73rd World Health Assembly, President Xi Jinping announced to the world that China would provide

US$2 billion over two years to help with COVID-19 response and with economic and social development in affected countries, especially developing countries. Xi Jinping also announced that COVID-19 vaccine development and deployment in China, when available, would be made a global public good. This will be one part of China's contribution to ensuring vaccine accessibility and affordability in developing countries. In addition to the medical supplies and assistance to more than 50 African countries and the African Union, and the seven Chinese medical expert teams which have already been sent to the African continent, China will further increase its assistance to African countries in COVID-19 response and continue to spare no efforts in providing support to African countries, sending urgently needed medical supplies, conducting medical technology cooperation and dispatching more medical expert groups and working groups. The assistance China has provided to the international community to its capacity has become effective reinforcement for weak points in the global struggle against public health crises.

Finally, China is a provider of global norms and technologies in COVID-19 response. Scientific norms, standards and technical guidance hold the key for the prevention and treatment of the disease across the world. In the face of the global crisis, China has shouldered responsibility as is due for a major power. It has provided information to WHO and relevant countries in a timely and transparent fashion, released the genome sequence at the earliest possible instance, shared control and treatment experience with the world without reservation and provided advanced technical support. China's successful experience in battling the disease has become an important reference point for other countries to jointly respond to global threats. As of May 31, China has shared its COVID-19 treatment experience with more than 200 countries and regions around the world, effectively reducing the number of confirmed local cases and mortality rates. The National Health Commission (NHC) has compiled China's diagnosis, treatment, prevention and control solutions into booklets, translated them into three languages and shared them with more than 180 countries and more than ten international and regional organisations. Together with WHO, the NHC has held an international briefing via video to share China's experience in COVID-19 response and discuss cases, the latest diagnosis and treatment solutions. These efforts have contributed to the global adoption of scientific prevention measures and provided the international community with valuable technical guidance on the prevention and treatment of the pandemic.

7.2.2 Features of China's public health diplomacy

First, China has carried out multidimensional cooperation to battle the pandemic. After the outbreak, China took a multi-pronged approach at the global, regional and bilateral levels to engage in joint response and promote global health security. At the global level, China has always advocated and practised multilateralism in prevention and treatment actions. At the Extraordinary G20 Leaders' Summit and at the opening of the 73rd World Health Assembly, President Xi Jinping repeatedly emphasised China's position and commitment to multilateralism. WHO is the most important multilateral institution in global health governance, and China is a staunch supporter of its leadership role in the global fight against COVID-19. China has pledged to join the Deferred Debt Relief Initiative for the Poorest Countries with the G20 partners to help countries which were hit the hardest and are economically strained overcome the current crisis. China also supports the Resolution on COVID-19 Response adopted at the 73rd World Health Assembly. These actions fully demonstrate China's commitment to multilateralism in the global fight against the pandemic. At the regional level, China upholds its principle of "extensive consultation, joint contribution and shared benefits" and actively promotes the establishment of a joint pandemic response mechanism in East Asia. The Special ASEAN Plus Three Summit on COVID-19, held on April 14, 2020, marked a good start in building a regional health governance platform in East Asia. At the bilateral level, China has acted quickly through bilateral channels to provide assistance within its capacity to more than 80 countries threatened by the pandemic, such as Italy, Serbia, Iran and Botswana. China's assistance to the international community demonstrates its sincerity and solidarity with the rest of the world.

Second, a wide range of actors in China have pitched in, making China's response to COVID-19 an international humanitarian operation unprecedented in scale. Apart from governmental efforts, civil society organisations, private foundations and companies have also risen to the challenge in a concerted manner. Chinese NGOs have tapped into their strengths and joined forces to explore the most effective response. They have demonstrated the Chinese spirit of cooperation and aa sense of humanitarianism. Together, they have endeavoured to build a community with a shared future for mankind and pushed forward international cooperation against the crisis. For example, during the pandemic, the China Foundation for Poverty Alleviation (CFPA) distributed free "food packages", worth a total of RMB 7 million, to poor children in Ethiopia, Nepal and Myanmar. The Blue Sky Rescue Team of the China Charity Federation assisted Cambodia in local disinfection work. The Beijing Pinglan Public Welfare Foundation, through its office in Lebanon, distributed "anti-epidemic packages" comprised of food, disinfectants, soap and other sanitation products to people stuck in refugee camps on the border between Lebanon and Syria. The Jack Ma Foundation and the Alibaba Foundation jointly donated over 100 million pieces of medical supplies, including masks, test kits, medical protective clothing and ventilators, to more than 150 countries around the world; the organisations also twice donated supplies to WHO. The first batch of urgently needed supplies included 2.2 million masks, 20,000 pieces of protective gear, 20,000 goggles and 50 ventilators. The second batch comprised 100 million medical masks, 1 million N95 masks and 1 million nucleic acid detection kits designated to support WHO's global pandemic efforts. Together, the Jack Ma Foundation and the Alibaba Foundation also pledged RMB 100 million to support vaccine and drug research and development. Alibaba Group used network technology to launch free online class software, an online medical consultation platform, an international doctor exchange platform

China's role in global health governance 211

and a volunteer platform. It has also instructed its logistics arm, Cainiao Network, to fly chartered cargo flights between China and foreign countries. China's tech giant Huawei donated medical supplies to New York City, the worst hit area in the United States.

At the same time, Chinese thinktanks and experts participated in international exchanges in various ways. For example, the Chinese Academy of Sciences released the 2019 Novel Coronavirus Resource database and built the Novel Coronavirus National Science and Technology Resource Service System and the COVID-19 Scientific Literature Sharing Platform. As of May 31, 2020, the three platforms had nearly 48 million downloads, and browsing and retrieval services recorded more than 370,000 users worldwide, giving timely intellectual support for the global response to the pandemic. Furthermore, the Chinese media launched new television programmes such as _COVID-19 Frontline_ and _China's Solutions to the Global COVID-19 Pandemic_ as platforms for international cooperation and exchanges. Overall, government agencies, NGOs and private businesses in China have together taken collective action to bring the pandemic under control and build a community of shared future for mankind.

Indeed, in the face of the global health crisis, no country has room in its foreign policy for isolationism. Only through mutual assistance can we achieve sustainable global health security. China and the rest of the world have become "mutually dependent" on each other amid the pandemic. Since the breakout of COVID-19, the high speed and massive scale of China's response are rarely seen in the world. China's speed, scale and efficiency all demonstrate the strengths and advantages of China's system China has set an example for other countries in terms of its effective prevention and control measures. As WHO Director-General Tedros Adhanom Ghebreyesus observed, "in many ways, China is actually setting a new standard for outbreak response".[7] China's multi-dimensional public health efforts as well as its contribution of multiple actors have made significant contributions to the fight against the pandemic. In the face of this serious crisis, humanity once again stands at a crossroads. China has taken a global perspective in its response and stands by its vision of building a community of shared future for mankind. China aims to actively strengthen solidarity and cooperation and vigorously promotes multilateral coordination. It will continue to adhere to the principles of scientific rationality and make global common interest a priority. China is committed to standing side by side with other peoples across the world in navigating these tough times, contributing its wisdom and solutions in fighting the pandemic and fully displaying its sense of responsibility as a major power.

Notes

1 See an interview with Dr Sue Desmond-Hellmann on the sidelines of the World Economic Forum in 2017. (2017, January 20). Retrieved from http://world.people.com.cn/n1/2017/0120/c1002-29039283.html.
2 See _China's President Xi Jinping Visits the World Health Organization_. (2017, January 19). Xinhua News. Retrieved from http://news.xinhuanet.com/mrdx/2017-01/19/c_135995263.htm.

212 *China's role in global health governance*

3 See *The 60th World Health Assembly: Joining Hands for a Bright Future*. (2007). Xinhua Net. Retrieved from http://news.xinhuanet.com/world/2007-05/17/content_6110968.htm.
4 See *Joint Statement of the Meeting of the Council of Heads of State of The Shanghai Cooperation Organization*. (2008). Retrieved from www.fmprc.gov.cn/mfa_eng/wjdt_665385/2649_665393/t513028.shtml.
5 See *China's Foreign Minister Wang Yi Delivers a Speech at UN Security Council Emergency Meeting on Ebola Virus outbreak*. Retrieved from www.chinanews.com/gn/2014/09-26/6631751.shtml.
6 Ibid.
7 See *WHO Director-General's Statement on IHR Emergency Committee on Novel Coronavirus*. (2020, January 30). Retrieved from www.who.int/dg/speeches/detail/who-director-general-s-statement-on-ihr-emergency-committee-on-novel-coronavirus-(2019-ncov).

References

Chan, M., Støre, J. G., & Kouchner, B. (2008). Foreign Policy and Global Public Health: Working Together towards Common Goals. *Bulletin of World Health Organization*, 86(7), 498.

Chen, Z., & Gao, Q. (2008). A Chinese Approach to Public Health: How to Ensure Access to Basic Health Care. *Qiushi*, 1, 35–38.

Horton, R. (2006). Iraq: Time to Signal a New Era for Health in Foreign Policy. *The Lancet*, 368(9545), 1395–1397.

Huang, Y. (2018). Emerging Power and Global Health Governance: The Case of BRICS Countries. In C. McInnes, K. Lee, & J. Youde (Eds.), *The Handbook of Global Health Politics*. Oxford: Oxford University Press.

Johns Hopkins Coronavirus Resource Centre. (2020). *Coronavirus COVID-19 Global Cases by the Centre for Systems Science and Engineering*. Retrieved from https://coronavirus.jhu.edu/map.html

Kaul, I. (2003). *Providing Global Public Goods: Managing Globalization*. Oxford: Oxford University Press.

Niblett, R. (2020, March 20). The End of Globalization as We Know It. *Foreign Policy*.

Partington, R., & Inman, P. (2020, March 2). Coronavirus Escalation Could Cut Global Economic Growth in Half. *The Guardian*.

Thompson, D. (2005). China's Soft Power in Africa: From the "Beijing Consensus" to Health Diplomacy. *China Brief*, 5(21), 3.

Wang, J. (2007). Convergence and Strategic Interactions of Sino-US Interest. *International Economic Review*, 4, 10–11.

WHO. (2020, June 2). *US $ 675 Million Needed for New Coronavirus Preparedness and Response Global Plan*. Retrieved from www.who.int/emergencies/diseases/novel-coronavirus-2019/donors-and-partners

WTO. (2020, April 8). *Trade Statistics and Outlook*. Retrieved from www.wto.org/english/news_e/pres20_e/pr855_e.pdf

8 Conclusion

Global governance is integrally connected to the supply of global public goods. Public health is "an important type of global public good" (Sandmo, 2006, p. 98). By overcoming various public health security threats, public health governance holds the key to the supply of global public goods for health. WHO, the international human rights regimes and WTO are the main actors in global health governance and are important agents in the provision of public goods. In previous chapters, we examined their weaknesses in current global health governance. By way of conclusion, we propose that the reason why these international mechanisms have failed to provide enough global public goods for health is that they lack publicness in both decision-making and the distribution of benefits. On a deeper level, their insufficiency has to do with the democratic deficits embedded in their structures, the North–South Divide in public health and their interest-driven orientation in global health governance.

8.1 International regimes and the triangle of publicness

The triangle of publicness is a model proposed by Inge Kaul, an expert in the United Nations Development Programme. Kaul believes that to achieve publicness in consumption of a good, people ought to ensure publicness is an element of decision-making and that benefits from the good are distributed equally among different social groups (see Figure 8.1). In other words, the efficiency of how a public good is supplied is dependent on whether the decision-making process is public to all and whether the benefits are allocated fairly. In the case of global health mechanisms, the efficiency of their provision of global public goods for health is determined by whether these mechanisms can achieve publicness in decision-making and in the distribution of benefits. Based on a critical analysis of these mechanisms in the preceding chapters, we see there are clear problems on both fronts of their publicness.

First, global health mechanisms lack publicity in decision-making, demonstrated through democratic deficits when member states are making global health policies. Stutzer and Frey (2005) believe that "world governance today is characterized by international organisations lacking democratic legitimacy and control by the citizens they claim to represent" (p. 325). International regimes provide

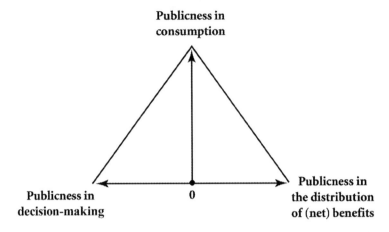

Figure 8.1 Triangle of Publicness

a platform through which member states cooperate with each other to produce a global public good. Therefore, decisions on how to make such public goods should be based on democratic and equal consultations among different members. According to UNDP (1997), "effective forms of democratic governance are characterized by participation, accountability and transparency" (p. 85). For regimes in global health governance, publicness in their decision-making is guaranteed only when these regimes present a wide basis of participation and achieve transparency and accountability. But the truth is, the regimes in global health governance inherently lack these interrelated qualities.

Regimes in global health governance lack wide participation. The provision of global public goods for health requires the support of effective global health policies, but "global policy-making needs to rely on the broadest-possible participation on a global scale" (Dallmayr, 2002, p. 154). The "global public nature" of health goods makes every country and region a "stakeholder" in health security. They have a right to participate in the decision-making process of relevant international regimes. However, not all of them are represented equally by international public health regimes. WTO, for instance, has more than 140 member states, but the decision-making power and the voice of the organisation are dominated by developed countries. As is noted, WTO is "intentionally designed to insulate against democratic pressure for change" (Wallach & Woodall, 2004, pp. 15–16). The same also goes for the BWC and international human rights regimes.

Accountability needs to be improved in the international regimes in global health governance. Accountability means that an organisation must be held responsible for its actions and impacts on all stakeholders. According to the Commission on Global Governance (1995), "accountable regulatory agencies are at the core of

Conclusion 215

the effective supply of global public goods" (p. 2). To be effective and legitimate, international regimes and global health governance must include all stakeholders and be accountable to them, rather than representing only the most powerful stakeholders. But the reality is just the opposite. For example, WTO's provisions on the protection of pharmaceutical patents are designed not to promote drug accessibility in developing countries but to protect the interests of multinational pharmaceutical companies in developed countries. As important stakeholders in global health governance, many developing countries find it hard to hold international regimes accountable when their public health interests are encroached upon.

Transparency is insufficient in international regimes in global health governance. An organisation's transparency is a prerequisite condition to ensure its accountability. "Transparency influences strategic interaction among parties to the treaty in the direction of compliance" (Chayes & Chayes, 1995, p. 22). In other words, how the norms and policies of an international mechanism are made must be open to all its members. Only in this way can this mechanism avoid problems of collective action and increase its compliance pull. WHO (2007) believes that "the solid foundation for global health security is cooperation, and this cooperation should be transparent" (p. 73). Unfortunately, "international mechanisms are neither democratic nor transparent" (Stiglitz, 2006, p. 163). It is particularly so in the decision-making process of global health mechanisms. WTO's "Green Room" process, which excludes members from certain meetings, illustrates how opaque the decision-making can be. WTO's decisions are reached through consensus. This may at first glance seem democratic. In practice, though, such consensus is only reached by major developed countries, and all others are asked to join it. Conversely, if one or only a few major developed countries reject a decision, even if most other countries have already agreed to it, such consensus would still be "one that has not been reached". American scholar Richard Steinberg (2002) compares WTO's "decision-making by consensus" to an "organised hypocrisy in the procedural context" (p. 342). According to a report on the WTO (2003), the fundamental reason why members are not put on the same footing is WTO's "lack of transparency and as well as the lack of participation or exclusion of a majority of Members in decision making processes" (p. 9). Democratic deficits generated in this manner would inevitably reduce the legitimacy of global health regulations and norms. In the long run, member would be less motivated and less incentivised to comply with these norms, ultimately resulting in the collective action problem.

Secondly, global health mechanisms lack publicity in the distribution of benefits. Globalisation is characterised by an asymmetry of gains and losses. The same goes for the globalisation of health issues. Aginam (2003) observes that:

> In the so-called age of globalization, marked by a phenomenal rise in the intrusive web of global interdependence, multilateral public health issues, are still solidly founded on governance mechanisms similar to the 19th century International Sanitary Conventions and Regulations.
>
> (p. 6)

216   *Conclusion*

In the 19th century, public health governance mechanisms were used mainly to protect Western populations from contagious diseases of the "uncivilized world", rather than to improve the health of the entire world. Today, global health governance mechanisms still mainly reflect the interests of developed countries rather than public health security concerns of developing countries. International mechanisms which largely "define and reflect the basic property right" in the international community have a right to determine when, how and which members can or can't receive the benefit and by how much of that benefit" (Su, 2001, p. 15). The same also goes for international public health mechanisms. These mechanisms are the products of power struggles in international politics and ultimately generate their benefits in the form of national interests. "Whether an infectious disease is included in the international agenda is not determined by the severity of its consequences but rather by whether demarcating the crisis as a health issue is in the interest of major powers in the international community" (Shiffman & Smith, 2007, p. 1370). The prevailing "international norms reflect Western values; International organisations and rules mainly serve the interests of developed countries" (Yang, 2007, p. 9). Since most global health mechanisms are set up and designed by Western countries, global health governance efforts inevitably reflect their intentions, values and national interests. All the global health mechanisms used today are led by Western developed countries in one way or another. These developed countries participate in the provision of global public goods for health more out of self-interest than of altruism. Calculation of interest rather than moral consideration provides the substance of their motivation. The United States, for example, started to link global health to self-interest as early as 1971. American House Representative Hugh L. Carey (1971) testified at a congressional hearing with the following words:

> In order to protect the safety of our own people, it is in our practical interest to find and fight diseases on foreign lands. Improved health overseas in all age brackets means expanding consumer markets and increased trade for US products.

In other words, whether and to what extent the United States provides global public goods for health depends on whether the nation can benefit from the action. If it cannot, it will simple "mind its own business". As another example, despite WHO's repeated warning against the high infections rates of HIV/AIDS in Africa in the 1980s, the United States and a few other Western countries acted as if nothing had happened. It was only recently that the United States started to put HIV/AIDS prevention on its agenda, but there have already been concerns that the United States' global AIDS prevention campaign is driven by a desire to advance its own pharmaceutical industry (McNeil, 2004). These examples show that compared with developing countries, the United States has reaped additional net national benefits in its provision of global public goods for AIDS prevention and treatment in Africa. Developing countries' consumption and enjoyment of such goods is only the spill-over effect of America's self-interest. In other words, there is no publicness in the distribution of benefits in the prevention and control of AIDS. At the same time, the "toolbox" attitude some powers take towards global health mechanisms is also an important reason for the absence of such publicness. For example, WHO, one of the main actors of global health governance, is one of the most representative organisations in the world. However, due to its emphasis on social rights and its frequent support for the rights of developing countries, it fails to receive full backing from developed countries. This is why "in the global health governance, especially since the 1990s, the role of WHO has been relatively weakened" (Hein & Kohlmorgen, 2008, p. 98). Developed countries instead give their support to other international mechanisms, such as WTO, the international human rights mechanisms and the World Bank, because these organisations better reflect their "voice" and interest. Developed countries' efforts to protect the intellectual property rights of pharmaceutical products through WTO is just one example of their preference. In fact, even in WHO, developed countries are constantly seeking ways to maximise their national interest. The IHR, for instance, are designed not so much to promote global health governance worldwide as to set up a quarantine line between the developed and developing world when infectious diseases occur in the latter. In Lawrence Gostin's (2007) words:

> Not only does the IHR lack a realistic funding mechanism, it was neither historically nor politically intended as a vehicle for improving health in poor countries. Its *raison d'être* is to control the international migration of diseases. And since most serious infectious diseases move from the Southern to the Northern Hemisphere, richer countries stand to benefit most from the regulations.
>
> (p. 998)

The same is also true for the BWC. Developed countries have ignored the BWC's emphasis on strengthening international cooperation on biotechnology but go to great lengths to exaggerate the importance of export control of biotechnology. Their pragmatism results in the absence of publicness in the distribution of global public goods for health.

From this analysis, it can be concluded that in the process of providing global public goods for health, the international regimes do not exhibit publicness in decision-making and the distribution of benefits. This undermines their legitimacy and worsens problems of collective action. The optimal provision of global public goods requires a well-functioning and open political negotiation and consultation process for decision-making. An adequate supply of global public goods for health requires the active involvement of most of the developing nations in the decision-making process. Developing countries must make their public health concerns, needs and voices heard when international norms and rules are made. Only in this way can global public goods for health be truly "public" and fair at the global level. If most developing countries cannot make their voices heard in global health decision-making and instead let a few developed countries dominate the decision-making in the supply of global public goods for health, then such

218 *Conclusion*

goods may become club goods or private goods of developed countries, deteriorating both capacity and motivation for developing countries to participate in global health regimes. In today's interrelated global health security landscape, no country should expect to build a Maginot Line of defence to stop diseases at its national borders. Otherwise, it would surely lead to a tragedy of the commons in global health governance.

8.2 Deeper political and economic reasons behind the insufficient provision of global public goods for health

The lack of publicness in decision-making and in distribution of benefits has its root causes in international politics and economy. It is also a reflection of imbalance in global development. A vicious cycle is formed when the shortage of global public goods for health in turn aggravates the global development imbalance. On the whole, there are several deep-seated reasons behind the insufficient supply of global public goods for health.

First, power imbalance. Power imbalance is a central subject of international political studies research. As David Held, a well-known American international political scientist, puts it, "any convincing view of global governance" cannot ignore the essential fact that power between countries are unequal" (Held & McGrew, 2002, p. 12). As global health threats increasingly transcend to international political issues, global health regimes cannot insulate themselves from power politics either. Fidler (2005) also believes that "the reality of global health today can hardly be explained without reference to the impact that power has on the health-foreign policy relationship" (p. 189). Today's global health regimes reflect rather than re-align the power structure in international relations. Take WHO as an example. An implicit rule is that the five permanent members of the UN Security Council would automatically become members of WHO's Executive Board. As some scholars have observed, "the work of international agencies such as WHO is very much determined by the power structure in the world" (Navarro, 2008, p. 152). The voice of international human rights regimes is similarly controlled by Western developed countries. It is even more so in the case of WTO. While developed countries can align the agenda of global health regimes to their national public health interest, developing countries have virtually collectively "lost their voice" in the formulation of these policies. The controversies surrounding intellectual property rights of medicines and their accessibility to developing countries best illustrates WTO's power imbalance. International relations tend to benefit the privileged and the powerful and make poor countries disproportionately bear the burden of infectious diseases. It is such kind of power politics that contributes to a "democratic deficit" in global health policies.

Secondly, global health regimes do not have a strong compulsory dispute resolution mechanism. Global health regimes are much like a form of "global contracts". Despite the less than democratic nature of these contracts, they still provide a platform for members to cooperate and a framework to produce global public goods for health. But in the absence of a strong enforcement mechanism,

Conclusion 219

low compliance has seriously affected the implementation of global health policies. As Hobbes famously says, "covenants, without the sword, are but words". Take WHO's International Health Regulations as an example. Although the newly revised version introduced an arbitration clause intended to resolve disputes between members, if a member state did not notify WHO of its internal outbreak nor allow WTO investigators in their country for verification, WHO could not do anything about such breach, thereby laying the seed for IHR's weak compliance. Similarly, in the absence of a compulsory mechanism in the international human rights regimes, the right to health has become more rhetoric than action. In short, due to such absence, there is a risk that global health cooperation might become less predictable, thus exacerbating the collective action problem that already exists in the supply of global public goods for health. On a deeper level, many member states still subscribe to the traditional concept of sovereignty. Mutua (1998) observes that "as a general rule, states are reluctant to couple a strong instrument with a powerful and effective enforcement body" (p. 216). Public health issues are still considered member states' internal issues, so member states unwilling to grant global health regimes have more power. This is just as Gostin (2004b) has observed, "for a long time, global health has been restricted by the old and rigid views of sovereignty, horizontal governance and entrenched power structures" (Heymann et al., 2002, p. 607). In fact, as public health security threats become more globalised, if national public health policies are still driven by the traditional view of public health sovereignty and if their scope is still restricted within national borders, the provision of global public goods for health is bound to fall into the trap of collective action.

Second, global health governance is driven by economic benefits. Today's global health cooperation still retains hallmarks of the public health diplomacy among European countries in the 19th century, which was mainly carried out to pursue economic benefits rather than human health improvement. This economic motive was also an important factor that made public health cooperation in the 19th century a mere formality. Global health regimes also reflect this "interest-driven orientation". It is stated that the IHR (2005) seek to "prevent, protect against, control and provide a public health response to the international spread of disease in ways that are commensurate with and restricted to public health risks, and which avoid unnecessary interference with international traffic and trade" (WHO, 2005). Yet when public health benefits conflict with trade benefits, the latter always prevails.[1] WHO's regulations on the intellectual property rights of medicines is also proof that the economic interest of Western developed countries is prioritised over global health and safety. It is "due to these competing priorities that the contemporary global infectious disease governance framework has become a rather weak global governance project" (Neubauer, 2005, p. 290). It should be noted that the developed countries' practice of putting pharmaceutical patent rights ahead of public health security has prompted radical backlash in some developing countries. For example, since 2006, Indonesia, back then the most affected nation by the avian influenza virus, has stopped sharing virus samples with WHO and other foreign laboratories on the grounds of "viral sovereignty" (Holbrooke, 2008).

220 Conclusion

Although the decision ignores the fact that a virus can now travel passport-free, it is understandably a measure of exasperation by a developing country. Global health governance can attain "the highest possible health by all peoples" only if it puts people first, effectively protects their right to health and makes people's health rather than economic gains the ultimate goal.

Finally, the present North–South Divide in public health is also accountable. As WHO (1948) put in its Constitution, "uneven development in different countries in the promotion of health and control of disease, especially communicable disease, is a common danger". Although recent advances in medical technology has promoted global public health, the health disparities between global North and South is widening. The "10/90 gap" between the North and the South in public health is still a grim reality facing global health governance (ibid., p. 1). American scholar Farmer (1997) likens this health gap to a "structural violence". Gostin and Taylor (2008) point out that, "the great inequality constitutes the most serious global health threat" (p. 54). If social, economic and political justice are increasingly the core concern of global governance regimes, then health equality must also become a core metric for the success of such governance. Unless global health regimes commit themselves to eliminating such inequality, their legitimacy would continue to be questioned, thereby making compliance a challenge and ultimately weakening the efficiency of global health governance. The North–South Divide in public health is the result of an unequal international political and economic order. Therefore, "global health victories will depend on how well international politics are played" (Erikson, 2008, p. 1230). Only when countries, especially developed ones, become aware of threats posed to global health security and work to improve the fairness and impartiality of the global health regimes as well as gradually solve the problem of global health capacity deficits can they expect to promote and reshape the structure of global health governance.

Gostin (2004a) argues that "global health governance is both old, outdated and structurally weak" (p. 2623). It is outdated because many member states are still constrained by traditional views of national security and sovereignty; it is weak because many of them still believe in traditional centralised national power and refuse to yield some sovereignty to the global health regimes. As a result, sovereignty and nationalism have surpassed values underpinning global health safety. In the face of the potential threats posed by infectious diseases and bioterrorism, it would be nothing short of foolish to still regard public health issues as "low-level politics". If public health problems are not properly handled, they will pose a grave threat to national, international and even global security. Only when they are taken as security issues, or securitised, can they become a priority in global governance. The process of global health governance is also a process to de-securitise these threats. In the context of irreversible globalisation, the claim "the health of every country depends on the health of other countries" is no longer empty words but a factual observation based on solid epidemiological science. As American scholar Christian Enemark (2005) puts it, "to cope with the security challenges posed by infectious diseases requires global health governance and global public goods for health" (p. 109). Global interdependence of public health security necessitates the need for global public goods for health. As the main actors in global health governance, global health regimes have played an irreplaceable role to provide such global public goods for health. However, their lack of publicness in decision-making and in the distribution of benefits has led them into the predicament of collective action, which in turn severely restricts their capacity in providing public health goods. In Held's (2004) point of view, "systematizing the provision of global public goods requires not just building on existing forms of multilateral institutions, but also extending and developing them in order to address questions of transparency, accountability and democracy" (p. 377). The same applies to the provision of public goods. Countries around the world must work to democratise public health policymaking based on principles of fairness and justice. They should also yield some sovereignty to strengthen these international regimes, in particular to improve WHO's enforceability, to finally overcome the problems associated with collective action. Another reason that leads to the collective action problem is that member states still differ in their understanding of the securitisation of global health threats and of the nature of public goods. They need to interact with each to construct a global consensus on these two aspects because "constructivism is the best theoretical starting point to help understand the dynamics of global health governance" (Kickbusch, 2003, p. 195) and "an ideal, single global health governance approach does not exist" (Gable, 2007, p. 541). Therefore, effective global health governance calls for participation from other actors. A multi-level approach is not only necessary but also inevitable in global health governance. Global health regimes cannot function without coordination and cooperation from national governments, NGOs and private partnerships. Public health threats posed by infectious diseases were, are and will continue to be a basic parameter and determinant affecting the course of human history. The world still has many public health challenges to tackle. As Jon Cohen (2006) put it, "to use a universal and time-tested aphorism to describe global infectious disease control, 'this is easier said than done'" (p. 167). This means countries around the world must work to reduce and overcome problems of collective action through various levels of public health diplomacy to achieve better global health governance.

Health is a fruitful and friendly arena for foreign diplomacy. As the largest developing country in the world today, China has elevated the Healthy China initiative to a national strategic level. It has held the National Health Conference, hosted the ninth Global Conference on Health Promotion and launched Healthy China 2030, an action plan intended to promote China's national health over the next 15 years. China is now working hard to build a community of shared future for mankind. This goal is reflected in China's global health governance efforts. China's proposal to build a "Healthy Silk Road" is a brand-new approach taken to achieve global health governance. As an important stakeholder in global health governance, China spares no efforts to improve its domestic public health system. Meanwhile, China endeavours to use public health diplomacy to provide more global public goods for health, thereby showing its friendship to the international community. These efforts will eventually prove to the world that a rising China is a contributor, rather than a threat, to world peace and development.

222 *Conclusion*

Note

1 Article 57 of the IHR (2005) stipulates that "States Parties recognize that the IHR and other relevant international agreements should be interpreted so as to be compatible, the provisions of the IHR shall not affect the rights and obligations of any State Party deriving from other international agreements." When the IHR conflict with WTO regulations, Article 57 of the IHR provides the legal basis to override WTO rules. In addition, given that WTO has a more advanced dispute settlement mechanism than WHO, if a member state of WTO feels that other states have adopted inappropriate restrictions in response to public health emergencies that have occurred on its territory, the said member may submit a dispute to WTO instead of WHO. WTO has shown a preference for trade issues over public health from previous disputes. The EU's imposition on beef imports containing artificial growth hormones is a good case in point. The WTO dispute settlement mechanism rejected the import restriction on the grounds of lack of scientific evidence.

References

Aginam, O. (2003). The Nineteenth Century Colonial Fingerprints on Public Health Diplomacy: A Postcolonial View. *Law, Social Justice & Global Development Journal*, 1(6).

Carey, H. L. (1971). *International Health Agency Act Hearings*. Hearings before the Subcommittee on International Organizations and Movements of the Committee on Foreign Affairs, House of Representative, 92nd Congress, first Session on H.R.10042. Washington, DC.

Chayes, A., & Chayes, A. H. (1995). *The New Sovereignty: Compliance with International Regulatory Agreements*. Cambridge, MA: Harvard University Press.

Cohen, J. (2006). The New World of Global Health. *Science*, 311(5758), 167.

Commission on Global Governance. (1995). *Our Global Neighbourhood: The Report of the Commission on Global Governance*. Oxford: Oxford University Press.

Dallmayr, F. R. (2002). Globalization and Inequality: A Plea for Global Justice. *International Studies Review*, 4(2), 137–156.

Enemark, C. (2005). Infectious Diseases and International Security: The Biological Weapons Convention and beyond. *The Nonproliferation Review*, 12(1), 107–125.

Erikson, S. L. (2008). Getting Political: Fighting for Global Health. *The Lancet*, 371(9620), 1229–1230.

Farmer, P. (1997). On Suffering and Structural Violence: A View from below. In A. Kleinman, V. Das, & M. Lock (Eds.), *Social Suffering*. Berkeley: University of California Press.

Fidler, D. P. (2005). Health as Foreign Policy: Between Principle and Power. *Whitehead Journal of Diplomacy and International Relations*, 6, 179–189.

Gable, L. (2007). The Proliferation of Human Rights in Global Health Governance. *The Journal of Law, Medicine & Ethics*, 35(4), 534–544.

Gostin, L. O. (2004a). International Infectious Disease Law: Revision of the World Health Organization's International Health Regulations. *Journal of the American Medical Association*, 291(21), 2623–2627.

Gostin, L. O. (2004b). The International Health Regulations and beyond. *The Lancet*, 4(10), 606–607.

Gostin, L. O. (2007). A Proposal for a Framework Convention on Global Health. *Journal of International Economic Law*, 10(4), 989–1008.

Gostin, L. O., & Taylor, A. L. (2008). Global Health Law: A Definition and Grand Challenges. *Public Health Ethics*, 1(1), 53–63.

Hein, W., & Kohlmorgen, L. (2008). Global Health Governance: Conflicts on Global Social Rights. *Global Social Policy*, 8(1), 80–108.

Held, D. (2004). Democratic Accountability and Political Effectiveness from a Cosmopolitan Perspective. *Government and Opposition*, 39(2), 364–391.

Held, D., & McGrew, A. (2002). *Governing Globalization*. Cambridge: Polity Press.

Heymann, D., Detels, R., McEwen, J., Beaglehole, R., & Tanaka, H. (2002). *Oxford Textbook of Public Health*. Oxford: Oxford University Press.

Holbrooke, R. C. (2008, August 21). "Sovereignty" That Risks Global Health. *Washington Post*.

Kickbusch, I. (2003). Global Health Governance: Some Theoretical Considerations on the New Political Space. In K. Lee (Ed.), *Health Impacts of Globalization: Towards Global Governance* (p. 195). New York: Palgrave Macmillan.

McNeil Jr, D. G. (2004, March 28). Plan to Battle AIDS Worldwide Is Falling Short. *New York Times*, p. A1.

Mutua, M. (1998). Looking Past the Human Rights Committee: An Argument for De-Marginalizing Enforcement. *Buffalo Human Rights Law Review*, 4, 211–216.

Navarro, V. (2008). Neoliberalism and Its Consequences: The World Health Situation since Alma Ata. *Global Social Policy*, 8(2), 152–155.

Neubauer, D. E. (2005). Globalization and Emerging Governance Modalities. *Environmental Health and Preventive Medicine*, 10(5), 286–294.

Sandmo, A. (2006). International Aspects of Public Goods Provision. In I. Kaul (Ed.), *Providing Global Public Goods: Managing Globalization* (C. Zhang et al., Trans., p. 98). Beijing: People's Publishing House.

Shiffman, J., & Smith, S. (2007). Generation of Political Priority for Global Health Initiatives: A Framework and Case Study of Maternal Mortality. *The Lancet*, 370(9595), 1370–1379.

Steinberg, R. H. (2002). In the Shadow of Law or Power? Consensus-Based Bargaining and Outcomes in the GATT/WTO. *International Organization*, 56(2), 339–374.

Stiglitz, J. E. (2006). Global Public Goods and Global Finance: Does Global Governance Ensure That the Global Public Interest Is Served? In J.-P. Touffut (Ed.), *Advancing Public Goods* (pp. 149–163). Northampton, MA: Edward Elgar Publishing Limited.

Stutzer, A., & Frey, B. S. (2005). Making International Organizations More Democratic. *Review of Law & Economics*, 1(3), 305–330.

Su, C. (2001). New Institutionalism and Old Institutionalism: Institutional Factors in International Politics. *Fudan Journal of International Politics Research*, 1, 15.

United Nations Development Programme. (1997). *Reconceptualizing Governance, Discussion Papers 2, Bureau for Development Policies*. New York.

Wallach, L., & Woodall, P. (2004). *Whose Trade Organization? A Comprehensive Guide to the WTO*. New York: New Press.

WHO. (1948). *Constitution of WHO*. Geneva: WHO.

WHO. (2005). *The International Health Regulations*. Geneva: WHO.

WHO. (2007). *The World Health Report 2007: A Safer Future: Global Health Security in the 21st Century*. Geneva: WHO.

WTO. (2003). *Memorandum on the Need to Improve Internal Transparency and Participation in the WTO*. Retrieved from www.ciel.org/wp-content/uploads/2015/05/Cancun_21July03_Memo.pdf

Yang, J. (2007). China's Soft Power: A Global Public Goods View. *International Issues Review*, 9.

Index

Page numbers in *italics* indicate figures; page numbers in **bold** indicate tables.

Ad Hoc Group (AHG): strengthening BWC 175–176, 182–183

Africa: Africans 18–19; HIV/AIDS in Africa 1, 26, 28, 142–143; medical teams from China to **205**; public health cooperation with China 203–207

Agenda for Peace, An (Boutros-Ghali) 21

Agenda for Sustainable Development (2030) 24, 33, 197

Aginam, Obijiofor 4

Agreement on Application of Sanitary and Phytosanitary Measures (SPS), WTO agreement 110, **111**, 112, 113, 114

Agreement on Technical Barriers to Trade (TBT), WTO agreement 110, **111**, 112, 113, 114

Agreement on Trade-Related Aspects of Intellectual Property Rights (TRIPS) 8, 9–10, 22; Article 7 of 116; Article 8(1) of 116; Article 27(2) of 116–117; Article 27(3) of 117; Article 31 of 117; Article 65 of 117; Article 66 of 117; China endorsing 196; compulsory licensing 128; declaration on 118–120; Doha Declaration 118–120; free trade and 124; preamble to 116; prices of medications 143; privatisation of global public goods 126–127; protocol amending 120–123; public health-related articles in 116–118; purpose of 115; scientific progress and 152; Uruguay Round of GATT 115, 116; WTO agreement 110, **111**, 112–114, 114

AIDS (acquired immune deficiency syndrome) 1, 3, 19; global spread of 21; *see also* HIV/AIDS

Alibaba Foundation 210

Alibek, Ken 186

American War of Independence 135

Annan, Kofi 29, 32, 133, 138

anthrax virus: attacks in United States 15, 26, 34, 68, 76–77, 121, 186–187; bioterrorism of 21, 177–178; Japan and 172; leak in Soviet Union 181; outbreak 1; public health crisis 194; Sverdlovsk incident (1979) 174, 190n6

antibiotics 20

Asia-Pacific Economic Cooperation (APEC) 23, 198–199

Aum Shinrikyo, sarin attack by 26

avian influenza/flu 15, 19; infectious disease 127, 196, 198–200, 203; pandemic 39–40; prevention and control 198; virus 219

Bangkok Charter for Health Promotion in a Globalized World 156

Ban, Ki-moon 33

Bartsch, Sonja 16

Bayer, Cipro story 121–122

Beaglehole, Robert 17

Beck, Ulrich 1

Beckford, Delroy S. 16

Beijing Pinglan Public Welfare Foundation 210

Belt and Road 197

benefits of scientific progress, ICESCR and right to 151–152

Berlinguer, G. 20

Bill & Melinda Gates Foundation **45**, 88, **88**, 195

Biological Weapons Convention (BWC) 2, 4, 171, 188–189, 190n5; annual reports 174, 190n10; Article 10 of 178–179; biosecurity dilemma 180, 185–187; collective action problems 185;

confidence-building measures (CBMs) 174, 176; conflicts between WHO and 76–79; deficiencies of 181–184; dilemmas leading to defects of 184–188; dual-use dilemma of biotechnology 187–188; emergence of bioterrorism 177–178; first international norm 47; historical background to development of 171–172; impact on public health responses 178–179; lacking binding verification mechanisms 181–182; lacking confidence-building measures 182–183; lacking organisational support for 183–184; links between public health and 176–180; means towards the end 179–180; post-Protocol period (2001–present) 176; pre-Protocol period (1981–1991) 173–174; Protocol period (1991–2001) 175–176; stages of development of 172–173; verification measures 175, 181–182, 190n14

biosecurity dilemma 180, 185–187

Biosecurity in the Global Age (Fidler and Gostin) 4

biotechnology, dual-use dilemma of 187–188

bioterrorism 3; discourse of 26

bird flu (H5N1) virus: epidemic 23–24, 26, 30, 33, 39–40, 86, 197; infectious disease 204; prevention and control 199

Black Death 19, 39, 109

Blix, Hans 184

Bloom, Barry 87

Blue Sky Rescue Team 210

Bobbio, Norberto 136

Bolton, John 176

Bonita, Ruth 17

Booth, Ken 21

Boston Globe (newspaper) 22

Boutros-Ghali, Boutros 21

Brandt Report 20

BRIC (Brazil, Russia, India, and China): annual themes of health minister meetings **202**; cooperation mechanism 201–202

Brower, Jennifer 6

Brundtland, Gro Harlem 87, 90–91, 95, 97

Buzan, Barry 10n1, 20

Caballero-Anthony, Mely 6

Cainiao Network 211

Carey, Hugh L. 216

Carlton University 4

Centres for Disease Control and Prevention 178

Chalk, Peter 6

Chan, Margaret 87, 92, 97, 196–197

China: Asia-Pacific Economic Cooperation (APEC) 198–199; bilateral public health diplomacy 202–207; BRICS cooperation mechanism 201–202; China-Africa public health cooperation 203–207; construction of global health security mechanisms 196–197; contribution to global health governance programs 197–198; cooperation between East Asia and 199–200; features of public health diplomacy 209–211; global health diplomacy 195–198; global health governance and 10, 194–207; health governance in 128–129; medical teams to African countries **205**; proposal for Healthy Silk Road 221; regional public health diplomacy 198–202; Shanghai Cooperation Organization (SCO) 200; Sino-US public health cooperation 203

China Charity Federation 210

China Foundation for Poverty Alleviation (CFPA) 210

Chinese Academy of Social Sciences 6

cholera: epidemic in India 57–59; EU banning fresh fish imports 99n16

Chyba, C. F. 180

Cipro, public health and 121–122

Clinton administration, AIDS 28

Codex Alimentarious 76, 110, 113

Cohen, Jon 221

Cold War 25, 26, 80, 143

collective action, problem of 36

Collective Action (Sandler) 185

Collective Goods and International Organizations (Russett and Sulivan) 36

Colorado College 4

Columbia University 6

Combating Infectious Diseases in East Asia (Caballero-Anthony) 6

Coming Plague, The (Garrett) 15

Conceicao, Pedro 38

confidence-building measures (CBMs), BWC and 174, 176

consensus principle, APEC's health agenda 198–199

Constitution of WHO (World Health Organization) 45; Article 2 of 65–66, 74; Article 7 of 78; Article 9 of 81, 82; Article 12 of 74, 162; Article 14 of 78; Article 15 of 74; Article 16 of 74; Article 19 of 66; Article 21 of 66; Article 23 of 67, 71; Article 31 of 71,

226 *Index*

75; Article 32 of 71; Article 35 of 75; Article 37–39 of 75; Article 42 of 71; Article 43 of 71, 75; Article 45 of 71, 72; Article 56 of 81; Article 76 of 99n13; preamble of 65, 70, 141

Contemporary Global Issue (Shaojun Li) 6

Convention Against Torture and Other Cruel, Inhuman or Degrading Treatment or Punishment, potential impact on public health **144**

Convention on the Elimination of All Forms of Discrimination Against Women, potential impact on public health **144**

Convention on the Prohibition of Biological Weapons 24

Convention on the Rights of the Child: potential impact on public health **144**; protecting right to health 158–159; right to health 158

Convention to Suppress the Slave Trade and Slavery (1926) 135

Cooper, Andrew F. 4

Cooper, Kent 145

Cooper, Sherry 40

Copenhagen School 9, 25

cordon sanitaire 56

Covenant of the League of Nations 14

COVID-19 8; China's response to 10, 210–211; China's role in prevention and treatment of 207–209; pandemic 1, 207

crisis in governance, term 16

Declaration of Alma-Ata on Primary Health Care 24, 48n5; North-South divide 163–164; potential impact on public health **144**; right to health 156

Declaration on the Right to Development 138; potential impact on public health **144**

Declaration on the TRIPS and Public Health 33, 34

Deferred Debt Relief Initiative for Poorest Countries 210

Deliberate Use of Biological and Chemical Agents to Cause Harm (WHO) 34

Democracy in America (Tocqueville) 146

Desmond-Hellmann, Sue 195, 211n1

disease: IHR defining 70; travel for international spread of 55

Doctors Without Borders 24

Doha Declaration 22, 46; TRIPS and public health 118–120

East Asia, public health cooperation with China 199–200

Ebola virus 1, 19, 205; crisis 94, 204–206; epidemic 32, 205; infectious disease 19, 148, 153; outbreak 206; outbreak in West Africa 1, 32; prevention and control **202**

Economic United Nations, World Trade Organization as 46

education, ICESCR and right to 151

efavirenz 115

Emerging Infections (Institute of Medicine) 19

Enemark, Christian 220

equality, ICCPR and right to 149–150

Europeans 18–19; European Union banning fresh fish from East African countries 99n16

Executive Board 95; of World Health Assembly 64

fair competition and trade principle, WTO 108

Fidler, David P. 3, 4

Financial Times (newspaper) 122

flexible regimes, of global health governance 23

Food and Agriculture Organization of the United Nations (FAO) 45, 66

Foreign Policy and Global Health (FPGH) 195

Fourie, Peter 30

Fox, Mark A. 18

Framework Convention on Tobacco Control 23, 87, 89

free-rider problem 35–36, 42, 43

free trade doctrine, WTO's 124–125

French revolution 135

Fudan University 22

Future of financing for WHO, The (Chan) 92

Gandhi, Indira 122

Garrett, Laurie 15

Gates, Bill 33

Gates Foundation 24

General Agreement on Tariffs and Trade (GATT) 107, 108, 111

General Agreement on Trade in Services (GATS), WTO agreement 110, **111**, 112, 114

Geneva Graduate Institute of International and Development Studies 29

Geneva Protocol 172; banning biological weapons 172; BWC as improvement

over 172–173; *see also* Biological
Weapons Convention (BWC)
German Institute of Global and Area
Studies (GIGA) 4
German Overseas Institute 6
Ghebreyesus, Tedros Adhanom 98, 211
GlaxoSmithKline 128
Global Fund to Fight AIDS, Tuberculosis
and Malaria 23, 24, 41, **45**, 88, **88**, 198
global governance 16; definition 16; rise of
22; *see also* global health governance
global health 1; literature view of 3–7;
problems 2; publicness of 2; trade and
9–10; UK Department of Health 17
global health governance 16; actors
and functions in **45**, 48n3; actors
in **88**; characteristics of global
public goods 39–42; definitions 16;
diversity of actors in 24–25; economic
benefits driving 219–220; factors
for rise of 17–22; features of 23–25;
flexibility of formal/informal regimes
23; global public goods 35–42;
high level of professionalism 25;
ICCPR and 145–150; ICESCR and
150–152; influence of globalisation
18–20; institutionalisation of 60–63;
international human rights mechanisms
in 160–166; international regimes
in 44–48; key concepts in 15–17;
multilateralism 23–24; necessity
of 25–35; negative impact of WTO
norms on 112–114; right to health
and 154–160; rise of 22; rise of non-
traditional security studies 20–22;
securitisation 25–35; significance of
international regimes 42–44; World
Health Organization (WHO) 9; WTO
agreements and 114–123; WTO's role in
123–129; *see also* Biological Weapons
Convention (BWC)
Global Health Governance (Aginam) 4
Global Health Governance (Hein) 6
*Global Health Governance and Fight
Against HIV/AIDS* (Hein) 4–5
Global Health Governance Program 93
Global Health Initiative (GHI) 88
global health security, UK Department of
Health 17
Global Health Security Conference 33
Global Health Support Programme
(GHSP) 23
Global Outbreak Alert and Response
Network (GOARN) 74

Global Polio Eradication Initiative 37
Global Program of Work, World Health
Organization 143
global public bads 22; globalisation and
17, 19–20
global public goods 35–42; characteristics
of 39–42; classification of 38;
definitions of 36–37; negative
externalities of public health crises
39–41; non-excludability of public
health security 41; non-rivalry of public
health security 41–42; notion of 35–36
Global Public Goods (Kaul) 37
Global Public Goods for Health (Smith) 5
global public health 16; WTO and 106–114
global security, public health threatening
31–32
*Global Threat of New and Re-emerging
Infectious Diseases* (Brower and
Chalk) 6
*Global Threat of New and Re-emerging
Infectious Diseases, The* (Rand) 22, 33
Global Trade Development Centre 16
Gong, Xiangqian 7
Gostin, Lawrence O. 4, 86, 217
governance 16
Governing Global Health (Cooper) 4
Group of Government Experts (GGE) 175

H1N1 virus 90
H5N1 *see* bird flu (H5N1) virus
Hamburg University 182
Ha Noi Declaration (2006) 23, 199
Hardin, Garrett 36, 114
Harvard University 134
Havana Charter, WTO 107
He, Fan 7
He, Yafei 98
health, WHO definition of 65
Health for All Strategy 99n15
Health Organisation of the League of
Nations (HOLN) 61–62, 98n7
Health Silk Road 197
Hein, Wolfgang 4, 16
Held, David 218
Helms-Biden Reauthorization Act 89
Henkin, Louis 133
hepatitis B 128, 151, 153
HIV/AIDS 1, 21; accessibility of
medicines 8; alarming spread around
world 40; compulsory licenses to
medicine 122; Doha Declaration and
118–119; epidemic in Africa 26, 28,
142–143; freedom of movement and

228   Index

147–148; global security threat 31–32; human rights crisis and 47; infectious disease 203; prevalence of 113; public health crisis 194; as threat to individual security 30; TRIPS Agreement and 115, 118–119, 121; UN fight against, 142

HIV/AIDS and Human Rights 149

Horton, Richard 195

Huiping, Xiong 163–164

Hu, Jintao 33, 199

Human Development Report, types of human security 29

human emancipation 21

human rights 133–134; justified restraints on, in public health governance 152–154; linkages between public health and 139, *141*, 141–143; major international declarations and covenants on **140**; Western liberal concept 137

Human Rights Committee (HRC) 162

human rights conventions 10, 47, 71, 163, 164, 197

Human Rights Council 133

human rights principles, IHR and 70–72

human security 16; global infectious diseases and 21–22

human welfare 106

hunger, ICESCR and right to be free from 150–151

Impact of Infectious Diseases on Economic Development and International Relations (Fan He) 7

India, infectious disease 40–41

Indiana University 3

Infectious Disease Control from the Perspective of International Law (Gong) 7

infectious diseases, global bads 17, 19–20

In Larger Freedom (Annan) 138

Institute for Health Metrics and Evaluation, University of Washington 96

integrated governance 69

intermediate global public goods 38

International Air Transport Association 39

International Alliance of National Public Health Institutes (IANPHI) 34

International Association of National Public Health Institutes 197

International Atomic Energy Agency (IAEA) 69, 76, 83, 84, 183

International Bill of Human Rights 47

International Bill of Rights 135

international collective goods, concept of 36

International Committee of Experts on Epidemiology and Quarantine 67

International Conference on Trade and Employment 107

International Convention on the Elimination of All Forms of Discrimination Against Women, right to health 157–158

International Convention on the Elimination of All Forms of Racial Discrimination, potential impact on public health **144**

International Court of Justice (ICJ) 80–81

International Covenant on Civil and Political Rights (ICCPR) 10, 133; global health governance and 145–150; international human rights and 161; North-South divide 165–166; potential impact on public health **144**; right to equality 149–150; right to freedom of association with others 146–147; right to freedom of information 145–146; right to freedom of movement 147–148; right to health 164; right to liberty 148–149; Siracusa Principles 153

International Covenant on Economic, Social and Cultural Rights (ICESCR) 10, 24, 133, 137–138; global health governance and 150–152; potential impact on public health **144**; right to be free from hunger 150–151; right to benefits of scientific progress 151–152; right to everyone to education 151; right to health 157, 163, 164; right to social security 150

International Fundraising Conference on Avian Influenza Prevention and Control 198

International Health Conference, Paris 14

International Health Organization, call for a new 62

International Health Regulations (IHR) 3; all-risks approach 70; Article 1 of 70; Article 3.1 of 70; Article 5 of 72; Article 7 of 188–189; Article 13 of 72; Article 14 of 189; Article 14(2) of 69–70; Article 32 of 143; Article 44 of 73; Article 57 of 222n1; background and birth of (2005) 67–68; conflicts between international regimes and 76; conflicts between WHO and BWC 76–79; failure to address non-compliance of developing countries 86–87; goals by 69–70; granting powers

to WHO 74–75; human rights principles of 70–72; information sources for 73–74; insufficient "compliance pull" of (2005) 85–86; national capacity for upholding global health governance 72–73; political conflicts exposed by (2005) 75–79; reporting public health emergencies 73; revision process 74; scope of 70; surveillance and response capacities 73; transformative features of (2005) 68–75; weaknesses of 85–87
international human rights: biases and discriminations in regimes 164–166; lacking mandatory enforcement 161–162; mechanisms in global health governance 160–166; North-South divide 161, 163–164; public health and 46–47; vagueness on right to health 162–163
International Human Rights Commission 161–162
international human rights regimes: development phases of 135–139; historical background on development of 134–135; links with public health 134–143; major declarations and covenants on human rights **140**; relationship between human rights and public health 139, 141–143
International Labour Organization 66, 99n9, 135
International Monetary Fund (IMF) 45, 107
International Red Cross Organization 23
international regimes: accountability in 214–215; actors of global health governance 42–48; decision making of 213–214; distribution of benefits 215, 217–218; globalisation and 215–217; lacking dispute resolution mechanism 218–219; participation of 214; transparency 215; triangle of publicness and 213–218
International Relations Studies 16
International Sanitary Bureau 60, 61
International Sanitary Conferences 45, 98n4; early (1851–1897) 55–59, **59**; miasma theory 57; purpose of first 56–57
International Sanitary Convention 55, 57, 60, 68
International Sanitary Regulations (1948) 68
International Task Force on Global Public Goods 38

International Veterinary Agency 15
intersubjectivity: definition 28; securitisation of global health 28, 33–35, *35*
Investing for Health (World Bank) 21
Isla, Nicolas 182
isolation policy 98n3

Jack Ma Foundation 210
Jacobson v. Massachusetts (1905) 148
Jameson, Wilson 84
Jamison, D. T. 106
Jefferson, Thomas 35
Jewkes, John 125
Johnson, Lyndon 146

Kaul, Inge 10, 37, 95, 213
Keefe, Tania 5
Keohane, Robert 22, 127
Kickbusch, Ilona 29
Kindleberger, Charles P. 36
Kissinger, Henry 80
Koivusalo, Meri 5
Kyoto Protocol 38

Lancet, The (journal) 195
League of Nations 14, 135
League of Nations Health Organization (HOLN) 14, 45; establishment of 61–62
Legionnaires' disease 19
Lewis, Stephen 125
Liberty, ICCPR and right to 148–149
Li, Bin 204
Li, Shaojun 6
Littlewood, J. 182
low politics 2

Maastricht Guidelines 156
Macroeconomics and Health (WHO) 88
Mahler, Halfdan 80
Mahley, Donald 175
Mahley, John 179
Making a Healthy World (Koivusalo and Ollila) 5
Man, the State, and War (Waltz) 7
Mann, J. M. 134
market access principle, WTO 108
market failure 126
market fundamentalism 124; term 130n4
Marrakesh Agreement 46, 111
Marx, Karl 134
mass murder by complacency 125
Merck & Company (MSD) 125
Merck, Georg 125

230 *Index*

Mexico Summit (2002) 23, 199
miasma theory 57
microbialpolitik, term 3
Monroe Doctrine 61
Monterey Institute of International Studies
187
Montreal Protocol 38
Moral Apprentices Act (1802) 155
More Secure World, A (UN Security
Council) 32, 34
most-favoured-nation (MFN) treatment,
WTO principle 108
multilateral health cooperation, purpose of
developing 56
multilateralism of global health
governance 23–24
multilateralization 14
mutual vulnerability 17, 19, 22, 31, 48n4

National Health Commission (NHC) 209
national security, defining 21, 30
national treatment principle, WTO 108
Native Americans 18–19
nelfinavir 115
New York Times (newspaper) 186
Nguyen, Michael 175
Nixon, Richard 172, 186
non-governmental organizations (NGOs) 5
North-South Divide: international human
rights and 161, 163–164; public health
10, 36, 125–126, 220; right to health
165–166

Office international d'hygiène publique
(OIHP) 60–61, 98n7; establishment of
60–61; United States as member of 61
Ollila, Eeva 5
Olson, Mancur 36
O'Neill, Jim 201
Open Society Justice Initiative 30
Organisation for the Prohibition of
Chemical Weapons (OPCW) 183
Organization for Economic Cooperation
and Development (OECD) **88**, 207
Osakwe, Christopher 81
Ottawa Charter for Health Promotion 156
Ottoman Empire 57, 58, **59**
Our Global Neighborhood (Global
Governance Commission) 16
Oxfam 115, 151

Pakistan, infectious disease 40–41
Pan-American Health Organization 61,
65, 163

Pan-American Sanitary Bureau 61
Panitchpakdi, Supachai 120
Patent Law: People's Republic of China
128
Pearson, Graham 175
Peloponnesian War 18
People, States, and Fear (Buzan) 20
Piot, Peter 142, 147
Plagues and Human (Wang and Meng) 6
Plagues and Politics (Price-Smith) 4
political neutrality 77
Politics of Global Health Governance
(Thomas and Weber) 6
Politics of Global Health Governance, The
(Zacher and Keefe) 5
President's Emergency Plan for AIDS
Relief (PEPFAR) 23, 88
Price-Smith, Andrew T. 4, 30
privatizing the market 126
Programme for Preparedness for
Deliberate Epidemics (PDE) 178
Protocol for the Prohibition of the Use in
War of Asphyxiating Poisonous or Other
Gases and of Bacteriological Methods of
Warfare 172; *see also* Geneva Protocol
Providing Global Public Goods (Kaul) 37
public health 1; Biological Weapons
Convention (BWC) and 176–180, *178*;
China 128–129; China's diplomacy
and COVID-19 response 207–211;
Cipro and 121–122; features of China's
diplomacy 209–211; impact of BWC
on resources 178–179; international
human rights and 10; justified restraints
on human rights 152–154; linkages
between human rights and 139, *141*,
141–143; securitisation of global health
35; threat to country's security 30–31;
threat to global security 31–32; as threat
to individual security 29–30; trade and
109; WTO and 109–112
Public Health Act (1848) 155
public health cooperation: Asia-Pacific
Economic Cooperation (APEC)
198–199; BRICS 201–202; China and
Africa 203–207; China and East Asia
199–200; China's bilateral 202–207;
Shanghai Cooperation Organization
(SCO) 200; Sino-US 203
public health gap, developed and
developing countries 125–126
*Public Health Response to Biological and
Chemical Weapons* (WHO) 34
public health security 9

Index 231

quarantines 56, 204; concept of 109; derivation 98n1; International Sanitary Conferences **59**, 60; measures 60, 66, 71, 73, 123, 147–149, 153; policies and 56–58; regulations 14

Red Cross 23, **45**, **88**
Regional Office for Africa (AFRO) 99n8
Regional Office for Europe (EURO) 99n8
Regional Office for South East Asia (SEARO) 99n8
Regional Office for the Eastern Mediterranean (EMRO) 99n8
Regional Office for the Western Pacific (WPRO) 99n8
research: case analysis 8; framework 9–10; historical analysis 8; levels of analysis 7; methods and contributions 7–9; qualitative analysis 7–8; quantitative analysis 8
right to health: components of *155*; definition of 154–155; development of 155–156; global health governance 154–160; goal at the international level 157–160; international human rights covenants 159–160; national recognition of *160*; phrase 162; Tower of Babel and 154, 167n24; vagueness of 162–163
right to know, term 145
Road Map Towards the Implementation of the United Nations Millennium Declaration (UN) 38
Rockefeller Foundation 24, **45**, **88**
Roemers, Ruth 162
Roll Back Malaria 87
Roman Empire 172
Rome Agreement 60
Rome Declaration 33
Romeo and Juliet (Shakespeare) 98n2
Russett, Bruce M. 36
Russian Revolution 135

St. Petersburg Summit (2006) 23
Sandler, Todd 36, 185
sarin attack, Tokyo subway 26
SARS (severe acute respiratory syndrome) 15, 19; freedom of information and 146; global health governance 67; IHR revision and 68, 74, 79; infectious disease 127, 148–149, 153, 198, 203; international public health 46; outbreak (2003) 1, 6, 8, 39, 196; public health crisis 194, 199–200; spread of 41–42; warnings and national sovereignty 83

SARS, Governance, and Globalization of Diseases (Fidler) 3
SARS Cooperation Action Plan 199
Schönteich, Martin 30
Secretariat, implementing work of WHO 64–65
securitization 10–11n1; content of theory 26–27; core concepts of 27–28; existential threats 27, 29–32; global health governance 25–35; global health issues 28–35; intersubjectivity 28, 33–35; speech act 27–28, 32–33; three-dimensional structure of health issues *35*
Security (Buzan) 26
Sen, Amartya 146
Shanghai Cooperation Organization (SCO) 200
Shanghai Summit (2001) 23
Siddiqi, Javed 5, 58, 61, 98n7
Siracusa Principles, ICCPR and 153
smallpox: as biological weapon 172, 187; control of 61; epidemic 19; global eradication of 41, 68; vaccination 148
Smith, Richard D. 5
Smithson, Amy 188
social emancipation 21
social security, ICESCR and right to 150
Soros, George 130n4
Steinberg, Richard 215
Stimson Centre 188
Stonathan 115
Stop TB Partnership 88
Strategic Preparedness and Response Plan, WTO 208
Suez Canal 55, 58–59
Sulivan, John D. 36
Sverdlovsk incident (1979), anthrax 174, 190n6

technical self-determination 82
terrorism: ever-growing threat of 171; *see also* Biological Weapons Convention (BWC)
Theory and Structures of International Political Economy, The (Sandler) 36
Thomas, Caroline 6
Thucydides 18
Thurow, Lester C. 113
Tianjin Communiqué 201, **202**
Tóth, Tibor 176
Tower of Babel 154, 167n24
trade: global health and 9–10; public health and 109
tragedy of the commons 42, 43–44, 114, 218

232   *Index*

Tragedy of the Commons, The (Hardin) 36
Treaty on the Non-Proliferation of Nuclear
 Weapons 184
triangle of publicness: international
 regimes and 213–218; model 10, 213,
 214; theory of 95
TRIPS Agreement *see* Agreement on
 Trade-Related Aspects of Intellectual
 Property Rights (TRIPS)
Tucker, Jonathan B. 187
typhus 61, 98n4

UNAIDS (Joint United Nations Program
 on HIV/AIDS) 33
United Nations (UN): Millennium
 Development Goals (MDGs) 4, 15, 24,
 73, 160, 204; WHO as agency of 55
United Nations Commission on Human
 Rights 133, 138, 162, 166n2
United Nations Convention on the Rights
 of the Child 133
United Nations Department of
 Disarmament Affairs (UNODA) 183
United Nations Development Programme
 29, **88**, 95, 213
United Nations Ebola Emergency
 Mission 32
United Nations Economic and Social
 Council (ECOSOC) 62, 166n2
United Nations Educational, Scientific and
 Cultural Organization (UNESCO) 135
United Nations Human Rights, website
 48–49n8
United Nations Human Rights Council 138
United Nations Mission for Ebola
 Emergency Response (UNMEER) 206
United Nations Relief and Rehabilitation
 Administration (UNRRA) 62
United Nations Security Council 32, 78,
 81, 95; Resolution 1540 of 188, 189
United Nations Special Commission
 (UNSCOM) 182
United Nations World Conference on
 Human Rights 139
Universal Declaration of Human Rights
 133, 136, 137; Article 12 157; Article 23
 158; Article 24 158–159; Article 25(1)
 157; freedom of association 146–147;
 freedom of information 145–146;
 freedom of movement 147–148;
 potential impact on public health **144**;
 right to health 155, 157–160; right to
 liberty 148–149

universal health coverage, priorities of
 99n21
University of Bradford 175
University of British Columbia 5
University of California 180
University of East Anglia 5
University of Hamburg 16
University of Michigan 187
University of Southampton 6
University of Washington 96
Uruguay Round 107, 115, 116
US (United States): Sino-US public
 health cooperation 203; United States
 Declaration of Independence 134
US Army Medical Research Institute for
 Infectious Diseases (USAMRID) 177
US National Security Council 25
US Rand Corporation 22, 33

Vasak, Karel 135
Vienna Declaration and Programme of
 Action 166–167n5
Virchow, Rudolph 2
von Senger, Harro 136

Walker, Gordon R. 18
Waltz, Kenneth 7, 29
Wang, Xudong 6
Wang, Yi 204, 206
Washington Post (newspaper) 186
weapons of mass destruction (WMD) 47,
 76–77, 171, 177; Biological Weapons
 Convention (BWC) 47; Weapons of
 Mass Destruction Commission 184
Weber, Martin 6
Wen, Jinbao 199–200
Western University 5
Westphalian system 3
Wheelis, Mark 180
WHO Action Program o Essential Drugs
 152
WHO and Public Health (Li Na et al) 6
WHO Reforms for a Healthy Future
 (Chan) 87, 92
Williams, Owain 123
Working Group of Governmental Experts
 on the Right to Development 138
World Bank 21, 30, 37, 45, 88, 107, 217
World Economic Forum 147
World Health and World Politics
 (Siddiqi) 5
World Health Assembly 46, 96; delegates
 of 63–64; Executive Board of 64; as

policymaking body of WHO 63; World Health Assembly Resolution 156
World Health Day 33, 62
World Health Forum 96
World Health Organization (WHO) 2, 4, 45; actors in global health governance **88**; background for reform of 87–91; background of 55–63; conflicts between BWC and 76–79; early International Sanitary Conferences (1851–1897) 55–59, **59**; establishment of 62–63; excessive reliance on extra-budgetary funding 89–91, *90*; Executive Board of 64, 80, 95; financial crisis of 89; functionalism orientation of 82–83; functions of 65–67; global health governance 9; Global Health Governance Program 93; governance structure of 63–67; hurdles to WHO reforms 94–97; institutionalisation of international health cooperation 60–63; lacking compulsory dispute settlement mechanism 81–85; limitations in global health governance 79–87; neglect for international law 83–85; objective of 65; politicisation of 79–81; power of "soft law" of 67–79; reform agenda 92–94; reforms of 87–97; Secretariat of 64–65, 80, 91; sensitivity to sovereignty 83; structural defect of 91; structure of 63–65; Triangle of Publicness theory 95; World Health Assembly of 63–64, 80; *see also* Constitution of WHO (World Health Organization); International Health Regulations (IHR)
World Health Report 2007 17

world pharmaceutical market **127**
World Trade Organization (WTO) 2, 4, 76, 88, 106; Agreement on Trade-Related Aspects of Intellectual Property Rights (TRIPS) 8, 9–10; background of 107; establishment of 46; free trade doctrine 124–125; global public health and 106–114; Green Room meetings 125, 215; health issues and relevant agreements **111**; limitations in global health governance 123–129; negative impact of norms on global health governance 112–114; power politics and double standards in 127–129; principles of 108; privatisation of global public goods 126–127; public health divide between developed and developing countries 125–126; public health issues and 109–112; purposes of 107–109; trade and public health 109
world trade services 130n3
World War I 61, 135, 172
World War II 61, 107, 133, 134, 143
Wright, Susan 187
Wu, Yi 196

Xi, Jinping 33, 196–197, 204, 208–209

Yamey, Gavin 87
Yaqing, Qin 85
Young, Oran 43
Yu, Keping 17

Zacher, Mark 5
zero-growth policy 89, 90

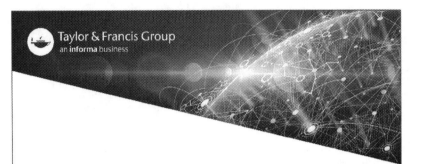

Printed in the United States
By Bookmasters